FOCUS ON LUNG CANCER RESEARCH

HORIZONS IN CANCER RESEARCH

Volume 1: Prostate Cancer
John N. Lucas (Editor)
ISBN 1-59454-100-0

Volume 2: Trends in Ovarian Cancer Research
A. P. Bardos (Editor)
ISBN 1-59454-023-3

Volume 3: Percutaneous Cryotherapy of Renal Cell Carcinoma under an Open MRI System
Junta Harada, Kazuo Miyasaka and Sajio Sumida (Editors)
ISBN 1-59454-169-8

Volume 4: Focus on Colorectal Cancer Research
Julia D. Martinez (Editor)
ISBN 1-59454-101-9

Volume 5: Focus on Leukemia Research
Rafael M. Romero (Editor)
ISBN 1-59454-093-4

Volume 6: Progress in Bladder Cancer Research
A. M. Mallory (Editor)
ISBN 1-59454-129-9

Volume 7: Trends in Prostate Cancer Research
John N. Lucas (Editor)
ISBN 1-59454-265-1

Volume 8: Tumor Budding in Colorectal Cancer Recent Progress in Colorectal Cancer Research
Tadahiko Masaki (Editor)
ISBN 1-59454-189-2

Volume 9: Trends in Breast Cancer Research
Andrew P. Yao (Editor)
ISBN 1-59454-134-5

Volume 10: Trends in Leukemia Research
Rafael M. Romero (Editor)
ISBN 1-59454-311-9

Volume 11: Liver Cancer: New Research
Felix Lee (Editor)
ISBN 1-59454-182-5

Volume 12: Focus on Lung Cancer
Robert L. Carafaro (Editor)
ISBN 1-59454-082-9

FOCUS ON LUNG CANCER RESEARCH

ROBERT L. CARAFARO
(EDITOR)

Nova Biomedical Books
New York

For permission to use material from this book please contact us:
Telephone 631-231-7269; Fax 631-231-8175
Web Site: http://www.novapublishers.com

LIBRARY OF CONGRESS CATALOGING-IN-PUBLICATION DATA:
Available Upon Request

ISBN: 1-59454-082-9

Published by Nova Science Publishers, Inc. ✢ New York

CONTENTS

PREFACE

Chronic inhalation of cigarette smoke is a major risk factor for the development of lung cancer. It has been suggested that genetic susceptibility may contribute to the risk, because only a small portion of smokers develops the disease. Developments in molecular biology have led to growing interest in investigation of biological markers, which may increase predisposition to lung carcinogenesis. The relationships of lung cancer to markers of genetic susceptibility genes, including metabolic genes, DNA repair genes, cell cycle control gene and addiction genes are summarized here in Chapter 1.

As reported in Chapter 2, enormous progress recently has been made in understanding the molecular and cellular biology of lung cancer. Genetic abnormalities of proto-*Oncogene*s and tumor suppressor genes are well known changes which are frequently involved in lung cancer pathogenesis. However, a major finding which comes more and more into focus is that epigenetic inactivation of certain tumor suppressor genes by aberrant promoter methylation frequently occurs in lung carcinomas. These findings point to potential novel therapies to re-activate gene expression.

The extracellular matrix (ECM) is a complex network of interstitial connective tissue filling the extracellular space of the submucosa, which functions by mechanically supporting the three dimensional structure of the cell body, maintaining tissue homeostasis, and it also affects various biologic cell functions. The matrix metalloproteinases (MMPs), a growing family of zinc-dependent neutral endopeptidases, are the key enzymes in the degradation of the ECM, which belong to the metzincin superfamily. The expression of MMPs is strictly regulated to maintain proper homeostasis in the normal stomal environment. On the other hand, during cancer progression, it is well recognized that MMPs promote tumor invasion and metastasis via ECM degradation. Chapter 3 reports on the findings of research on the pathogenic contribution of MMPs to lung cancer.

In the last few decades cancer research has generated an enormous amount of information regarding the molecular biologic processes that take place in cancer tissue, one of which is the formation of new blood vessels, angiogenesis. More than 100 papers have been published so far, studying various components of angiogenesis and their relation to lung cancer. Chapter 4 reviews the existing literature in the field of angiogenesis and lung cancer and provides a new model based on recent publications.

Through a systematic review of the literature presented in Chapter 5, the laboratory variables that, in addition to performance status and to stage or extent of the disease, would allow a more accurate stratification of lung cancer patients who participate in chemotherapy trials, with or without radiotherapy. Of 1143 publications retrieved, the authors exclusion and inclusion criteria allowed them to include 26 studies in their review, of which 12 evaluated small-cell lung (SCLC) cancer patients, and 14 evaluated non-small-cell lung (NSCLC) cancer patients. The authors recommendations are more in agreement with the recommendations made in the clinical practice guidelines that use evidence-based methods than with the guidelines that do not.

As reported in Chapter 6, despite limited clinical evidence to support its efficacy, cannabis is widely used for the relief of pain and spasticity by people suffering from multiple sclerosis or spinal cord injury. Although cannabis is not associated with an increased cancer risk when it is used orally, when cannabis burns in a cigarette or pipe it generates a number of pro-carcinogenic substances. Cannabis smokers who do not use tobacco have been reported to show a number of pathological abnormalities in the lungs that are indicative of the early stages of the development of cancer. While the evidence to date does not prove conclusively that cannabis smoking can cause lung cancer, it does suggest that the risk of cancer is high. If cannabis is to be used for therapeutic purposes, it would therefore be best if its active ingredients were delivered orally or by aerosol spray.

In: Focus on Lung Cancer Research
Editor: Robert L. Carafaro, pp. 1-49
ISBN 1-59454-082-9

Chapter I

GENETIC POLYMORPHISM OF ENZYMES INVOLVED IN XENOBIOTIC METABOLISM AND THE RISK OF LUNG CANCER: A REVIEW

Chikako Kiyohara[1,*], Kouichi Yoshimasu[2], Taro Shirakawa[3] and Julian M. Hopkin[4]

[1] Department of Preventive Medicine, Division of Social Medicine, Graduate School of Medical Sciences, Kyushu University, Maidashi 3-1-1, Higashi-ku, Fukuoka, 812-8582, Japan

[2] Department of Neuropsychiatry , Graduate School of Medical Sciences, Kyushu University, Maidashi 3-1-1, Higashi-ku, Fukuoka, 812-8582, Japan

[3] Department of Health Promotion and Human Behavior, Kyoto University Graduate School of Public Health, Yoshida-konoe, Kyoto 606-8501, Japan

[4] Experimental Medicine Unit, University of Wales, Swansea SA2 8PP, UK

ABSTRACT

Chronic inhalation of cigarette smoke is a major risk factor for the development of lung cancer. It has been suggested that genetic susceptibility may contribute to the risk, because only a small portion of smokers develops the disease. Developments in molecular biology have led to growing interest in investigation of biological markers, which may increase predisposition to lung carcinogenesis. Therefore the high risk genotype of an individual could be determined easily. As there are the great number of carcinogen-activating and -detoxifying enzymes, the variation in their expression and the complexity of exposures to tobacco carcinogens, the existence of multiple alleles at loci of those enzymes may result in differential susceptibilities of individuals. Genetic

---

* Correspondence: Chikako Kiyohara, Department of Preventive Medicine, Division of Social Medicine, Graduate School of Medical Sciences, Kyushu University, Maidashi 3-1-1, Higashi-Ku, Fukuoka 812-8582, Japan. Tel: +81 92 642 6113, Fax: +81 92 642 6115 E-mail: chikako@phealth.med.kyushu-u.ac.jp

difference is also known for substances in tobacco smoke absorption, their metabolism and for interactions with receptors. The relationships of lung cancer to markers of genetic susceptibility genes, including metabolic genes, DNA repair genes, cell cycle control gene (p53 tumor suppressor gene) and addiction genes are summarized here. As lung cancer is a multifactorial disease, an improved understanding of the interplay of environmental and genetic polymorphisms at multiple loci may help identify individuals who are at increased risk for lung cancer. Hopefully, in the future we will be able to screen for lung cancer susceptibility by using specific biomarkers.

INTRODUCTION

Lung cancer death is major cause of death in the developed countries. Although chronic inhalation of cigarette smoke is a major risk factor for the development of lung cancer, it appears important to examine genetic susceptibility to the disease.

Cigarette smoke contains several thousand chemicals, of which about 50 compounds are known carcinogens, including polycyclic aromatic hydrocarbons (PAHs), aromatic amines and N-nitroso compounds. Some of these compounds are reactive carcinogens, but most are procarcinogens, which need to be activated by phase I enzymes such as those encoded by the cytochrome P450 (*CYP*) supergene family, and converted into reactive carcinogens. All these reactive carcinogens can bind to DNA and form DNA adducts capable of inducing mutations and initiating carcinogenesis. *CYPs* are a multigene superfamily of mixed function monooxygenases. Based on sequence homology, the *CYP* superfamily is divided into 10 subfamilies, *CYP1-CYP10*. Subfamilies *CYP1*, *CYP2*, *CYP3* and *CYP4* are primarily involved in drug metabolism [1].

Following phase I reaction, phase II enzymes such as glutathione S-transferases (GSTs) are responsible for detoxification of activated forms PAH epoxides. GSTs are constitutively found in a wide variety of tissues, with different characteristic patterns of GST isozymes. *GSTs* also form a superfamily of genes consisting of five distinct families, named alpha, mu, pi, theta and sigma [2, 3]. The major isoforms, which involve the metabolic activation of carcinogens derived from tobacco smoke or detoxification of those activated carcinogens, are listed in Tables 1 [1, 4, 5] and 2 [6 – 9].

Since advances in molecular biology have allowed many allelic variants of several drug-metabolizing enzymes to be characterized at the molecular level, specific nucleotide changes have been identified as the basis for altered protein structure and/or function. Therefore, the high risk genotype of an individual could be determined easily. The existence of multiple alleles at loci of those enzymes may result in differential susceptibilities of individuals [10]. Since genetic polymorphisms have been found for both phase I and phase II enzymes, risk assessment could be increased in sensitivity if polymorphisms in both phases of enzymes are taken into consideration as biomarkers for susceptibility to cancer. It is likely that an individual with the high risk genotype (either a genotype coding for a more active phase I enzyme or a less efficient phase II enzyme, or both of those) might be at higher risk of cancer than that with the opposite genotype (combination).

Table 1. Selected human phase I enzymes and examples of human tissue and carcinogens in tobacco smoke activated by them [1, 4, 5]

Gene	Chromosomal location	Tissue expression	Activation of constituents in tobacco smoke
CYP1A1	15q22-q24	Lung, skin, placenta, lymphocytes	PAHs
CYP2D6	22q13.1	Lung, liver, intestine, prostate	TSNAs
CYP2E1	10q24.3-qter	Lung, liver, brain, kidney	TSNAs
CYP2A6	19q13.2	Lung, nasal, pharyngeal	TSNAs
CYP2C9	10q24.1-q24.3	Liver, intestine	PAHs
CYP2C19	10q24.1-q24.3	Liver, prostate	PAHs
*mEPHX1**	1q42.1	Lung, liver, kidney, testis, lymphocytes	PAHs
*NQO1**	16q22	Lung, liver, kidney, brain	PAHs, HCAs
MPO	17q21-23	Neutrophils, monocytes, macrophages	PAHs, HCAs, AAs

PAH: polycyclic aromatic hydrocarbon
TNSA: tobacco specific nitrosoamine
HCA: heterocyclic amine
AA: arylamine
*; The enzyme has a dual role in the detoxification and activation of procarcinogens.

Table 2. Selected human phase II enzymes and examples of human tissue and carcinogens in tobacco smoke inactivated by them [6 – 9]

Gene	Chromosoma l location	Tissue expression	Detoxification of metabolites
*GSTM1**	1p13.1	Lung, prostate, brain, breast, lymphocytes, colon, small intestine, esophagus, stomach, thymus, heart, skeletal muscle, kidney, spleen, testis, uterus, aorta, adrenal gland	PAHs
*GSTT1**	22q11.23	Lung, liver, erythrocytes, brain, kidney, spleen, small intestine, skeletal muscle, heart	Halomethanes
*GSTP1**	11q13	Lung, placenta, stomach, esophagus, bladder, skin, breast, colon, oral cavity	PAHs
*mEPHX1***	1q42.1	Lung, liver, kidney, testis, lymphocytes	PAHs
*NQO1***	16q22	Lung, liver, kidney, brain	PAHs

*; GSTs are constitutively found at high levels in a wide variety of tissues with different characteristic patterns of GST isozyme expression.
**; The enzyme has a dual role in the detoxification and activation of procarcinogens.

Another potentially important source of inter-individual variability in relation to the development of lung cancer is metabolism involved in tobacco-derived carcinogens other than PAHs, DNA repair capacity, cell cycle control function, and smoking behavior (Table 3). The relationship between genetic polymorphisms and lung cancer was discussed with special emphasis on several genes of the listed genes in Table 3.

Table 3. Candidate genes involved in the risk of lung cancer

Category	Candidate genes
Phase I metabolic genes	*CYP1A1, CYP1A2, CYP2A6, CYP2D6, CYP2E1, CYP2C9,CYP2C19, ADH2, mEPHX1*, NQO1*, NQO2*
Phase II metabolic genes	*ADH3, MPO, mEPHX1*, GSTM1, GSTT1, GSTP1, NAT2, ALDH2, SOD2, NQO1*,NQO2, SULT1A1, SULT1A2, SULT1A3*
DNA repair genes	*XRCC1, XRCC3, XPD, XPF, ERCC1*
Cell cycle control genes	*TP53, HRAS*
Addiction genes	*CYP2A6, CYP2D6, DRD2, DRD4, DRD5, nAChR, SLC6A3, 5-HTT*

CYP, cytochrome P450; ADH, alcohol dehydrogenase; MPO, myeloperoxidase; mEPHX1, microsomal epoxide hydrolase; GST, glutathione S-transferase; NAT; N-acethyltransferase; ALDH, aldehyde dehydrogenase; SOD, superoxide dismutaseO; NQO, SULT, sulfotransferase; XRCC; DR, dopamine receptor; nAChR, neuronal nicotine acetylcholine receptor; SLC6A3, dopamine transporter; 5-HTT, serotonin transporter

*; The enzyme has a dual role in the detoxification and activation of procarcinogens.

1. *CYP1A1* POLYMORPHISMS

Human *CYP1A* gene locus has two distinct members, CYP1A1, which is predominantly expressed in extrahepatic tissues, including the lung, lymphocytes and placentas, and the liver specific CYP1A2. Substrates for and inducers of CYP1A1 include PAHs such as benzo(a)pyrene (BP), whereas CYP1A2 is active in the metabolism of aromatic amines. Cancer risk associated with PAHs is mediated in part by aryl hydrocarbon hydroxylase (AHH), which is used as an indicator of the phenotype of *CYP1A1*. Since AHH is responsible for the activation of PAHs in cigarette smoke, it may be important for the causation of lung cancer [1[.

To date, four genetic polymorphisms have been described in human *CYP1A1* gene [11 – 14], which is located on chromosome 15q22-q24. A related family member, *CYP1A2*, is located approximately 25 kb away from *CYP1A1* on chromosome 15. The polymorphism detected first, which was ascribed to the presence (*CYP1A1*2* allele) or absence (wild-type *CYP1A1*1* allele) of the *Msp* I site, was a thymine to cytosine transition 1197 bp downstream of exon 7 (3801T=>3801C) [11]. The second Ile-Val polymorphism occurred in the heme-binding region (Ile462Val, 2455A=>2455G) [12]. The third polymorphism results from a single base change adenine to guanine in the 3' noncoding region approximately 300 bp upstream from the polyadenylation site (3205T=>3205C, *CYP1A1*4* allele) [13]. This mutation leads to cleavage of the normal 2.3 kb *Msp* I restriction fragment into 1.3 and 1.0 kb fragments. This race-specific polymorphism has been found in African-Americans but not in

Caucasians and Asians. A novel mutation (*CYP1A1*5*) was 2 bases upstream of the Ile-Val polymorphism (Thr461Asn, 2453C=>2453A) [14].

The *Msp* I polymorphism can be classified into 3 genotypes, predominant homozygous alleles (genotype A), heterozygote (genotype B) and homozygous rare alleles (genotype C) [11]. The genotype C is closely related to high inducible CYP1A1 phenotypic activity [15]. An overrepresentation of genotype C was observed in lung cancer patients compared with controls in Asian populations [16 -19] but was not observed in non-Asian populations [20 – 30]. This might be sparsity of the allele in Caucasians. Healthy individuals with genotype C are most common among Asians (14 %) and least common among Caucasians (1.2 %) with African-Americans (5.9 %) intermediate between these groups [31]. Similarly, the Val/Val genotype in Ile-Val polymorphism results in a reduced catalytic enzyme activity [15] and was shown to be associated with lung cancer in a Japanese population [12, 32]. The Ile-Val polymorphism was less common than the *Msp* I polymorphism [12, 21, 23, 23]. This polymorphism is closely linked to *Msp* I polymorphism not only in a Japanese population [12] but also in Northern Europeans [20].

As for the third polymorphism in the *CYP1A1* gene, no linkage was observed with either the *Msp* I or Ile-Val polymorphism. In African-Americans, the frequency of heterozygotes was 15.2-19.4% in controls and the homozygous variant was rare even in cases [12, 33-35]. This race specific polymorphism has been associated with an increased risk of adenocarcinoma [35] whereas other studies [33, 36] did not confirm the report. As suggested by Talioli et al. [34, 35], the third restriction length fragment polymorphism (RFLP), which might be a useful tool to identify African-Americans at increased risk for lung cancer, does not appear to hold promise. The fourth *Msp* I RFLP may not represent a susceptibility factor for lung cancer [14].

The interindividual difference in genetically determined susceptibility to squamous cell carcinoma of the lung has been investigated in relation to cigarette smoking dose [16]. The total amount of cigarettes consumed over ones lifetime was compared among three genotypes in the first *Msp* I polymorphism. The patients with genotype C contracted lung cancer after fewer cigarettes than those with other genotypes. Individuals with genotype C were at significantly higher risk with an odds ratio (OR) of 7.31 (95% confidence interval (CI) =2.13-25.12) at a low dose level of cigarette smoking and the difference in susceptibility between genotypes was reduced at high doses [16].

A meta-analysis of published studies was undertaken by Houlston to clarify the effect of variation within the *CYP1A1* gene defined by the *Msp* I and Ile-Val polymorphisms [37]. The ORs for the genotypes C and Val/Val were found to be 1.27 (95% CI=0.91-1.77) and 1.62 (95% CI=0.93-2.82), respectively. His results have provided little support for the role of those polymorphisms in the development of lung cancer. Recently, a pooled analysis of 22 case-control studies based on the database of the International Projects on Genetic Susceptibility to Environmental Carcinogens (GESC) was conducted [38]. A clear association between *CYP1A1 Msp* I polymorphism and lung cancer was observed among Caucasians (age- and gender-adjusted OR = 2.36, 95% CI = 1.16 - 4.81) while the lack of association was observed among Asians in contrast with the above-mentioned meta-analysis [37]. The major reason for the discrepancy may depend on the different datasets. Design specificities or unknown effect modifiers may exist in the Asian studies. *CYP1A1* polymorphisms are attractive with respect to biologically plausible susceptibility factors. As stated earlier, the frequency of both *Msp* I and Ile-Val polymorphisms varies among ethnic groups. The findings in the Japanese population studies to date reveal high risks of lung cancer for the *CYP1A1-Msp* I polymorphism. However, direct applicability to screening strategies in lung cancer in high prevalence area like Japan awaits further studies.

2. *CYP2D6* Polymorphism

More than 30 commonly prescribed drugs are substrates for CYP2D6, including those that act on the cardiovascular and central nervous system. This major polymorphism that inactivates the *CYP2D6* gene leads to profound changes in drug pharmacokinetics and can therefore have severe clinical consequences, leading to marked drug side effects and even, in extreme cases, death [39].

Phenotyping analysis is carried out by administration of the probe drug debrisoquine and subsequent urine analysis at 8-hour intervals to determine the ratio between the parent compound debrisoquine and the primary metabolite 4-hydroxydebrisoquine. This ratio varies 10,000-fold in the Caucasian population [40].

The *CYP2D6* gene is located on chromosome 22q13.1. A number of alleles have now been characterized at the *CYP2D6* locus. The phenotypic consequence of many of these allelic variants remains to be established. The first genetic polymorphism in the metabolism of drugs associated with the expression of *CYP2D6* in humans was 4-hydroxylation of the antihypertensive drug debrisoquine [41]. The genetic polymorphism of the *CYP2D6* is an autosomal recessive trait [42] expressed in three major phenotypes, commonly termed ultra-rapid metabolizers (UM), extensive metabolizers (EM) and poor metabolizers (PM) [43, 44]. A minority of individuals have been shown to inherit multiple copies of the wild-type *CYP2D6* gene [45]. These UM require doses of medication that vastly exceed the normal range in order to achieve a therapeutic effect [46]. The interindividual variations in the activity of CYP2D6 are closely linked to mutant alleles encoding the *CYP2D6* gene [47]. Inactivating mutations at the *CYP2D6* gene are *CYP2D6*3* (deletion of A2549 in exon 5), *CYP2D6*4* (1846G=>1846A at splicing site), *CYP2D6*5* (complete deletion of the wild-type allele *CYP2D6*1*), *CYP2D6*6A* (deletion of T1707 in exon 3) and *CYP2D6*16* (a hybrid of 5'-CYP2D7/CYP2D6-3' gene with breakpoints between the end of intron 7 and the start of exon 9 for both genes involved) while decreased enzyme activity is seen with *CYP2D6*9* (deletion of Lys281) and *CYP2D6*10A* (Pro34Ser, 100C=>100T in exon 1 and Ser486Thr, 4180G=>4180C in exon 9). Carriers with one wild-type allele and one inactivating allele are predicted as HEM [48]. The *CYP2D6**3, *CYP2D6**4 and *CYP2D6**5 alleles account for the majority (greater than 90%) of the PM phenotype [47]. The phenotype-genotype concordance, which predicts the metabolic phenotype by genetic analyses, was found to be between 93.4% and 100% [49].

The genetically determined capacity of the CYP2D6 is suspected to be involved in the activation of tobacco-specific nitrosamines, such as 4-(methylnitrosamino)-1-(3-pyridyl)-1-butanone (NNK). Interindividual differences in the metabolic capacity of the CYP2D6 may be expected to be a key factor in susceptibility to develop several types of cancers where environmental chemicals are implicated [50, 51]. There have been a series of studies on the association of a genetic polymorphism at the *CYP2D6* gene with lung cancer susceptibility. All case-control studies have been performed in Caucasians with the exception of the study of London et al. [52], which was performed in African-Americans. Among controls, Caucasian populations have a PM frequency of between 6-10% [49, 52-63], whereas African-Americans have only a 3% frequency [63] and Asians less than 1% [64, 65].

A meta-analysis of the published findings as of 1992 has demonstrated an overall OR of 0.44 (95% CI = 0.29-0.63) for lung cancer patients with the PM phenotype [66]. Also, the overall OR for genotyped *CYP2D6* (accounted only for the *CYP2D6*4* allele) was 1.0 (95% CI = 0.7 - 1.5) [59]. The PM genotype determined by the presence of the inactivating allele was not significantly associated with decreased [48, 52-55, 62] or increased [57, 58, 60, 61] risk of lung cancer. Many of these studies have been contradictory either because of the small numbers of patients studied or because of the limitations and controversy surrounding the pharmacogenetic assay used to identify the affected individuals. For the *CYP2D6**9 allele, Agundez et al. [57] reported that the *CYP2D6**9 mutant allele was 6-fold more frequent among lung cancer patients than controls. However, Legrand et al. [63] reported that the *CYP2D6**9 allele was present in 4.9% of controls and 6% of lung cancer patients and that this mutant allele might not be an risk factor for lung cancer in a French population.

The effect of tobacco smoking on lung cancer risk might rise with increasing CYP2D6 activity, and the effect of CYP2D6 activity might rise with increasing tobacco consumption. The significant interaction between CYP2D6 activity and smoking dose was observed [67]. Among individuals with high CYP2D6 activity, heavy smokers showed a 5-fold increased risk compared with light smokers.

The relation between the *CYP2D6* polymorphism and lung cancer remains conflicting and inconclusive. There is some biological plausibility to more efficient activation of N-nitroso compounds such as NNK in tobacco smoke by the EM genotype, but the absence of any reports of that activity in the lung as the target organ is problematic for the *CYP2D6*-lung cancer hypothesis. While there is a possible molecular epidemiologic association between the prevalence of the EM genotype and lung cancer, the association, if it exists, may be weak.

3. *CYP2E1* POLYMORPHISM

CYP2E1 is involved in metabolic activation of carcinogenic tobacco-specific N-nitrosamines (including N-nitrosoethylmethylamine (NDMA), N-nitropyrrolidine), aniline, benzene and other low-molecular-weight compounds. The CYP2E1 is constitutively expressed in liver and can also be induced by chemicals such as ethanol and acetone in humans [59, 68, 69]. Protein levels and catalytic activities of CYP2E1 have been shown to vary among individuals [70, 71]. Although the genetic basis of such differences has not been fully clarified, RFLPs in *CYP2E1* gene by *Dra* I (intron 6) [72, 73], *Rsa* I (intron 5) [73] and *Rsa* I/*Pst* I (5'-flanking region) [74, 75], and *Taq* I (intron 7) [76] have been reported.

The *CYP2E1* gene is located on chromosome 10q24.3 - qter. The relation between the *CYP2E1 Dra* I polymorphism and lung cancer was first reported in a Japanese population by Uematsu et al. [73]. The *Dra* I RFLP is caused by a base pair change (*CYP2E1*6* allele,

7632T => 7632A) in intron 6 of the *CYP2E1* gene. They divided the *Dra* I RFLP polymorphism into three genotypes; heterozygotes (CD) and two forms of homozygotes (CC and DD). Since this polymorphism is caused by a base pair change of the *CYP2E1* gene, it is unlikely that this change directly affects the variability of the gene expression. Although it could be a marker in linkage disequilibrium with an active site, its effect on the CYP2E1 phenotype is still unclear [74]. Racial variation in the frequency of this polymorphism has been reported [31]. A rare allele (C) frequency for Asians (9.4 %) was higher than that for Caucasians (0.8 %). In a Japanese population, the distribution of *Dra* I genotypes in lung cancer patients was significantly different from that of healthy controls [73]. The frequency of genotype CD in lung cancer patients was higher than in controls, while the genotypes CC and DD were lower. In Finnish [77] and Swedish [78] populations, there is a much lower allele frequency for C in controls (0.09) and no association between lung cancer risk and *Dra* I polymorphism was seen. There is no clear evidence that this polymorphism is related to lung cancer risk.

The polymorphism in the 5' flanking region at -1053bp (C=>T) is found to be in linkage with another point mutation at -1293bp (G =>C) [74, 78, 79]. The *Rsa* I/*Pst* I RFLP has two alleles c1 (wild-type *CYP2E1*1* allele) and c2 (*CYP2E1*3* allele). The racial differences in allelic frequency have been reported by Kato et al. [79]. Kato et al. [79] reported that the allelic frequencies of this polymorphism were markedly different in Japanese, African-Americans, and Caucasians. The *Rsa* I rare allele c2 was present at a frequency of 0.02 in Caucasians, 0.02 in African-Americans and 0.27 in Japanese ($P<0.05$). Stephens et al. [80] also reported the ethnic-differences in allelic frequency of *Rsa* I RFLP. A rare c2 allele frequency for Taiwanese, African-Americans and European-Americans was 0.28, 0.01 and 0.04, respectively. High frequencies of the c2 and C alleles in the *CYP2E1* gene have consistently been found in several Asian populations [31, 81, 82], in contrast to other ethnic groups [78, 83]. This polymorphism might be functionally important because it is located at a putative binding site for the transcription factor HNF-1 and has been associated with higher levels of *CYP2E1* transcription. Recently, an increase in transcriptional activity, mRNA and protein expression *in vitro* was observed in the c2/c2 genotype [84]. It is conceivable that the *CYP2E1 Rsa* I/*Pst* I polymorphism might contribute to differences in susceptibility to lung cancer. The c2 rare allele has been demonstrated to be less common among Swedish lung cancer patients [78] and this difference is more pronounced when adenocarcinoma patients are excluded from the cancer group. In the Finnish study, Hirvonen et al. [77] failed to show any association of this polymorphism with lung cancer. London et al. [85] suggested that the rare c2 allele was not associated with an increased risk of lung cancer. This polymorphism did not also affect lung cancer risk in one Japanese population [81] whereas the c2/c2 genotype was associated with an increased risk of squamous cell carcinoma (OR=2.45, 95% CI=0.92-6.48) in another Japanese population [82]. Wu et al. [86] reported that individuals who lack a c2 allele might be at higher risk for developing lung cancer in Mexican-Americans, but not in African-Americans. Using the combined genotypes c1/c2 and c2/c2 as the reference, the OR for c1/c1 genotype was 14.0 (95% CI=1.9-101.5) among Mexican-Americans. Moreover, they suggested a greater than multiplicative interaction between cigarette smoking and the *CYP2E1* c1/c1 genotype by stratified analysis. The OR for the c1/c1 genotype and pack-years of smoking (≥30 vs. 0, dichotomized categories) was 45.8

(95% CI=5.7-368.7) in the overall population. In that case, the interaction term was not statistically significant probably due to the small sample size that also resulted in the wide CI. A major reason for this disagreement might be an ethnic difference in allelic frequency of the polymorphism and the small sample size. Larger studies might be necessary to rule out a modest association between the *CYP2E1 Rsa* I polymorphism and lung cancer risk.

Given the low gene frequency in the European- and African-American population studies to date and the relatively modest ORs associated with these polymorphisms, demonstration of a *CYP2E1*-lung cancer relation would require case and control groups of greater than 1,000 subjects each. These study magnitudes have not been reported in the molecular epidemiology literature as it relates to lung cancer. The low estimates of attributable risk imply that the *CYP2E1* polymorphisms at this time must be considered unlikely as strong determinants of lung cancer risk in the Caucasian and African-American populations. In addition, since all polymorphisms are located in non-coding regions of *CYP2E1*, a novel polymorphism(s) in *CYP2E1* would be a promising tool for the detection of the genetic susceptibility to lung cancer.

4. *GST* POLYMORPHISMS

Following the phase I reaction, phase II enzymes such as glutathione S-transferases are responsible for detoxification of activated forms of PAH epoxides. The GSTs activities are inherited in an autosomal dominant fashion [87] and a 100- to 200-fold difference in cytosolic GSTs in lymphocytes from healthy subjects [88, 89]. *GST* genes form a superfamily of at least 13 genes consisting of five distinct families, named alpha (*GSTA*), sigma (*GSTS*), mu (*GSTM*), pi (*GSTP*) and theta (*GSTT*). Certain genes within the *GSTM*, *GSTT* and *GSTP* subfamilies (*GSTM1*, *GSTT1* and *GSTP1*) are polymorphic in humans and the levels of individual enzymes expressed can be influenced by induction and by genetic polymorphism. Since these polymorphisms are considered in terms of risk from certain potentially carcinogenic chemicals, they are currently being investigated as possible cancer risk modifiers. The *GSTM1, GSTT1* and *GSTP1* genes locate on chromosomes 1p13.3, 22q11.23 and 11q13, respectively. The phenotypic absence of GSTM1 and GSTT1 activity is due to homozygosity for deletion of these genes, termed the null genotype [7, 87]. Genetic polymorphism at the *GSTP1* locus results from a single base pair substitution in exon 5 (Ile104Val, 313A=>313G) and exon 6 (Ala113Val, 341C=>341T) [90]. *In vitro* cDNA expression study suggests that these amino acid substitutions reduce enzyme activity [91]. For *GSTA* genes, one study has reported an RFLP in *GSTA2* [92] but whether there is a genetic basis for this variation and its implications is unclear. Less is known about the association between *GSTA2* and newly found *GSTS* genes, and lung cancer risk. Most interest in the possible consequences of *GSTs* polymorphisms has therefore focused on the polymorphisms at the *GSTM1, GSTT1* and *GSTP1* gene loci. The homozygous deletion of the *GSTM1* gene was shown to occur in approximately 50% of the population of various ethnic origins [10] while the homozygous deletion of the *GSTT1* gene is distributed at between 10% and 64% of various ethnic groups [10]. The frequency of the *GSTT1* null genotype in Caucasian populations is 30% or less but the null type genotype frequency in Asian populations may be similar to that of *GSTM1*. Individuals homozygous for the 105 valine allele (the mutant allele) are most common among African-Americans (19%) and least common among Japanese (0-3.1%) with Caucasians (6.5-11.7%) intermediate between these groups [93].

The association between *GSTM1* polymorphism and lung cancer risk has been controversial in the published literatures. The reason for the discrepancies in the *GSTM1* findings is unclear. One problem may be the relatively weak influence of any one genotype on disease risk and the unequal distribution of confounding factors such as polymorphisms at other relevant loci in cases and controls. Differences in exposure to carcinogens such as cigarette smoke are also likely to be important with the effects of such variables exaggerated in studies of small numbers of subjects.

McWilliams et al. [94] combined 12 case-control studies and determined lung cancer risk. They concluded that *GSTM1* deficiency is a moderate risk factor for lung cancer development with an OR of 1.41 (95% CI=1.23-1.61) using Mantel-Haenszel methods for stratified data. The association appeared stronger for Japanese (OR=1.6, 95% CI=1.2-2.1) than for Caucasians (OR=1.2, 95% CI=1.0-1.4). The studies, which determined GSTM1 status by phenotyping (3 studies) or genotyping (8 studies) yielded a summary OR of 1.8 (95% CI=1.3-2.5) or 1.3 (95% CI=1.2-1.6), respectively. A recent meta-analysis based on genotyping studies (19 studies) showed that *GSTM1* deficiency conferred a 1.13-fold increase in the risk of lung cancer (95% CI=1.04-1.25) [95]. Pooling the 4 studies that were based on phenotyping methods, the OR was higher (OR=2.12, 95 % CI=1.43-3.13) than those based on genotyping methods.

Individuals deficient in the *GSTM1* have been reported to be at high risk for smoking related lung cancer [87, 96-99]. Smokers with the GSTM1 enzyme have approximately one-third of the risk for lung carcinoma of smokers without the enzyme [96, 100, 101]. A recent study also suggested that the effect of the nulled *GSTM1* gene on susceptibility to lung cancer may be more evident in heavy smoker patients [102] whereas others found nonsignificant association of the *GSTM1* null genotype with lung cancer [103 – 105].

Individuals with the *GSTT1* null genotype have been reported to have a nonsignificant risk for lung cancer [102, 103, 105 – 110] while a statistically significant OR of 1.41 for the *GSTT1* null genotype was reported by Spitz et al. [104]

There is less information on the role of the *GSTP1* gene as a cancer risk modifier. Given that *GSTP1* is the most abundant isoform in the lungs [111], it is anticipated to be of particular importance in the detoxification of inhaled carcinogens. Six published studies have reported that *GSTP1* polymorphism in exon 5 did not increase the risk of lung cancer [102, 109, 111-114].

Since the *GSTM1* and *GSTT1* genes are involved in the detoxification of tobacco-smoke-derived carcinogens, individuals with concurrent lack of these genes are expected to be at particular risk of developing lung cancer. A significant association was also observed for concurrent lack of the *GSTM1* and *GSTT1* genes and susceptibility to squamous cell carcinoma [110]. For that cell type, the risk was 2.3-fold (95% CI=1.0-5.3) when compared with that of individuals having other genotype combinations. In contrast, that genotype combination did not affect the risk for other histological types of lung cancer. Kelsey et al. [107] and Kiyohara et al. [103] also showed significant increased ORs for the association of lung cancer and the presence of both null polymorphisms. However, these findings are in contrast to these of previous studies, in which no association between the concurrent lack of these genes and susceptibility to lung cancer was observed [106, 108 – 110]. The significant increased risk for lung cancer has appeared for individuals with concurrently high levels of smoking and the combined *GSTM1* and *GSTT1* null genotypes compared with those with at least one null and low levels of smoking [109].

Epidemiological studies examining the protective association of cruciferous vegetables within smoking strata have had mixed results. Isothiocyanates (ITCs) are nonnutrient compounds in cruciferous vegetables with anticarcinogenic properties. ITCs are effective inhibitors of tumorigenesis in animal model systems [116]. One proposed mechanism for their protective action is through direct inhibition of their catalytic activities, with induction of phase II enzymes. ITCs are potent inhibitors of NNK metabolism [117]. The protective effect of ITCs was seen primarily among individuals with homozygous deletion of *GSTM1* (OR=0.36, 95% CI=0.20-0.63) and particularly with deletion of both *GSTM1* and *GSTT1* (OR=0.28, 95% CI=0.13-0.57) [118]. A large joint effect of both null genotypes and low ITC intake (OR=0.18, 95% CI=0.06-0.58) was observed by Spitz et al. [104].

The biological plausibility of the protective effect of GST through its conjugating activity is compelling. However, for a polymorphism as prevalent as the *GSTM1* null genotype, any overriding influence on the process of carcinogenesis should have been easily detectable in molecular epidemiologic studies, but the findings described above are less than compelling. The findings do suggest that the *GSTM1* null genotype and the concurrent lack of *GSTM1* and *GSTT1* are modestly associated with susceptibility to lung cancer. Although some of the inconsistencies reported in the role of *GST* genotypes in lung cancer risk could be due to unexpected confounding from dietary factors such as ITCs (diet-gene interaction), the overall role of *GST* polymorphisms in modifying the lung cancer risk may therefore be more limited than has been so far anticipated.

5 Combination of Susceptibility Genotypes

PAHs require metabolic activation by phase I enzymes to their ultimate forms (reactive intermediates) and these intermediates are then subjected to detoxification by phase II enzymes. Thus, genetically determined susceptibility to lung cancer may depend on the metabolic balance between phase I and phase II enzymes. It is important to identify individuals genetically who are at high risk of lung cancer in terms of polymorphisms of genes for encoding phase I enzymes and phase II enzymes. Nakachi et al. [118] reported that individuals with genotype C combined with nulled *GSTM1* were at significantly high risk with an OR of 16.00 (95% CI=3.76-68.02) for squamous cell carcinoma, at a low dose level of cigarette smoking. In a similar manner, the role of the combined genotypes *CYP1A1* and *GSTM1* as a possible modulator of smoking related lung cancers was studied in relation to the tobacco smoke level in Japanese patients aged below 70 years with squamous or small cell carcinomas of the lung [119]. Among male smoking patients, the overall proportion of the *GSTM1* null genotype was slightly higher than among healthy male smoker controls (56.7% versus 48.1%, P=0.17). Little difference was observed between smoker patients and corresponding controls in the overall frequencies of genotype C (16-18%). However, when subjects were categorized by both *Msp* I polymorphism in the *CYP1A1* gene and the *GSTM1* polymorphism, the *GSTM1* null genotype became markedly more expressed in patients with genotype C when compared with the corresponding smoker controls (81.3% versus 39.4%, P<0.01). When ORs were estimated using nonsmoking patients and healthy controls as a reference, the relative risk for developing lung cancer was found to increase in a cigarette dose-dependent manner across all combinations of genotypes. Furthermore, a 7- to 8-fold variation in risk was found among the various combinations; 3.2 in individuals with combined *GSTM1* non-null and genotype C and 21.9 in those with combined *GSTM1* null and genotype C when the smoking dose was high. These results suggest that individuals with genotype C are relatively resistant to tobacco-related lung cancers when combined with the *GSTM1* non-null genotype, but are highly susceptible when combined with the *GSTM1* null genotype.

In Caucasian populations, a combined risk of squamous cell carcinoma was indicated for patients, diagnosed before 66 years of age, carrying both the *GSTM1* null genotype and a rare *CYP1A1 Msp* I homozygous allele (OR=3.0, 95% CI=1.2-7.2) [23]. However, there were few patients with that combined genotype to analyze. The infrequency of this particular combined genotype suggests that it will not likely be applicable to screening European populations. In patients with inducible *CYP1A1*, the expressing *GSTM1* gene appeared to have a protective effect against contracting bronchial lung cancer, since 88% of the lung tumors in this patient group were peripheral, whereas almost equal numbers of peripheral and bronchial tumors were observed in those patients lacking the gene [120]. Neither the *CYP1A1 Msp* I heterozygous genotype alone nor the *GSTM1* null genotype alone were associated with a significant increase in lung cancer risk, although having both genetic traits was associated with a 2-fold increase in risk (95% CI=1.0-3.4) [27]. The presence of at least one copy of the *CYP1A1 Msp* I variant allele was found to be associated with a 2.4-fold (95% CI=1.2-4.7) increase in the risk of squamous cell carcinoma when this gene was considered singly and a 3.1-fold (95% CI=1.2-7.9) increase when combined with a *GSTM1* deletion [121]. The effect of the *GSTM1* null genotype on lung cancer has not been modified by the *CYP1A1* genotype in a French population [109].

The findings on combination phases I and II carcinogen bioactivation polymorphisms are controversial. Combination bioactivation polymorphisms are attractive with respect to biologically plausible susceptibility factors. The findings in Japanese population studies to date reveal high ORs for lung cancer. However, only 10 to 24% of Japanese lung cancer patients display these combination polymorphisms. For non-Asian populations, the relevance of the *CYP1A1 Msp* I and *GSTM1* polymorphisms to lung cancer is questionable, given their low prevalence in both lung cancer and general populations. Combined *CYP1A1* and *GSTM1* genotype is thus a potential predictor of genetic susceptibility to smoking-related lung cancers in populations where *CYP1A1* alleles are common.

6 OTHER *CYP* POLYMORPHISMS

CYP2A6 mediates 7-hydroxylation of coumarin, a component of cigarette smoke and activates several nitrosamines in tobacco smoke, including NNK [122]. The catalytic selectivity of CYP2A6 appears to overlap with that of CYP2E1. The location of this isoform is in extrahepatic tissues such as lung, nasal and pharyngeal. The *CYP2A6* gene is located on chromosome 19q13.2. Four variants have been identified, namely *CYP2A6*2* (Ile160His, 479T=>479A in exon 3), *CYP2A6*3* (gene conversion between wild-type *CYP2A6*1A* allele and the neighboring *CYP2A7*), *CYP2A6*4A-4D* (the four deletion alleles *CYP2A6* gene) and *CYP2A6*5* (Gyl479Val, 1436G=>1436T in exon 9). The *CYP2A6*2* allele detected by *Xcml* may be associated with reduced activity [123]. Originally, the *CYP2A6*3* allele identified by *Dde* I was expected to reduce activity because of its sequence similarity to *CYP2A7*, which codes for the inactive enzyme [124]. Very recently, improvements have been made to the original genotyping methods [125] and *CYP2A6*3* was shown to be lacking in different populations [126 – 128]. One reason for the original misclassification turned out to be due to the very common *CYP2A6*1B* allele (normal enzymatic activity) exhibiting a gene conversion between the 3'-flanking regions of the *CYP2A6* and *CYP2A7* genes [125]. Four *CYP2A6*4* alleles cause a lack of enzymatic activity [125]. The *CYP2A6*5* allele also abolish the catalytic activity of the encoded enzyme due to a point mutation. The frequency of the major *CYP2A6* alleles in healthy controls has been observed among various populations. The allelic frequencies of CYP2A6*2 were rather low in both Caucasian (2.3-3.0%) and Chinese (0-0.7%) populations, whereas the CYP2A6*4 alleles were fairly common in Chinese (8.6-15.1%) and rare in Caucasian (0.5-1.0%) [129, 130]. A small study showed that a decreased risk of lung cancer (OR=0.5, 95% CI=0.1-2.1) was observed among individuals with both the *CYP2A6**2 and *CYP2A6**3 alleles [131]. The whole gene deletion was associated with a decreased risk of lung cancer among a Japanese population [132]. Likewise, individuals with at least one *CYP2A6*4* allele were at a 2-fold (95% CI=1.2-3.2) increased risk of lung cancer compared with those without the *CYP2A6*4* allele [130].

Members of *CYP2C* gene subfamily are constitutively expressed. *CYP2C9* metabolizes PAH-type tobacco carcinogens such as BP [1] and catalyzes the hydroxylation of several medications, including warfarin, tolbutamide and phenytoin [133]. The *CYP2C9* gene is located on chromosome10q24. Two mutant alleles, *CYP2C9*2* (Arg144Cys, 430C=>430T) and *CYP2C9*3* (Ile359Leu, 1075A=>1075C) have been described [134] and appear to decrease activity [135]. Thus, these allelic variants may decrease the risk of lung cancer although individuals homozygous for either *CYP2C9*2* or *CYP2C9*3* are relatively uncommon [136]. A slightly increased risk of lung cancer has been observed with the presence of the *CYP2C9*2* allele among Caucasians [137, 138], whereas the *CYP2C9*3* allele was not significantly associated with a decreased lung cancer risk [134, 138]. Although the functional significance *in vivo* of both allelic variants has been demonstrated for drug metabolism, *CYP2C9**2 for wafarin [139] and *CYP2C9*3* for tolbutamide [133], there is no evidence to address whether either allele influences CYP2C9 activity for BP metabolism. It is possible that they might differentially influence activity towards BP and thus lung cancer risk. There is some biological plausibility to less efficient activation of PAHs such as BP in tobacco smoke by the mutant genotypes, but any difference of in the patterns of association observed for *CYP2C9*2* and *CYP2C9*3* alleles in relation to lung cancer risk are compatible to chance.

CYP2C19 activities have been exemplified by mephenytoin hydroxylation [140, 141] and the *CYP2C19* gene locates on chromosome10q24. The PM phenotype is explained to a great extent by two mutant alleles [142], *CYP2C19*2* (681G=>681A, a mutation in exon 5 causing an aberrant splice site) and *CYP2C19*3* (636G=>636A, a point mutation in exon 4 introducing a premature stop codon). The *CYP2C19*2* is mainly found in Asians [142]. The combined *CYP2C19* genotypes (*CYP2C19*2/*2*, *CYP2C19*2/*3* or *CYP2C19*3/*3*) correspond to that predicted for the CYP2C19 PM phenotype. The CYP2C19 PM phenotype comprises 3-5% of Caucasians, but 18-23% of Asians [143]. A very small study conducted among Japanese showed that the PM phenotype was associated with an increased risk of squamous cell carcinoma of the lung. There is a possibility that the role of CYP2C9 and CYP2C19 is in the detoxification of tobacco-derived carcinogens.

Some studies have suggested a relation between lung cancer and the occurrence of a rare allele, although future research is needed to establish a significant relation.

7 *NQO* Polymorphism

NAD(P)H quinone oxidoreductase 1 (NQO1), formerly referred to as DT-diaphorase, is a cytosolic enzyme catalyzing the two-electron reduction of quinone substrates. NQO1 either metabolically activates or detoxifies carcinogens present in cigarette smoke. BP is one of the most important carcinogens and the formation of BP quinone-DNA adduct is prevented by NQO1 [144]. In contrast, carcinogenic heterocyclic amines present in smoke are metabolically activated by NQO1 [145]. Therefore this enzyme is thought to be involved in both metabolic activation and detoxification of carcinogenic agents that could be involved in lung carcinogenesis. The *NQO1* gene is located on chromosome 16q22. Recently, a polymorphism of the gene encoding *NQO1* has been described. The polymorphic variant of the gene (Pro187Ser, a C to T transition at base pair 609) is associated with reduced NQO1 activity [146 – 149]. The three genotypes of this gene are the homozygous wild-type C/C (normal activity), the heterozygous C/T genotype (mild activity) and the homozygous rare allele T/T genotype (2-4 % of normal activity).

There have been several studies examining the relationship between the *NOQ1* polymorphism and lung cancer risk, but the conclusions have been contradictory. Rosvold et al. [150] reported that the rare allele was observed to be approximately twice as common in Caucasian cases as in controls. Lewis et al. [151] also reported that the variant allele was associated with a nonsignificant increased risk of lung cancer and a significant increased risk (OR=3.80, 95% CI=1.19-12.1) of small cell lung cancer. They concluded that the variant *NQO1* allele may play in activating genotoxins. In contrast, some studies [152, 153 – 155] have shown that the allele is inversely associated with lung cancer risk. Recently, a large study showed that no difference for the genotype distribution between lung cancer cases and controls [156]. However, there was a gene-environment interaction between the genotype and smoking: current smokers with the T/T genotype had a smaller cancer risk that those with C/C genotype (OR=0.38, 95% CI=0.19-1.00).

As shown in Table 4, a nonsignificant protective overall OR of 0.85 (95% CI=0.69 - 1.05) was reported by Kiyohara et al. [157]. Therefore, it is still unclear whether variant *NQO1* genotype is associated with a decreased risk of lung cancer.

Table 4. The overall ORs of selected genetic polymorphisms

Polymorphism	Cases/Controls	OR (95% CI)	Analysis	Reference
Phase I metabolic polymorphism				
CYP1A1 (T3801C)	3473	1.27 (0.91 - 1.77)	Meta	37
CYP1A1 (Ile462Val)	2290	1.62 (0.93 -2.82)	Meta	37
CYP1A1 (T3801C)	2451/3358	2.36 (1.16-4.81)	Pooled	38
NQO1 (Pro187Ser)	1584/2184	0.85 (0.69 - 1.05)	Meta	157
mEPHX1 (Try113His)	1010/1616	0.96 (0.66 - 1.39)	Meta	157
mEPHX1 (His139Arg)	1010/1616	1.44 (1.03 - 2.00)	Meta	157
Combined genotypes	1818/2563	0.96 (0.68 - 1.34)	Meta	157
Phase II metabolic polymorphism				
GSTM1	1593/2135	1.41 (1.23 - 1.60)	Meta	94
GSTM1	9045	1.13 (1.03 - 1.25)	Meta	95
MPO (G-463A)	1266/1748	0.63 (0.45 - 0.87)	Meta	157
Ohter polymorphism				
XRCC (Arg399Gln)	613/1055	1.02 (0.54 - 1.93)	Meta	157
XPD (Lys751Gln)	672/1047	1.50 (1.09 - 2.07)	Meta	157
p53 (Arg72Pro)	3305/3639	1.16 (0.99 - 1.38)	Meta	157

NQO2 is a polymorphic gene that encodes an enzyme with similar activity to *NQO1*. *NQO2* might be more important than *NQO1* in determining lung cancer risk. As the role of NQO1 may be different among different histology and different ethnic groups, a larger study group is warranted to evaluate the effect of smoking amount on those parameters.

8 *mEPHX1* Polymorphism

Microsomal epoxide hydrolase (mEPHX1) is an important phase II biotransformation enzyme and it is highly expressed in several human tissues including the lung, where it catalyzes the hydrolysis of various epoxides and reactive epoxide intermediates into less reactive and more water soluble dihydrodiols, which are then excreted from the body [158 – 160]. Hence, mEPHX1 is a protective enzyme involved in general oxidative defenses against a number of environmental substances [160 – 162]. However, mEPHX1 is also involved in the xenobiotic activation of tobacco carcinogens. Combined with CYP, mEPHX1 can metabolize PAHs into highly mutagenic and carcinogenic diol epoxides [163 – 165]. Thus, the activation or inactivation effects of mEPHX1 depend on the specific compounds being metabolized.

The *mEPHX1* gene is located on chromosome 1q42.1. There are two polymorphisms that affect enzyme activity in the human *mEPHX1* gene. One variant is characterized by substitution of histidine for tyrosine in exon 3 (Tyr113His, T=>C) and the other is substitution of arginine for histidine in exon 4 (His139Arg, A=>G), conferring low and high enzymatic activity, respectively [166].

Lower activity *mEPHX1* genotypes were associated with decreased lung cancer risk in several studies. French study found that lower activity of *mEPHX1* exon 3 genotype (His/His) was a protective factor for lung cancer [167]. Three Caucasian studies [152, 160, 168], two Chinese studies [169, 170] and a study of Wu et al. among African-Ameri cans and Mexican-Americans [171] found, however, no significant relationship between *mEPHX1* exon 3 genotype and lung cancer risk. A significant protective effect of low activity *mEPHX1* exon 3 genotype was observed among African-Americans [152] and Spaniards [168]. In Table 4, the calculated OR for *mEPHX1* exon 3 genotype of 0.96 (95% CI=0.66-1.39) was shown [157].

For *mEPHX1* exon 4 polymorphism, 6 of 7 studies could not found a significant association and the direction of the association was different among them [152, 160, 167, 168, 170, 171]. However, the exon 4 polymorphism associated with a significantly increased risk of lung cancer among Chinese and Mexican-Americans [169, 171]. The overall OR among the 7 case-control studies with 9 different ethnic populations was 1.44 (95% CI=1.03-2.00), which was significantly different than 1.0 (Table 4, [157]).

When combine polymorphisms exon 3 and exon 4, low activity genotype was significantly associated with a decreased risk of lung cancer among French Caucasian [167]. However, other studies among Caucasian populations [152, 160, 168] and among African-Americans [152] did not confirm the association. Although a Taiwanese study also found that low mEPHX1 activity genotype was not associated with decreased risk of lung cancer (OR=1.03, 95% CI=0.66-1.61), low activity genotype was significantly associated with a decreased risk of squamous cell carcinoma (OR=0.51, 95% CI=0.27-0.96) [172]. The relationship between *mEPHX1* genotypes and lung cancer risk has not been studied in a large number of subjects. Recently, no relationship between the low activity genotype and lung cancer risk was found by a large American study [173]. It also indicated that cumulative cigarette smoking exposures play pivotal roles in the association between both *mEPHX1* polymorphisms and lung cancer risk, altering the direction of risk (in the case of combined low activity genotype in both exon 3 and exon 4 polymorphisms) from a risk factor (OR=1.59, 95% CI=0.80-3.14) in nonsmokers to a protective factor (OR=0.45, 95% CI=0.22-0.93) in heavy smokers [173]. The 6 case-control studies in 7 different ethnic populations of lung cancer and the combined genotype included 4381 subjects (1818 lung cancer cases and 1563 controls). The overall OR of 0.96 (95% CI=0.68-1.34) was shown in Table 4 [157].

Differences in associations between ethnic subgroups or between study populations can result from linkage disequilibrium with additional allelic variants that modulate overall enzyme activity and may be present in different frequencies in the different groups or linkage disequilibrium with another gene that is causally related to lung cancer. Joint effects among *mEPHX1* genotype, other genetic polymorphisms and cigarette smoking should be investigated in additional studies.

9 *MPO* POLYMORPHISM

Neutrophil recruitment into lung tissue occurs after exposure to variety of insults known to increase lung cancer risk, including tobacco smoke particles, infection, asbestos and ozone [174 – 176]. Following immunological and/or chemical insults, neutrophils release myeloperoxidase (MPO) and undergo a respiratory burst, which is characterized by a massive increase in oxygen consumption and a consequent NADPH-dependent production of superoxide and other free radicals [174]. MPO is present in the primary granules of neutrophils and catalyzes the production of the potent bacteriotoxic oxidizing agent hypochlorous acid (a one and two-electron oxidant that can attack endogenous molecules including DNA) from hydroxyl radicals and chloride ions. A significant proportion (25-40 %) of the hydrogen peroxide formed by activated neutrophils may be converted to hypochlorous acids [177, 178]. MPO metabolically activates a wide range of tobacco smoke mutagens and environmental pollutants to DNA-damaging metabolites, including aromatic amines [179], the promutagenic derivatives of PAHs [180 – 182] and heterocyclic amines [183]. The *MPO* gene is located on chromosome 17q21-23. A G to A transition at position –463 in the promoter region of the *MPO* gene, which leads to the loss of a SP1 transcription binding site in an Alu hormone-responsive element [184], has been shown to reduce *MPO* mRNA expression [185]. It is possible that possession of two copies of the A allele of the *MPO* gene reduces the risk of lung. The wild-type G allele is present in 75 % of Caucasians [186 – 188].

Although the five studies found material associations between *MPO* genotype and lung cancer risk, estimates of the nature and extent of the association varied considerably between studies. Possession of the A/A genotype (8-10 % of the population) was associated with a decreased risk of lung cancer in Caucasians (OR=0.30, 95% CI=0.10-0.93) and 39% reduction (not statistically significant) in African Americans compared with those with two G alleles [186]. A second study [187] of populations with Caucasians, Japanese or Hawaiian ethnicity reported an overall 50 % reduction in risk (95% CI=0.2-1.3) for those with the A/A genotype compared with those with the G/G genotype. In a case-control study in the Berlin area [56], possession of one or two A alleles was suggested as being a protective factor for cancer of the lung (OR=0.58, 95% CI=0.38-0.88) and larynx (OR=0.63, 95 % CI=0.43-0.92) but not for cancer of the pharynx (OR=0.82, 95% CI=0.57-1.17). A smaller Caucasian study [189] has reported an overall reduction in risk of 48% for those possessing the A allele (95% CI=0.30-0.90). In a case-control study nested within a Finnish clinical trial [190], no evidence of an overall association between lung cancer risk and *MPO* genotype was observed, although the A/G or A/A genotype was associated with an increased risk of lung cancer among a subset of men of >64 years old (OR=2.92, 95% CI=1.33-6.43). The overall

OR from the 5 case-control studies of lung cancer among 8 ethnic groups was 0.63 (95% CI=0.45 - 0.87) [157].

The consistency of agreement between these studies, except for Hawaiian analysis [187], and the overall OR form the meta-analysis, suggests an important role for *MPO* in lung cancer etiology, possibly through activation of carcinogens and/or production of free radicals in or near the target cells.

10 DNA Repair Genes

1) ERCC and XRCC

Physiologically, the DNA repair capacity should be correlated with the level of proteins involved in DNA repair activity, which is controlled at the transcriptional level [191]. Therefore, it is conceivable that the baseline transcriptional level of DNA repair genes reflects a cellular ability to meet repair demand once the cells are stimulated by carcinogen exposure. One major DNA repair pathway capable of removing a variety of structurally unrelated DNA lesions, including those induced by tobacco carcinogens, is nucleotide excision repair (NER). This complex DNA repair process consists of approximately 30 proteins involved in sequential damage recognition, chromatin remodeling, incision of the damaged DNA strand on both sides of the lesion, excision of the oligonuleotide containing the damage and gap-filling DNA synthesis followed by strand ligation [192]. For example, smoking-related bulky adducts induced by benzo(a)pyrene or other PAHs and arylamines are removed effectively by the NER pathway [193]. In xeroderma pigmentosum (XP), patients have an extraordinarily higher rate of skin cancer because of a genetically determined defect in NER [191]. Other cancer-prone patients who have deficient DNA repair also have a higher rate of internal cancer [194].

Three rare, autosomal recessive inherited human disorders are associated with impaired NER activity: XP, Cockayne Syndrome (CS) and trichothiodystrophy (TTD) [195]. XP has been studied most extensively. Seven different human NER genes, which correct seven distinct genetic XP complementation groups (XPA, XPB, XPC, XPD, XPE, XPF and XPG) have been identified [195].

A number of genes that correct defective human NER have been designated as excision repair cross-complementing (*ERCC*) genes. The human gene responsible for XP groups B, D, F and G are identified as *ERCC3*, *ERCC2*, *ERCC4* and *ERCC5*, respectively. *ERCC1* has not been found to be involved in any XP, CS or TTD [196] because defects in *ERCC1* resulting from mutations or deletions of this cause early death before the disease develop [197]. *ERCC6* is identical to CSB and mutations in this gene are involved in CS [198]. Concerning DNA repair genes, eleven genes have been reported to date (nine NER genes (*ERCC1-6*, *XPA*, *XPE*, and *XPF*), a gene involved in double-strand break repair/recombination genes (X-ray cross-complementing group 3, *XRCC3*), and a gene functioning in base excision repair and the repair of radiation-induced damage (*XRCC1*)).

Polymorphisms in DNA repair genes may be associated with differences in the repair efficiency of DNA damage and may influence an individual's risk of lung cancer because the variant genotype in those polymorphisms might destroy or alter repair function. Reduced

DNA repair capacity has been shown to be associated with a 5.7-fold (95% CI=2.1-15.7) increased risk of developing lung cancer [199]. The overall 2.1-fold (95% CI=1.5-3.0) increased risk of lung cancer was consistent with their previous small pilot study [200]. Reduced gene expression levels of *ERCC5* (OR=2.32, 95% CI=1.22-4.43), *ERCC6* (OR=2.49, 95% CI=1.28-4.84) and *XPC* (OR=2.19, 95% CI=1.15-4.18) was significantly associated with an increased risk of lung cancer whereas *ERCC1* and *ERCC3* were not associated with lung cancer risk [201]. They postulated that lower DNA repair capacity in lung cancer patients may be the consequence of low expression of the NER genes. Ratnasinghe et al. [202] investigated three *XRCC1* polymorphisms (Arg194Trp, Arg280His and Arg399Gln) and found that only Arg280His allele was associated with an increased risk of lung cancer (OR=1.8, 95% CI=1.0-3.4). Divine et al. [203] reported that possessing the Gln/Gln genotype in *XRCC1* Arg399Gln polymorphism was significantly associated with an increased risk of adenocarcinoma of the lung among non-Hispanic (OR=3.25, 95% CI=1.2-10.7) and Hispanic (OR=1.40, 95 % CI=0.3-5.9) populations. This polymorphism was nonsignificnatly associated with decreased risk of lung cancer in both African-Americans (OR=0.6, 95% CI=0.2-2.3) and Caucasians (OR=0.6, 95% CI=0.3-1.3) while the codon 194 polymorphism was associated with increased risk (OR=2.3, 95% CI=0.2-25) among African-Americans [204]. In that study, neither the cases nor the controls with the genotype Trp/Trp was observed among Caucasians. *XRCC3* Thr241Met polymorphism was not associated with the risk of lung cancer among Caucasian and African-Americans [205]. For *XPD* Asp312Asn polymorphism, the Asp/Asp genotype has been found to have almost twice the risk of lung cancer when the Asp/Asn + Asn/Asn combined genotype served as reference [206]. The lung cancer risk was moderately associated with *XPD* Lys715Gln polymorphism among Caucasians [205, 207] while an OR was 1.03 among African-Americans [205]. Spitz et al. [207] reported that OR for variant Lys751Gln genotype was 1.36 (95% CI=0.84-2.20). For individuals with homozygous for the variant genotype at either locus, a statistically significant risk was seen (OR=1.84, 95% CI=1.11-3.04).

Both reduced NER gene expression [201] and low DNA repair capacity [199, 200] was associated with an increased risk of lung cancer while almost polymorphisms described here were not. As DNA repair capacity might be modified by the tumor burden, a causal relationship between lung cancer and DNA repair capacity could not be determined in case-control studies. It is important to investigate precisely the biological significance of the polymorphisms involved in DNA repair. The direct relationship between DNA repair capacity and expression level of the NER genes or those polymorphisms needs to be determined in future cohort studies.

2) Glutathione Peroxidase 1 and Human 8-Oxoguanine-DNA Glycosylase 1

In view of its abundance and mutagenicity, a number of defense mechanisms operate to minimize 8-hydroxyguanine (oh^{8}Gua) accumulation within the genome. oh^{8}Gua is a major DNA lesion produced by oxygen-radicals [208]. Primary defense mechanisms include antioxidants and enzymes such as glutathione peroxidase [209, 210]. Glutathione peroxidases reduce organic peroxides and hydrogen peroxides through the coupled oxidation of reduced glutathione. Glutathione peroxidase 1 (GPX1) is the major cytosolic form of this enzyme, but other isozymes are found in the plasma and phospholipid membranes [211]. The cytosolic form of human GPX1 belongs to a family of selenium–dependent peroxidases that include another cytosolic forms, hGXP2 [212], the plasma-based hGXP3 [213] and the phospholipids hydroperoxidase hGPX4 [214]. Polymorphisms in *GPX1* are characterized by a variable polyalanine repeat and the six-alanine repeat form (ALA6, instead of ALA5 or ALA7 with the wild-type proline) also contains a proline to leucine substitution at codon 198 towards the C-terminus [211]. Recently, this polymorphism showed no functional effect on erythrocyte GPX1 activity [215]. In addition, the presence of the ALA6 allele (the Leu allele was nonsignificnatly associated with reduced levels of oh^{8}Gua levels [216]. Although biochemical characterization of the human GPX1 enzymes encoded by the distinct genotype of the GPX1 polymorphism is till unclear, constitutive genotype may play a significant role in determining oh^{8}Gua levels within tissue DNA.

The formation of oh^{8}Gua in DNA causes G to T transversion, since oh^{8}Gua pairs with adenine as well as cytosine [217, 218]. The human 8-oxoguanine-DNA glycosylase 1 (*hOGG1*) gene encodes base excision repair proteins for oh^{8}Gua in double-stranded DNA [219]. The OGG1 protein possesses the ability to excise oh^{8}Gua paired with cytosine [219]. The *hOGG1* Ser326Cys polymorphism was initially identified by Kohno et al. [220]. Preliminary evidence from *E. coli* complementation assay suggested that the *hOGG1* Cys isoform exhibited reduced oh^{8}Gua repair activity [220]. However, Hardie et al. [221] suggested that differences in oh^{8}Gua glycosylase activity within *hOGG1* polymorphic variants were insufficient to impact on tissue oh^{8}Gua levels because levels of oh^{8}Gua did not vary with *hOGG1* genotype.

Both *GPX1* and *hOGG1* locate to regions of chromosome 3p (3p21 and 3p25/26, respectively) which are subjects to frequent and early loss of heterozygosity during lung cancer development [211, 222, 223].

A Japanese study indicated the Ser allele frequency was similar between controls (0.59) and lung cancer cases (0.59) but this polymorphism related to risk of squamous cell carcinoma when combined subjects with at least one Ser allele (OR=3.01, 95% CI=1.33-6.83) [224]. A Caucasian study also reported that the distributions of *hOGG1* Ser allele were not different between Caucasian lung cancer patient (0.74) and general population (0.76) [221]. The *hOGG1* Ser allele was more prevalent in Caucasians (Hungarian 0.81, English 0.76) than Asians (Japanese 0.59, Chinese 0.39) [221, 224]. The differences of this polymorphism among populations will influence the interpretations and strategies for its use as potential tool for estimation of a particular individual risk. No major difference in *hOGG1* genotype distribution was observed between lung cancer cases and controls [216, 225]. To date, three case-control studies were reported and none of them showed significant effects on lung cancer susceptibility. The *hOGG1* gene alone is probably not major contributor to lung cancer susceptibility.

A significant association between *hGPX1* genotype and lung cancer risk was observed [223]. The ORs for heterozygote and for homozygous variants were 1.8 (95% CI=1.2-2.8) and 2.3 (95% CI=1.3-3.8), respectively. The generalization of these results, however, may be somewhat restricted because the study was conducted among a Caucasian male smoker population. It should be attempt to examine the association between the *hGPX1* polymorphisms and lung cancer risk in other ethnic groups.

11 *P53* POLYMORPHISM

The *p53* tumor suppressor gene is one of the most commonly mutated genes in all types of human cancer [226, 227]. Recent studies of the function of the wild-type *p53* demonstrated that its antiproliferative effect is mediated by stimulation of a 21-kDa protein (p21cip/waf) that inhibits cyclin-dependent kinase activity and, thereby, cell division [228, 229]. This negative cell cycle controller effect may explain why the wild-type *p53* gene can suppress the transformation of malignant cells *in vitro* [230, 231]. Analysis of somatic tissue from many human cancers has shown that the wild-type *p53* allele frequently is lost and a mutant allele retained, providing a growth advantage for malignant cells [232 – 234]. The mutation of the *p53* gene can damage its DNA-binding properties and cell cycle control and in cell proliferation [235]. Somatic p53 mutations are found more frequently in squamous cell carcinoma than in adenocarcinoma, although this may be a function of higher exposures to tobacco in patients with squamous cell carcinoma [236].

The *p53* gene is located on chromosome 17p13. This gene is a key and potent mediator of cellular response against genotoxic insults [237]. The Pro allele of the *p53* polymorphism has been linked epidemiologically to smoking-related lung and bladder cancers in some studies. However, the exact biological mechanisms for an increased risk by the Pro allele are not fully understood.

To date, several polymorphisms in the *p53* gene has been reported. A germline polymorphism of *p53* with a single-base change at codon 72 (Arg72Pro , G=>C) that causes an amino acid replacement of arginine by proline has been reported to be associated with lung cancer.

Weston et al. [238] reported a small increased frequency of the Pro allele in adenocarcinomas among Caucasian, but a later study [239] by this same group did not confirm this finding in a different set of cancer cases and controls. They reported that the frequency of the Pro/Pro genotype was similar in lung cancer cases and controls. The Pro/Pro genotype was found to be overrepresented in a study of Japanese lung cancer, especially in Kreyberg I but not in adenocarcinoma [240]. Fan et al. [241] also found that the frequency of the Pro/Pro genotype was significantly higher in adenocarcinoma cases than controls. An enhanced risk of adenocarcinoma was reported for African-Americans with the Pro/Pro genotype [242]. A Swedish study has suggested that the codon 72 alleles may not be functionally involved in lung cancer but, rather, may be a marker in linkage disequilibrium with other cancer susceptibility sites on the *p53* gene [243]. No difference in the prevalence of the codon 72 *p53* polymorphism between lung cancer cases and controls has been found [244 – 247]. Murata et al. [247] reported that the genotypic frequencies of the *p53* gene in lung cancer patients were largely different between smokers and non-smokers ($p<0.001$). Biros et al. [248] found that another polymorphism *Msp* I may modify the susceptibility to lung cancer as a single factor rather than in combination with *BstU* I polymorphism. In a Caucasian population [249], when compared with the wild-type Arg/Arg genotype the adjusted OR of lung cancer for the Pro/Pro genotype was 1.29 (95% CI=0.9-1.8). The adjusted OR for adenocarcinoma and squamous cell carcinoma were1.33 (95% CI=0.9-2.0) and 0.75 (95% CI=0.4-1.5), respectively. As shown in Table 4, the overall OR was 1.16 (95% CI=0.99-1.38) [157]. A small and marginally significant increased risk of lung cancer was observed in a meta-analysis. Adenocarcinoma and squamous cell carcinoma, which are called non-small cell lung cancer, are distinct etiological entities that should be analyzed separately. Nine studies [240 - 247, 249] contained information on histology in a form suitable for pooled analysis. The *p53* polymorphism was associated with and ORs of 1.22 (95%CI=0.88-1.69) for adenocarcinoma and 0.98 (95%CI=0.71-1.23) for squamous cell carcinoma [157]. An overall OR from 4 studies [240, 241, 244, 246] for small cell carcinoma was 1.32 (95% CI=0.81-2.14) [157]. Restricting the analyses to the studies of Caucasian subjects, the major ethnic group, the OR of lung cancer associated with the *p53* polymorphism was 1.08 (95% CI=0.88-1.69) [157]. In non-Caucasian populations (African-Americans, Mexican-Americans, Japanese, Chinese and Hawaiian), the OR of this polymorphism was 1.15 (95% CI=0.89-1.49) [157]. There was no evidence of significant heterogeneity in either subgroup. Future analyses stratified by histology or ethnicity should be considered in future studies of the *p53* polymorphisms.

12 Genetic Influences on Smoking Behavior

The vast majority of cigarette smokers are daily smokers and, of these, the majority are nicotine-dependent smokers by DSM-IV criteria [250]. The only known way to reduce lung cancer risk in smokers is complete cessation, but most smokers are unable or unwilling to quit. Twin studies consistently have indicated important genetic influences on multiple aspects of smoking behavior, including both initiation and cessation [251]. To identify the genes involved in smoking behavior may lead to prevent the development of lung cancer.

1) Receptor Genes

Postsynaptic dopamine receptors can be classified as D1 class (D1 and D5) or D2 class (D2, D3 and D4) [252]. An intriguing aspect of dopamine receptor function is that, under normal conditions, concomitant stimulation of dopamine receptors of the D1 and D2 classes is required for manifestation of many of the behavioral and electrophysiological effects of dopamine [253 – 255]. This phenomenon has been referred to as requisite D1/D2 synergism [255]. There are differences between the DRD2 and DRD4, however such as in dopamine affinity (greater for the DRD4 in the low-affinity receptor state) and in the levels of protein expression [256]. There also is a difference for the binding of the dopamine agonist clozapine, which is an order of magnitude higher for the DRD4 compared with the DRD2 [257 – 260]. Clozapine is used for the treatment of schizophrenia, a disease that has a hypothesized underlying defect in the dopamine reward system.

Evidence for genetic determinants affecting the smoking phenotype has steadily accumulated both from studies of substance abuse in animals and from analysis of the contributions of genetics and personality to substance abuse in humans [261, 262]. Two recent linkage studies in humans [263, 264] have indicated regions of the genome in which loci affecting nicotine dependence and ever smoking may be found with further work. However, an appreciation of the neurotransmitter-related mechanisms involved in reward circuits in the human brain had suggested many candidate loci potentially associated with smoking behavior [265].

The hunt for genes associated with smoking behavior has been underway for many years. Among the candidate genes the *DRD2* gene is of particular interest and has been the focus of a great number of studies. The human *DRD2* gene has been mapped to a locus on human chromosome 11q23 and several polymorphisms of the gene have been reported [266]. Interindividual differences in the structure and expression of this gene result in alternation in dopamine availability to tobacco smoking. A polymorphism, an uncommon *Taq* I A restriction fragment length polymorphism (RFLP), (A1 or A2 allele) located in the 3'-flanking region of the *DRD2* gene [267]. Next, Hauge et al. [268] found that the more 5' *Taq* I B RFLP (B1 or B2 allele) is closer to the regulatory and structural coding regions of the gene. The A1 allele has been shown to be associated with low DRD2 density in human brain, compared with the A2 allele [269]. It has been hypothesized that such persons who have a reduced DRD2 density have a deficit in their reward system and experience an enhanced reward when exposed to dopaminergic agent, thereby making them more prone to nicotine dependence [270, 271]. Therefore, the A1 allele (or low DRD2 density) has been reported to be significantly associated with increased risk of alcoholism [272, 273], abuse of various drugs [274 – 276] and obesity [277, 278].

Bierut et al. [279] reported that genetic variation in the *DRD2* locus did not play a significant role in increasing the risk of smoking although the dopamine system may play a significant role in nicotine dependence. Recently, Spitz et al. [280] found that the *Taq* I B RFLP was a better maker for smoking behavior than *Taq* I A RFLP. There is substantial linkage disequilibrium between the A1 and B1 allelic variants [281, 282]. Three studies have shown a relationship between either *Taq* I A or *Taq* I B RFLP and genetic predisposition to smoking behavior [270, 280, 283] while no association was confirmed in another study [284]. Surprisingly, the A2 allele was associated with smoking behavior among Japanese [282]. The *DRD2* work is quite controversial. A considerable variation in the prevalence of the A1 allele (0.09-0.75) has been reported by Barr and Kidd [285] Several studies have also reported that various populations have the A1 allele frequencies of 0.12-0.24 among Caucasian [280], 0.36 among Japanese [282], 0.37 among African-American [286] and 0.42 among Mexican-American [286]. The prevalence of the A1 allele is higher among the colored than Caucasian. Ethnic variation of this gene may explain why those studies have been inconsistent. A low frequency of the variant allele may fail to establish the association due to low statistical power.

There is an imperfect 48-bp variable number of tandem repeat (VNTR) polymorphism involving 18 amino acids in the third exon of the *DRD4*. The relationship of the *DRD4* exon3 VNTR polymorphism to smoking behavior has received little attention to date. George et al. [287] found that there was an extremely high incidence (70 - 90%) of cigarette smoking among alcoholics with the repeated *DRD4* polymorphism. An association between the *DRD4* gene exon 3 polymorphism and smoking was also reported in African-Americans [288]. Further studies are needed to determine the role of the D4 receptor polymorphism.

The DRD5 binds dopamine 10 times more avidly than the DRD1 [289]. Genetic linkage and association data suggest that the *DRD5* may be positional candidate gene. Vanyukov et al. [290] reported a significant association between the microsatellite polymorphism D5

$(CT/GT/GA9)_n$ located about 55 kb from the *DRD5* gene with a heterogeneous set of psychoactive substance dependencies. However, *DRD5* was not substantially related to smoking initiation and progression to nicotine dependence [291].

Nicotine is considered the most addictive component in tobacco product [292]. Nicotine, via binding to neuronal nicotinic receptors, enhances dopamine release and neurotransmission in the mesolimbic dopamine system. Neuronal nicotine acetylcholine receptor (*nAChR*) family is believed to be most relevant to nicotine dependence and consists of 12 distinct genes encoding nine α-subunits and three ß-subunits. Dopaminergic neurons express α3, α4, α5, α6, α7, ß2 and ß3 subunits [293]. The identification and characterization of polymorphisms in the α_4 subunit of the *nAChR* is an area of active research [294 – 296]. Although several polymorphisms of this gene have been reported, there is no study on smoking behavior and those polymorphisms. No significant associations of the *nAChR* ß2 to smoking behavior or level of nicotine dependence were found [297]. Although the role of α6 subunit in the etiology of nicotine dependence remains unknown, this subunit was implicated in the stimulation effect of nicotine on habituated locomotion [298]. A6 subunit was suggested to be a useful tool to understand the mechanisms of nicotine dependence in mice [299]. On the whole, *nAChR* subunits have been performed on smoking have been negative. Future research in this field might focus on the establishment of new polymorphic sites in those subunits, with importance for function. Functionally important polymorphic alleles involved in smoking behavior might provide valuable tools for the understanding of nicotine dependence.

2) Transporter Genes

The serotoninergic system may be implicated in habitual smoking because nicotine increases brain serotonin secretion and nicotine withdrawal had the opposite effect [300, 301]. The serotonin transporter (5-HTT) is a plausible candidate for smoking predisposition because a polymorphism in the 5'-flanking region of this gene is associated with its transcriptional efficacy [302, 303]. There are two common alleles, a 44-bp insertion (L allele) or deletion (S allele). The S allele is associated with decreased transcriptional activity compared with the L allele. Serotonin transporter activity has been shown to decrease *in vivo* in the S/S genotype in comparison to activity in the L/S + L/L genotypes. Because the selective serotonin reuptake inhibitor fluoxetine antagonizes the ability of nicotine to evoke hyppocampal noradrenaline release *in vitro* [304], it is expected that the S allele would protect against habitual smoking and/or promote successful smoking cessation. Ishikawa et al. [305] suggested that individuals with the S/S genotype were less inclined to smoke and/or can more easily stop smoking than others. Smoking behavior was influenced by an interaction between neuroticism and the *5-HTT* genotype [306, 307].

Dopamine transporter (SLC6A3), determinable with a high affinity radioligand $[^{123}I]$-2ß-carnometoxy-3ß (4-iodophenyl)tropane, is relatively stable and, thus, a good indicator for the dopaminergic system [308, 309]. The *SLC6A3* gene has been shown to influence smoking behavior [310, 311]. However, these observations were not replicated in another subsequent study using non-volunteer white community sample [312]. These candidate genes studies need to be repeated in larger sample.

A rather large number of candidate genes for smoking behavior have been identified to date; however, few studies have found the association between these genes and smoking behavior. As population rates of smoking decline in response to social pressures, genetic influences may be particular strong among the remaining smokers. Understanding the genetic influences on smoking initiation may allow targeting of prevention strategies to individuals at high risk. It is likely that additional gene polymorphisms of relevance to smoking behavior will be identified during the next several years.

CONCLUSION

Molecular epidemiology has contributed to a growing awareness of the importance of relatively common genetic and acquired susceptibility factors in modulating risks associated with exposure to environmental carcinogens. Because lung cancer is largely preventable disease, the future challenge of molecular epidemiology is to analyze individuals who are exposed to carcinogens for a combination of genotypes associated with susceptibility to lung cancer. It is evident that use of more precisely measurable intermediary risk markers, like mutation in metabolic genes, DNA adducts and cytogenetic damage rather than lung cancer as an end point, will allow the identification of combinations of cancer-relevant genes that affect lung cancer outcome. Such associations could then be verified in epidemiological studies designed to address the association to be confirmed. Thus, further progress is expected from studies in which biomarkers for carcinogen exposure, early biological effects and susceptibility are integrated, which should allow establishment of the risk profiles of individuals and subgroups in given exposure situations.

IARC [313, 314] provided state-of the art reviews of the application of biomarkers and the design and analysis of molecular epidemiological studies. The prerequisites for proper study design and conduct include: (1) clear definition of representative study populations and controls; (2) a sample size adequate to provide enough statistical power; (3) proper documentation (or measurement) of exposure; (4) avoidance of confounding because of use of study subjects of mixed ethnic background; and (5) study only genetic polymorphisms that have been shown to lead to altered phenotypic expression.

Similarly, in order to avoid some of the problems associated molecular epidemiologic studies, Todd [315] has addressed the issue of guidelines for the interpretation of results from those studies of multifactorial diseases. They expect that those studies should contain large sample size, an independent replication followed by initial study, biological plausibility and physiologically meaningful data supporting a functional role of the polymorphism in question. The initial studies showed a substantially increased/decreased risk of developing lung cancer in individuals with specific genotypes.

Although some genetic polymorphisms discussed here have not shown significant increases/decreases in risk, individuals with differing genotypes may have different susceptibilities to lung cancer. A positive association between development of lung cancer and the mutant homozygous genotype of *CYP1A1* gene has been reported in several Japanese populations but such an association has not been observed in African-Americans. The relation between *CYP2D6* and lung cancer remains conflicting and inconclusive. Several polymorphisms have been identified at the *CYP2E1* locus. No definitive link between the polymorphisms of *CYP2E1* and the risk of lung cancer has, however, been identified. The role of other *CYP2* isoforms in lung carcinogenesis has not been sufficiently investigated. *GSTs* form a superfamily of genes consisting of five distinct families, named *GSTA*, *GSTM*, *GSTP*, *GSTT* and *GSTS*. The role of *GSTM, GSTT1* or *GSTP1* polymorphism in modifying the lung cancer risk may be more limited than has been so far anticipated. The results of meta-analyses indicate that the Arg/Arg genotype of *mEPHX1* exon 4 polymorphism was significantly associated with a decreased risk of lung cancer and the *MPO* polymorphism was a significant risk factor in the development of lung cancer. Those polymorphisms appear to be stronger candidates for lung cancer susceptibility genes although publication bias is always a possible limitation of combining data from various sources as in a typical meta-analysis or laboratory techniques for analysis of genotyping are different. Most of the PCR-based techniques currently used for such assignments have standardized and the quality control may not be necessarily required. The others polymorphisms, the risk estimates, although nonsignificant, are insufficiently precise to exclude a moderate risk, and larger studies are needed to obtain more precise risk estimates. There include polymorphisms in *NQO1*, DNA repair genes and *p53*. It is more likely, however, that the majority in variation in lung cancer susceptibility is due to genes that have not to be identified or tested. Candidate genes have involved immune function and cell cycle control. Alth ough a number of candidate genes for smoking behavior have been identified to date, the associations between them are on the ground of insufficient evidence. As stated above, the etiology of lung cancer cannot be explained by allelic variability at a single locus. Instead, the major burden of lung cancer in the population probably results from complex interaction between many genetic and environmental factors over time. An improved understanding of the interplay of environmental and genetic polymorphisms at multiple loci may help identify individuals who are at increased risk for lung cancer.

Conversely, the use of multiple comparisons in any given study raises the specter of finding an association by chance alone, if enough biomarkers and relationships are examined. Therefore, rigorous thresholds for statistical significance in such studies, far below the p=0.05 level, have been proposed and warrant integration into study design and reports [316].

Although the overall risk for developing cancer in individuals with at each 'at risk' genotype may be small, lung cancer is such common malignancy that even a small increase in risk translates to a large number of excess lung cancer cases at the population level. Therefore, polymorphisms, even which were not significantly associated with lung cancer, should be an important public health issue. In addition, a susceptibility factor in one population may not be a factor in another. There are differences in the prevalence of some metabolic polymorphisms such as *CYP1A1*, *CYP2D6* and *CYP2E1*, among the various ethnic groups [317]. In a population, where the prevalence of 'at risk' genotype in given polymorphism is very low, the 'at risk' allele or 'at risk' genotype was too infrequent to assess the risk it might confer to an individual; at a population level, the attributable risk must be small simply because it is an infrequent allele.

Knowledge of the prevalence and distribution of common genetic susceptibility factors and the ability to identify susceptible individuals or subgroups will have substantial preventive implications, in particular if more data are collected to show that people with certain high-risk genotypes are more susceptible to low levels of exposure. It is conceivable that such subjects could be : (1) more easily persuaded to avoid hazardous exposure like tobacco use; (2) targeted intensive smoking cessation programs; (3) be enrolled in chemoprevention trials; and (4) be involved in cancer screening programs that are nor appropriate for the general population. However, before results of individual screening for genetic traits can be used efficiently to implement preventive measures, more cancer-predisposing genes need to be studied and gene-environment and gene-gene interactions elucidated.

Rapid advances in high-throughout gene analysis by DNA chip technology will spread up the identification of new mutations in predisposing cancer genes. The main task, however, will be to characterize the functional significance of these gene variants in humans. Such efforts are under way, e.g., the Human Genome Project by Human Genome Organisation, which will come to its completion in the near future, or the Environmental Genome Project pursued by the National Institute for Environmental Health Services in the United States [318].

To this purpose, future studies involving larger control and case populations, precisely and uniformly defined clinical classification of lung cancer and better exposure histories will undoubtedly lead to a more thorough understanding of the role of various genes in lung cancer development.

REFERENCES

[1] Kamataki T. Metabolism of xenobiotics. In: Omura, T, Ishimura, Y, Fuijii-Kuriyama, Y, editors. *Cytochrome P-450*. 2nd Edition. Tokyo; Kodansha Ltd., 1993: 141-58.

[2] Mannervik B, Awasthi YC, Board PG, Hayes JD, Di Ilio C, Ketterer B, Listowsky I, Morgenstern R, Muramatsu M, Pearson WR. Nomenclature for human glutathione transferases. *Biochem J* 1992; 282: 305-6.

[3] Meyer DJ, Gilmore KS, Coles B, Dalton K, Hulbert PB, Ketterer B. Structural distinction of rat GSH transferase subunit 10. *Biochem J* 1991; 274: 619.

[4] Klebanoff SJ. Myeloperoxidase: occurrence and biological function. In: J Everse, J, Everse, KE, Grisham, MB,editors. *Peroxidases in Chemistry and Biology*. Vol. 1. Boca Raton, FL.; CRC Press, Inc., 1991: 1-35.

[5] Talalay P, De Long MJ, Prochaska HJ. Identification of a common chemical signal regulating the induction of enzymes that protect against chemical carcinogenesis. *Proc Natl Acad Sci (USA)*. 1988; 85: 8261-5.

[6] Mannervik B, Danielson UH. Glutathione transferases stracture and catalytic activity. *CRC Crit Rev Biochem* 1976; 23: 281-334.

[7] Pemble S, Schroeder KR, Spencer SR, Meyer DJ, Hallier E, Bolt HM, Ketterer B, Taylor JB. Human glutathione S-transferase theta (GSTT1): cDNA cloning and the characterization of a genetic polymorphism. *Biochem J.* 1994; 300: 271-6.

[8] Hayes JD, Pulford DJ. The glutathione S-transferase supergene family: regulation of GST and the contribution of the isoenzymes to cancer chemoprotection and drug resistance. *Crit Rev Biochem Mol Biol* 1995; 30: 445-600.

[9] Omiecinski CJ, Aicher L, Holubkov R, Checkoway H. Human peripheral lymphocytes as indicators of microsomal epoxide hydrolase activity in liver and lung. *Pharmacogenetics* 1993; 3:150-8.

[10] Kiyohara C. Genetic polymorphism of enzymes involved in xenobiotic metabolism and the risk of colorectal cancer. *J Epidemiol* 2000; 10: 349-60.

[11] Kawajiri K, Nakachi K, Imai K, Yoshii A, Shinoda N, Watanabe J. Identification of genetically high risk individuals to lung cancer by DNA polymorphisms of the cytochrome P450IA1 gene. *FEBS Lett* 1990; 263: 131-3.

[12] Hayashi S, Watanabe J, Nakachi K, Kawajiri K. Genetic linkage of lung cancer-associated MspI polymorphisms with amino acid replacement in the heme binding region of the human cytochrome P450IA1 gene. *J Biochem* 1991; 110: 407-11.

[13] Crofts F, Cosma GN, Currie D, Taioli E, Toniolo P, Garte SJ. A novel CYP1A1 gene polymorphism in African-Americans. *Carcinogenesis* 1993; 14: 1729-31.

[14] Cascorbi I, Brockmoller J, Roots I. A C4887A polymorphism in exon 7 of human CYP1A1: population frequency, mutation linkages, and impact on lung cancer susceptibility. *Cancer Res* 1996; 56: 4965-9.

[15] Kiyohara C, Hirohata T, Inutsuka T. The relationship between aryl hydrocarbon hydroxylase(AHH) activity and polymorphisms of the CYP1A1 gene. *Jpn J Cancer Res* 1996; 87: 18-24.

[16] Nakachi K, Imai K, Hayashi S, Watanabe J, Kawajiri K. Genetic susceptibility to squamous cell carcinoma of the lung in relation to cigarette smoking dose. *Cancer Res* 1991; 51: 5177-80.

[17] Ikawa S, Uematsu F, Watanabe K, Kimpara T, Osada M, Hossain A, Sagami I, Kikuchi H, Watanabe M. Assessment of cancer susceptibility in humans by use of genetic polymorphisms in carcinogen metabolism. *Pharmacogenetics* 1995; 5: S154-S160.

[18] Lin P, Wang SL, Wang HJ, Chen KW, Lee HS, Tsai KJ, Chen CY, Lee H. Association of CYP1A1 and microsomal epoxide hydrolase polymorphisms with lung squamous cell carcinoma. *Br J Cancer* 2000; 82: 852-7.

[19] Kim KS, Ryu SW, Kim YJ, Kim E. Polymorphism analysis of the CYP1A1 locus in Koreans: presence of the solitary m2 allele. *Mol Cells* 1999; 9: 78-83.

[20] Tefre T, Ryberg D, Haugen A, Nebert DW, Skaug V, Brogger A, Borresen AL. Human CYP1A1 (cytochrome P(1)450) gene: lack of association between the Msp I restriction fragment length polymorphism and incidence of lung cancer in a Norwegian population. *Pharmacogenetics* 1991; 1: 20-5.

[21] Hirvonen A, Husgafvel-Pursiainen K, Karjalainen A, Anttila S, Vainio H. Point-mutational MspI and Ile-Val polymorphisms closely linked in the CYP1A1 gene: lack of association with susceptibility to lung cancer in a Finnish study population. *Cancer Epidemiol Biomarkers Prev* 1992; 1: 485-9.

[22] Shields PG, Caporaso NE, Falk RT, Sugimura H, Trivers GE, Trump BF, Hoover RN, Weston A, Harris CC. Lung cancer, race, and a CYP1A1 genetic polymorphism. *Cancer Epidemiol Biomarkers Prev* 1993; 2: 481-5.

[23] Alexandrie AK, Sundberg MI, Seidegard J, Tornling G, Rannug A. Genetic susceptibility to lung cancer with special emphasis on CYP1A1 and GSTM1: a study

on host factors in relation to age at onset, gender and histological cancer types. *Carcinogenesis* 1994; 15: 1785-90.

[24] Drakoulis N, Cascorbi I, Brockmoller J, Gross CR, Roots I. Polymorphisms in the human CYP1A1 gene as susceptibility factors for lung cancer: exon-7 mutation (4889 A to G), and a T to C mutation in the 3'-flanking region. *Clin Invest* 1994; 72: 240-8.

[25] Jacquet M, Lambert V, Baudoux E, Muller M, Kremers P, Gielen J. Correlation between P450 CYP1A1 inducibility, MspI genotype and lung cancer incidence. *Eur J Cancer* 1996; 32A: 1701-6.

[26] Bouchardy C, Wikman H, Benhamou S, Hirvonen A, Dayer P, Husgafvel-Pursiainen K. *CYP1A1* genetic polymorphism, tobacco smoking and lung cancer risk in a French Caucasian population. *Biomarkers* 1997; 2: 131-4.

[27] Garcia-Closas M, Kelsey KT, Wiencke JK, Xu X, Wain JC, Christiani DC. A case-control study of cytochrome P450 1A1, glutathione S-transferase M1, cigarette smoking and lung cancer susceptibility (Massachusetts, United States) *Cancer Causes Control* 1997; 8: 544-53.

[28] Sugimura H, Suzuki I, Hamada GS, Iwase T, Takahashi T, Nagura K, Iwata H, Watanabe S, Kino I, Tsugane S. Cytochrome P-450 lA1 genotype in lung cancer patients and controls in Rio de Janeiro, Brazil. *Cancer Epidemiol. Biomarkers Prev* 1994; 3: 145-8.

[29] Ishibe N, Wiencke JK, Zuo ZF, McMillan A, Spitz M, Kelsey KT. Susceptibility to lung cancer in light smokers associated with CYP1A1 polymorphisms in Mexican- and African-Americans. *Cancer Epidemiol Biomarkers Prev* 1997; 6: 1075-80.

[30] Taioli E, Ford J, Trachman J, Li Y, Demopoulos R, Garte S. Lung cancer risk and CYP1A1 genotype in African Americans. *Carcinogenesis* 1998; 19: 813-7.

[31] Garte S, Gaspari L, Alexandrie AK, Ambrosone C, Autrup H, Autrup JL, Baranova H, Bathum L, Benhamou S, Boffetta P, Bouchardy C, Breskvar K, Brockmoller J, Cascorbi I, Clapper ML, Coutelle C, Daly A, Dell'Omo M, Dolzan V, Dresler CM, Fryer A, Haugen A, Hein DW, Hildesheim A, Hirvonen A, Hsieh LL, Ingelman-Sundberg M, Kalina I, Kang D, Kihara M, Kiyohara C, Kremers P, Lazarus P, Le Marchand L, Lechner MC, van Lieshout EM, London S, Manni JJ, Maugard CM, Morita S, Nazar-Stewart V, Noda K, Oda Y, Parl FF, Pastorelli R, Persson I, Peters WH, Rannug A, Rebbeck T, Risch A, Roelandt L, Romkes M, Ryberg D, Salagovic J, Schoket B, Seidegard J, Shields PG, Sim E, Sinnet D, Strange RC, Stucker I, Sugimura H, To-Figueras J, Vineis P, Yu MC, Taioli E. Metabolic gene polymorphism frequencies in control populations. *Cancer Epidemiol Biomarkers Prev* 2001;10: 1239-48.

[32] Kiyohara C, Nakanishi Y, Inutsuka S, Takayama K, Hara N, Motohiro A, Tanaka K, Kono S, Hirohata T. The relationship between CYP1A1 aryl hydrocarbon hydroxylase activity and lung cancer in a Japanese population. *Pharmacogenetics* 1998; 8: 315-23.

[33] London SJ, Daly AK, Fairbrother KS, Holmes C, Carpenter CL, Navidi WC, Idle JR. Lung cancer risk in African-Americans in relation to a race-specific CYP1A1 polymorphism. *Cancer Res* 1995; 55: 6035-7.

[34] Taioli E, Trachman J, Chen X, Toniolo P, Garte SJ. A CYP1A1 restriction fragment length polymorphism is associated with breast cancer in African-American women. *Cancer Res* 1995; 55: 3757-8.

[35] Taioli E, Crofts F, Trachman J, Demopoulos R, Toniolo P, Garte SJ. A specific African-American CYP1A1 polymorphism is associated with adenocarcinoma of the lung. *Cancer Res* 1995; 55: 472-3.

[36] Kelsey KT, Wiencke JK, Spitz MR. A race-specific genetic polymorphism in the CYP1A1 gene is not associated with lung cancer in African Americans. *Carcinogenesis* 1994; 15: 1121-4.

[37] Houlston RS. CYP1A1 polymorphisms and lung cancer risk: a meta-analysis. *Pharmacogenetics* 2000; 10: 105-14.

[38] Vineis P, Veglia F, Benhamou S, Butkiewicz D, Cascorbi I, Clapper ML, Dolzan V, Haugen A, Hirvonen A, Ingelman-Sundberg M, Kihara M, Kiyohara C, Kremers P, Le Marchand L, Ohshima S, Pastorelli R, Rannug A, Romkes M, Schoket B, Shields P, Strange RC, Stucker I, Sugimura H, Garte S, Gaspari L, Taioli E. CYP1A1 T3801 C polymorphism and lung cancer: a pooled analysis of 2451 cases and 3358 controls. *Int J Cancer* 2003; 104: 650-7.

[39] Kroemer HK, Mikus G, Eichelbaum M. Clinical relationship of pharmacogenetics. In: Kroemer, HK, Mikus, G, Eichelbaum, M editors. *Handbook of Experimental Pharmacology*. Berlin; Springer-Verlag, 1994: 265-88.

[40] Woolhouse NM, Andoh B, Mahgoub A, Sloan TP, Idle JR, Smith RL. Debrisoquin hydroxylation polymorphism among Ghanaians and Caucasians. *Clin Pharmacol Ther* 1979; 26: 584-91.

[41] Mahgoub A, Idle JR, Dring LG, Lancaster R, Smith RL. Polymorphic hydroxylation of Debrisoquine in man. *Lancet* 1977; 2: 584-6.

[42] Johansson I, Lundqvist E, Bertilsson L, Dahl ML, Sjoqvist F, Ingelman-Sundberg M. Inherited amplification of an active gene in the cytochrome P450 CYP2D locus as a cause of ultrarapid metabolism of debrisoquine. *Proc Acad Nat Sci (USA)* 1993; 90: 11825-9.

[43] Gonzalez FJ, Skoda RC, Kimura S, Umeno M, Zanger UM, Nebert DW, Gelboin HV, Hardwick JP, Meyer UA. Characterization of the common genetic defect in humans deficient in debrisoquine metabolism. *Nature* 1988; 331: 442-6.

[44] Skoda RC, Gonzalez FJ, Demierre A, Meyer UA. Two mutant alleles of the human cytochrome P-450db1 gene (P450C2D1) associated with genetically deficient metabolism of debrisoquine and other drugs. *Proc Acad Nat Sci (USA)* 1988; 85: 5240-3.

[45] Bertilsson L, Dahl ML, Sjoqvist F, Aberg-Wistedt A, Humble M, Johansson I, Lundqvist E, Ingelman-Sundberg M. Molecular basis for rational megaprescribing in ultrarapid hydroxylators of debrisoquine. *Lancet* 1993; 341: 363.

[46] Inaba T, Jurima M, Kalow W. Family studies of mephenytoin hydroxylation deficiency. *Am J Human Genet* 1986; 38: 768-72.

[47] Daly AK, Brockmoller J, Broly F, Eichelbaum M, Evans WE, Gonzalez FJ, Huang JD, Idle JR, Ingelman-Sundberg M, Ishizaki T, Jacqz-Aigrain E, Meyer UA, Nebert DW,

Steen VM, Wolf CR, Zanger UM. Nomenclature for human CYP2D6 alleles. *Pharmacogenetics* 1996; 6: 193-201.

[48] Ramachandran S, Lear JT, Ramsay H, Smith AG, Bowers B, Hutchinson PE, Jones PW, Fryer AA, Strange RC. Presentation with multiple cutaneous basal cell carcinomas: association of glutathione S-transferase and cytochrome P450 genotypes with clinical phenotype. *Cancer Epidemiol Biomarkers Prev* 1999; 8: 61-7.

[49] Laforest L, Wikman H, Benhamou S, Saarikoski ST, Bouchardy C, Hirvonen A, Dayer P, Husgafvel-Pursiainen K. CYP2D6 gene polymorphism in caucasian smokers: lung cancer susceptibility and phenotype-genotype relationships. *Eur J Cancer* 2000; 36: 1825-32.

[50] Gonzalez FJ. Genetic polymorphism and cancer susceptibility: fourteenth Sapporo Cancer Seminar. *Cancer Res* 1995; 55: 710-5.

[51] Nebert DW. Polymorphism of human CYP2D genes involved in drug metabolism: possible relationship to individual cancer risk. *Cancer Cells* 1991; 3: 93-6.

[52] London SJ, Daly AK, Leathart JB, Navidi WC, Carpenter CC, Idle JR. Genetic polymorphism of CYP2D6 and lung cancer risk in African-Americans and Caucasians in Los Angeles County. *Carcinogenesis* 1997; 18: 1203-14.

[53] Sugimura H, Caporaso NE, Shaw GL, Modali RV, Gonzalez FJ, Hoover RN, Resau JH, Trump BF, Weston A, Harris CC. Human debrisoquine hydroxylase gene polymorphisms in cancer patients and controls. *Carcinogenesis* 1990; 11: 1527-30.

[54] Roots I, Brockmoller J, Drakoulis N, Loddenkemper R. Mutant genes of cytochrome P-450IID6, glutathione S-transferase class Mu, and arylamine N-acetyltransferase in lung cancer patients. *Clin Invest* 1992; 70: 307-19.

[55] Wolf CR, Smith CA, Bishop T, Forman D, Gough AC, Spurr NK. CYP2D6 genotyping and the association with lung cancer susceptibility. *Pharmacogenetics* 1994 ;4: 104-6.

[56] Hirvonen A, Husgafvel-Pursiainen K, Anttila S, Karjalainen A, Pelkonen O, Vainio H. PCR-based CYP2D6 genotyping for Finnish lung cancer patients. *Pharmacogenetics* 1993; 3: 19-27.

[57] Agundez JA, Martinez C, Ladero JM, Ledesma MC, Ramos JM, Martin R, Rodriguez A, Jara C, Benitez J. Debrisoquin oxidation genotype and susceptibility to lung cancer. *Clin. Pharmacol. Ther.* 1994; 55: 10-14.

[58] Tefre T, Daly AK, Armstrong M, Leathart JB, Idle JR, Brogger A, Borresen AL. Genotyping of the CYP2D6 gene in Norwegian lung cancer patients and controls. *Pharmacogenetics* 1994; 4: 47-57.

[59] Rannug A, Alexandrie AK, Persson I, Ingelman-Sundberg M. Genetic polymorphism of cytochromes P450 1A1, 2D6 and 2E1: regulation and toxicological significance. *J Occup Environ Med* 1995; 37: 25-36.

[60] Dolzán V, Rudolf Z, Breskvar K. Human CYP2D6 gene polymorphism in Slovene cancer patients and healthy controls. *Carcinogenesis* 1995; 16: 2675-8.

[61] Stücker I, Cosme J, Laurent P, Cenee S, Beaune P, Bignon J, Depierre A, Milleron B, Hemon D. CYP2D6 genotype and lung cancer risk according to histologic type and tobacco exposure. *Carcinogenesis* 1995; 16: 2759-64.

[62] Shaw GL, Falk RT, Frame JN, Weiffenbach B, Nesbitt JC, Pass HI, Caporaso NE, Moir DT, Tucker MA. Genetic polymorphism of CYP2D6 and lung cancer risk. *Cancer Epidemiol Biomarkers Prev* 1998; 7: 215-9.

[63] Legrand M, Stucker I, Marez D, Sabbagh N, Lo-Guidice JM, Broly F. Influence of a mutation reducing the catalytic activity of the cytochrome P450 CYP2D6 on lung cancer susceptibility. *Carcinogenesis* 1996; 17: 2267-9.

[64] Katoh T, Higashi K. Ethnic differences of the primary gene defect at the cytochrome P-450 2D6. *J UOEH* 1992; 14: 205-9.

[65] Chida M, Yokoi T, Kosaka Y, Chiba K, Nakamura H, Ishizaki T, Yokota J, Kinoshita M, Sato K, Inaba M, Aoki Y, Gonzalez FJ, Kamataki T. Genetic polymorphism of CYP2D6 in the Japanese population. *Pharmacogenetics* 1999; 9: 601-5.

[66] Amos CI Caporaso NE, Western A. Host factors in lung cancer risk: a review of interdisciplinary studies. *Cancer Epidemiol Biomarkers Prev* 1992; 1: 505-13.

[67] Tyndale R, Aoyama T, Broly F, Matsunaga T, Inaba T, Kalow W, Gelboin HV, Meyer UA, Gonzalez FJ. Identification of a new variant CYP2D6 allele lacking the codon encoding Lys-281: possible association with the poor metabolizer phenotype. *Pharmacogenetics* 1991; 1: 26-32.

[68] Guengerich FJ. Interindividual variation in biotransformation of carcinogens: Basis and relevance. In: Groopman J, Skipper P, editors. *Molecular dosimetry and human cancer.* Boston: CRC Press, 1991: 27-45.

[69] Nebert DW. Genes encoding drug-metabolizing enzymes: possible role in human disease. In: Woodhead, AD, Bender, MA, Leonad, TC editors. *Phenotypic variation in populations: relevance to risk assessment.* New York; Plenum Press, 1988: 45-46.

[70] Wrighton SA, Thomas PE, Molowa DT, Haniu M, Shively JE, Maines SL, Watkins PB, Parker G, Mendez-Picon G, Levin W. Characterization of ethanol-inducible human liver N-nitrosodimethylamine demethylase. *Biochemistry* 1986; 25: 6731-65.

[71] Yoo JS, Guengerich FP, Yang CS. Metabolism of N-nitrosodialkylamines by human liver microsomes. *Cancer Res* 1988; 48: 1499-1504.

[72] Uematsu F, Kikuchi H, Ohmachi T, Sagami I, Motomiya M, Kamataki T, Komori M, Watanabe M. Two common RFLPs of the human CYP2E gene. *Nucleic Acids Res* 1991; 19: 2803.

[73] Uematsu F, Kikuchi H, Motomiya M, Abe T, Sagami I, Ohmachi T, Wakui A, Kanamaru R, Watanabe M. Association between restriction fragment length polymorphism of the human cytochrome P450IIE1 gene and susceptibility to lung cancer. *Jpn J Cancer Res* 1991; 82: 254-6.

[74] Watanabe J, Hayashi S, Nakachi K, Imai K, Suda Y, Sekine T, Kawajiri K. Kawajiri PstI and RsaI RFLPs in complete linkage disequilibrium at the CYP2E gene. *Nucleic Acids Res* 1990; 18: 7194.

[75] Hayashi S, Watanabe J, Kawajiri K. Genetic polymorphisms in the 5'-flanking region change transcriptional regulation of the human cytochrome P450IIE1 gene. *J Biochem* 1991; 110: 559-65.

[76] McBride OW, Umeno M, Gelboin HV, Gonzalez FJ. A Taq I polymorphism in the human P450IIE1 gene on chromosome 10 (CYP2E). *Nucleic Acids Res* 1987; 15: 10071.

[77] Hirvonen A, Husgafvel-Pursiainen K, Anttila S, Karjalainen A, Vainio H. The human CYP2E1 gene and lung cancer: DraI and RsaI restriction fragment length polymorphisms in a Finnish study population. *Carcinogenesis* 1993; 14: 85-8.

[78] Persson I, Johansson I, Bergling H, Dahl ML, Seidegard J, Rylander R, Rannug A, Hogberg J, Sundberg MI. Genetic polymorphism of cytochrome P4502E1 in a Swedish population. Relationship to incidence of lung cancer. *FEBS Lett* 1993; 319: 207-11.

[79] Kato S, Shields PG, Caporaso NE, Hoover RN, Trump BF, Sugimura H, Weston A, Harris CC. Cytochrome P450IIE1 genetic polymorphisms, racial variation, and lung cancer risk. *Cancer Res* 1992; 52: 6712-5.

[80] Stephens EA, Taylor JA, Kaplan N, Yang CH, Hsieh LL, Lucier GW, Bell DA. Ethnic variation in the CYP2E1 gene: polymorphism analysis of 695 African-Americans, European-Americans and Taiwanese. *Pharmacogenetics* 1994; 4: 185-92.

[81] Watanabe J, Yang JP, Eguchi H, Hayashi S, Imai K, Nakachi K, Kawajiri K. An Rsa I polymorphism in the CYP2E1 gene does not affect lung cancer risk in a Japanese population. *Jpn. J. Cancer Res* 1995; 86: 245-8.

[82] Oyama T, Kawamoto T, Mizoue T, Sugio K, Kodama Y, Mitsudomi T, Yasumoto K. Cytochrome P450 2E1 polymorphism as a risk factor for lung cancer: in relation to p53 gene mutation. *AntiCancer Res* 1997; 17: 583-7.

[83] Ingelman-Sundberg M, Johansson I, Persson I, Yue QY, Dahl ML, Bertilsson L, Sjoqvist F. Gentic polymorphism of cytochrome P450: interethnic differences and relationship to incidence of lung cancer. *Pharmacogenetics* 1992; 2: 264-71.

[84] Tsutsumi M, Wang JS, Takase S, Takada A. Hepatic messenger RNA contents of cytochrome P4502E1 in patients with different P4502E1 genotypes. *Alcohol Alcohol* 1994; 29: s29-s32.

[85] London SJ, Daly AK, Cooper J, Navidi WC, Idle JR. Lung cancer risk in relation to the CYP2E1 Rsa I genetic polymorphism among African-Americans and Caucasians in Los Angeles County. *Pharmacogenetics* 1996; 6: 527-33.

[86] Wu X, Shi H, Jiang H, Kemp B, Hong WK, Delclos GL, Spitz MR. Associations between cytochrome P4502E1 genotype, mutagen sensitivity, cigarette smoking and susceptibility to lung cancer. *Carcinogenesis* 1997; 18:967-73.

[87] Seidegard J, De Pierre JW, Birberg W, Pilotti A, Pero RW. Characterization of soluble glutathione transferase activity in resting mononuclear leukocytes from human blood. *Biochem Pharmacol* 1984; 33: 3053-8.

[88] Seidegard J, DePierre JW, Pero RW. Hereditary interindividual differences in the glutathione transferase activity towards trans-stilbene oxide in resting human mononuclear leukocytes are due to a particular isozyme(s). *Carcinogenesis* 1985; 6: 1211-6.

[89] Harries LW, Stubbins MJ, Forman D, D, Howard GC, Wolf CR. Identification of genetic polymorphisms at the glutathione S-transferase Pi locus and association with susceptibility to bladder, testicular and prostate cancer. *Carcinogenesis* 1997; 18: 641-4.

[90] Ali-Osman F, Akande OA, Antoun G, Mao J, Boulamwin J. Molecular cloning, characterization, and expression in Escherichia coli of full-length cDNAs of three

human glutathione S-transferase Pi gene variants. Evidence for differential catalytic activity of the encoded proteins. *J Biol Chem* 1997; 272: 10004-12.

[91] Zimniak P, Nanduri B, Pikula S, Bandorowicz-Pikula J, Singhal SS, Srivastava SK, Awasthi S, Awasthi YC. Naturally occurring human glutathione S-transferase GSTP1-1 isoforms with isoleucine and valine in position 104 differ in enzymic properties. *Eur J Biochem* 1994; 224: 893-9.

[92] Board PG, Webb GC, Coggan M. Isolation of a cDNA clone and localization of the human glutathione S-transferase 3 genes to chromosome bands 11q13 and 12q13-14. *Ann Hum Genet* 1989; 53: 205-13.

[93] Yamamura K, Kiyohara C, Nakanishi Y, Takayama K, Hara N. Lung cancer risk and genetic polymorphism at the glutathione S-transferase P1 locus in male Japanese. *Fukuoka Acta Med* 2000; 91: 203-6.

[94] McWilliams JE, Sanderson BJ, Harris EL, Richert-Boe KE, Henner WD. Glutathione S-transferase M1 (GSTM1) deficiency and lung cancer risk. *Cancer Epidemiol Biomarkers Prevent* 1995; 4: 589-94.

[95] Houlston RS. Glutathione S-transferase M1 status and lung cancer risk: a meta-analysis. *Cancer Epidemiol Biomarkers Prev* 1999; 8: 675-82.

[96] Seidegard J, Pero RW, Markowitz MM, Roush G, Miller DG, Beattie EJ. Isoenzyme(s) of glutathione transferase (class Mu) as a marker for the susceptibility to lung cancer: a follow up study. *Carcinogenesis* 1990; 11: 33-6.

[97] Ketterer B, Harris JM, Talaska G, Meyer DJ, Pemble SE, Taylor JB, Lang NP, Kadlubar FF. The human glutathione S-transferase supergene family, its polymorphism, and its effects on susceptibility to lung cancer. *Environ. Health Perspect.* 1992; 98: 87-94.

[98] Heckbert SR, Weiss NS, Hornung SK, Eaton DL, Motulsky AG. Glutathione S-transferase and epoxide hydrolase activity in human leukocytes in relation to risk of lung cancer and other smoking-related cancers. *J Natl Cancer Inst* 1992; 84: 414-22.

[99] Zhong S, Howie AF, Ketterer B, Taylor J, Hayes JD, Beckett GJ, Wathen CG, Wolf CR, Spurr NK. Glutathione S-transferase mu locus: use of genotyping and phenotyping assays to assess association with lung cancer susceptibility. *Carcinogenesis* 1991; 12: 1533-7.

[100] Nazar-Stewart V, Motulsky AG, Eaton DL, White E, Hornung SK, Leng ZT, Stapleton P, Weiss NS. The glutathione S-transferase mu polymorphism as a marker for susceptibility to lung carcinoma. *Cancer Res* 1993; 53: s2313-s2318.

[101] Seidegard J, Pero RW, Miller DG, Beattie EJ. A glutathione transferase in human leukocytes as a marker for the susceptibility to lung cancer. *Carcinogenesis* 1986; 7: 751-3.

[102] Lan Q, He X, Costa DJ, Tian L, Rothman N, Hu G, Mumford JL. Indoor coal combustion emissions, GSTM1 and GSTT1 genotypes, and lung cancer risk: a case-control study in Xuan Wei, China. *Cancer Epidemiol Biomarkers Prev* 2000; 9: 605-8.

[103] Kiyohara C, Yamamura K, Nakanishi Y, Takayama K, Hara N. Polymorphism in *GSTM1*, *GSTT1*, and *GSTP1* and susceptibility to lung cancer in a Japanese population, *Asian Pacific J Cancer Prev* 2000; 1: 293-8.

[104] Spitz MR, Duphorne CM, Detry MA, Pillow PC, Amos CI, Lei L, de Andrade M, Gu X, Hong WK, Wu X. Dietary intake of isothiocyanates: evidence of a joint effect with glutathione S-transferase polymorphisms in lung cancer risk. *Cancer Epidemiol Biomarkers Prev* 2000; 9: 1017-20.

[105] London SJ, Yuan JM, Chung FL, Gao YT, Coetzee GA, Ross RK, Yu MC. Isothiocyanates, glutathione S-transferase M1 and T1 polymorphisms, and lung-cancer risk: a prospective study of men in Shanghai, China. *Lancet* 2000; 356: 724-9.

[106] Deakin M, Elder J, Hendrickse C, Peckham D, Baldwin D, Pantin C, Wild N, Leopard P, Bell DA, Jones P, Duncan H, Brannigan K, Alldersea J, Fryer AA, Strange RC. Glutathione S-transferase GSTT1 genotypes and susceptibility to cancer: studies of interactions with GSTM1 in lung, oral, gastric and colorectal cancers. *Carcinogenesis* 1996; 17: 881-4.

[107] Kelsey KT, Spitz MR, Zuo ZF, Wiencke JK. Polymorphisms in the glutathione S-transferase class mu and theta genes interact and increase susceptibility to lung cancer in minority populations (Texas, United States). *Cancer Causes Control* 1997; 8: 554-9.

[108] To-Figueras J, Gene M, Gomez-Catalan J, Galan MC, Fuentes M, Ramon JM, Rodamilans M, Huguet E, Corbella J. Glutathione S-transferase M1 (GSTM1) and T1 (GSTT1) polymorphisms and lung cancer risk among Northwestern Mediterraneans. *Carcinogenesis* 1997; 18: 1529-33.

[109] Jourenkova N, Reinikainen M, Bouchardy C, Husgafvel-Pursiainen K, Dayer P, Benhamou S, Hirvonen A. Effects of glutathione S-transferases *GSTM1* and *GSTT1* genotypes on lung cancer risk in smokers. *Pharmacogenetics* 1997; 7: 515-8.

[110] Saarikoski ST, Voho A, Reinikainen M, Anttila S, Karjalainen A, Malaveille C, Vainio H, Husgafvel-Pursiainen K, Hirvonen A. Combined effect of polymorphic GST genes on individual susceptibility to lung cancer. *Int J Cancer* 1998; 77: 516-21.

[111] Anttila S, Hirvonen A, Vainio H, Husgafvel-Pursiainen K, Hayes JD, Ketterer B. Immunohistochemical localization of glutathione S-transferases in human lung. *Cancer Res* 1993; 53: 5643-8.

[112] Harris MJ, Coggan M, Langton L, Wilson SR, Board PG. Polymorphism of the Pi class glutathione S-transferase in normal populations and cancer patients. *Pharmacogenetics* 1998; 8: 27-31.

[113] To-Figueras J, Gene M, Gomez-Catalan J, Pique E, Borrego N, Carrasco JL, Ramon J, Corbella J. Genetic polymorphism of glutathione S-transferase P1 gene and lung cancer risk. *Cancer Causes Control* 1999; 10: 65-70.

[114] Katoh T, Kaneko S, Takasawa S, Nagata N, Inatomi H, Ikemura K, Itoh H, Matsumoto T, Kawamoto T, Bell DA. Human glutathione S-transferase P1 polymorphism and susceptibility to smoking related epithelial cancer; oral, lung, gastric, colorectal and urothelial cancer. *Pharmacogenetics* 1999; 9: 165-9.

[115] Kihara M, Kihara M, Noda K. Lung cancer risk of the GSTM1 null genotype is enhanced in the presence of the GSTP1 mutated genotype in male Japanese smokers. *Cancer Lett* 1999; 137: 53-60.

[116] Wattenberg LW. Inhibitory effects of benzyl isothiocyanate administered shortly before diethylnitrosamine or benzo[a]pyrene on pulmonary and forestomach neoplasia in A/J mice. *Carcinogenesis* 1987; 8: 1971-3.

[117] Morse MA, Eklind KI, Amin SG, Hecht SS, Chung FL. Effects of alkyl chain length on the inhibition of NNK-induced lung neoplasia in A/J mice by arylalkyl isothiocyanates. *Carcinogenesis* 1989; 10: 1757-9.

[118] Nakachi K, Imai K, Hayashi S, Kawajiri K. Polymorphisms of the CYP1A1 and glutathione S-transferase genes associated with susceptibility to lung cancer in relation to cigarette dose in a Japanese population. *Cancer Res.* 1993; 53: 2994-9.

[119] Kihara M, Kihara M, Noda K. Risk of smoking for squamous and small cell carcinomas of the lung modulated by combinations of CYP1A1 and GSTM1 gene polymorphisms in a Japanese population. *Carcinogenesis* 1995; 16: 2331-6.

[120] Anttila S, Hirvonen A, Husgafvel-Pursiainen K, Karjalainen A, Nurminen T, Vainio H. Combined effect of CYP1A1 inducibility and GSTM1 polymorphism on histological type of lung cancer. *Carcinogenesis* 1994; 15: 1133-5.

[121] Le Marchand L, Sivaraman L, Pierce L, Seifried A, Lum A, Wilkens LR, Lau AF. Associations of CYP1A1, GSTM1, and CYP2E1 polymorphisms with lung cancer suggest cell type specificities to tobacco carcinogens. *Cancer Res* 1998; 58: 4858-63.

[122] Tiano HF, Wang RL, Hosokawa M, Crespi C, Tindall KR, Langenbach R. Human CYP2A6 activation of 4-(methylnitrosamino)-1-(3-pyridyl)-1-butanone (NNK): mutational specificity in the gpt gene of AS52 cells. *Carcinogenesis* 1994; 15: 2859-66.

[123] Hadidi H, Zahlsen K, Idle JR, Cholerton S. A single amino acid substitution (Leu160His) in cytochrome P450 CYP2A6 causes switching from 7-hydroxylation to 3-hydroxylation of coumarin. *Food Chem Toxicol* 1997; 35: 903-7.

[124] Rautio A, Gullsten H, Pelkonen O. Expression and function CYP2A genes in humans. *Exp Toxicol Pathol* 1998; 50: 133-4.

[125] Oscarson M, McLellan RA, Gullsten H, Agundez JA, Benitez J, Rautio A, Raunio H, Pelkonen O, Ingelman-Sundberg M. Identification and characterisation of novel polymorphisms in the CYP2A locus: implications for nicotine metabolism. *FEBS Lett* 1999; 460: 321-7.

[126] Oscarson M, McLellan RA, Gullsten H, Yue QY, Lang MA, Bernal ML, Sinues B, Hirvonen A, Raunio H, Pelkonen O, Ingelman-Sundberg M. Characterisation and PCR-based detection of a CYP2A6 gene deletion found at a high frequency in a Chinese population. *FEBS Lett* 1999; 448: 105-110.

[127] Chen GF, Tang YM, Green B, Lin DX, Guengerich FP, Daly AK, Caporaso NE, Kadlubar FF. Low frequency of CYP2A6 gene polymorphism as revealed by a one-step polymerase chain reaction method. *Pharmacogenetics* 1999; 9: 327-32.

[128] Kitagawa K, Kunugita N, Katoh T, Yang M, Kawamoto T. The significance of the homozygous CYP2A6 deletion on nicotine metabolism: a new genotyping method of CYP2A6 using a single PCR-RFLP. *Biochem Biophys Res Commun* 1999; 262: 146-51.

[129] Raunio H, Rautio A, Gullsten H, Pelkonen O. Polymorphisms of CYP2A6 and its practical consequences. *Br J Clin Pharmacol* 2001; 52: 357-63.

[130] Tan W, Chen GF, Xing DY, Song CY, Kadlubar FF, Lin DX. Frequency of CYP2A6 gene deletion and its relation to risk of lung and esophageal cancer in the Chinese population. *Int J Cancer* 2001; 95: 96-101.

[131] London SJ, Idle JR, Daly AK, Coetzee GA. Genetic variation of CYP2A6, smoking, and risk of cancer. *Lancet* 1999; 353: 898-9.

[132] Kamataki T, Nunoya K, Sakai Y, Kushida H, Fujita K. Genetic polymorphism of CYP2A6 in relation to cancer. *Mutat Res* 1999; 428: 125-130.

[133] Brian WR, Srivastava PK, Umbenhauer DR, Lloyd RS, Guengerich FP. Expression of a human liver cytochrome P-450 protein with tolbutamide hydroxylase activity in Saccharomyces cerevisiae. *Biochemistry* 1989; 28: 4993-9.

[134] Ozawa S, Schoket B, McDaniel LP, Tang YM, Ambrosone CB, Kostic S, Vincze I, Kadlubar FF. Analyses of bronchial bulky DNA adduct levels and CYP2C9, GSTP1 and NQO1 genotypes in a Hungarian study population with pulmonary diseases. *Carcinogenesis* 1999; 20: 991-5.

[135] Sullivan-Klose TH, Ghanayem BI, Bell DA, Zhang ZY, Kaminsky LS, Shenfield GM, Miners JO, Birkett DJ, Goldstein JA. The role of the CYP2C9-Leu359 allelic variant in the tolbutamide polymorphism. *Pharmacogenetics* 1996; 6: 341-9.

[136] Nasu K, Kubota T, Ishizaki T. Genetic analysis of CYP2C9 polymorphism in a Japanese population. *Pharmacogenetics* 1997; 7: 405-9.

[137] London SJ, Daly AK, Leathart JB, Navidi WC, Idle JR. Lung cancer risk in relation to the CYP2C9*1/CYP2C9*2 genetic polymorphism among African-Americans and Caucasians in Los Angeles County, California. *Pharmacogenetics* 1996; 6: 527-33.

[138] London SJ, Sullivan-Klose T, Daly AK, Idle JR. Lung cancer risk in relation to the CYP2C9 genetic polymorphism among Caucasians in Los Angeles County. *Pharmacogenetics* 1997; 7: 401-4.

[139] Furuya H, Fernandez-Salguero P, Gregory W, Taber H, Steward A, Gonzalez FJ, Idle JR. Genetic polymorphism of CYP2C9 and its effect on warfarin maintenance dose requirement in patients undergoing anticoagulation therapy. *Pharmacogenetics* 1995; 5: 389392.

[140] Srivastava PK, Yun CH, Beaune PH, Ged C, Guengerich FP. Separation of human liver microsomal tolbutamide hydroxylase and (S)-mephenytoin 4'-hydroxylase cytochrome P-450 enzymes. *Mol Pharmacol* 1991; 40: 69-79.

[141] Goldstein JA, Faletto MB, Romkes-Sparks M, Sullivan T, Kitareewan S, Raucy JL, Lasker JM, Ghanayem BI. Evidence that CYP2C19 is the major (S)-mephenytoin 4'-hydroxylase in humans. *Biochemistry* 1994; 33: 1743-1752.

[142] De Morais SM, Wilkinson GR, Blaisdell J, Meyer UA, Nakamura K, Goldstein JA. Identification of a new genetic defect responsible for the polymorphism of (S)-mephenytoin metabolism in Japanese. *Mol Pharmacol* 1994; 46: 594-8.

[143] Ieiri I, Kubota T, Urae A, Kimura M, Wada Y, Mamiya K, Yoshioka S, Irie S, Amamoto T, Nakamura K, Nakano S, Higuchi S. Pharmacokinetics of omeprazole (a substrate of CYP2C19) and comparison with two mutant alleles, C gamma P2C19m1 in exon 5 and C gamma P2C19m2 in exon 4, in Japanese subjects. *Clin Pharmacol Ther* 1996; 59: 647-53.

[144] Joseph P, Jaiswal AK. NAD(P)H:quinone oxidoreductase1 (DT diaphorase) specifically prevents the formation of benzo[a]pyrene quinone-DNA adducts generated by cytochrome P4501A1 and P450 reductase. *Proc Natl Acad Sci (USA)* 1994; 91: 8413-7.

[145] De Flora S, Bennicelli C, D'Agostini F, Izzotti A, Camoirano A. Cytosolic activation of aromatic and heterocyclic amines. Inhibition by dicoumarol and enhancement in viral hepatitis B. *Environ Health Perspect* 1994; 102 (Suppl 6): 69-74.

[146] Jaiswal AK, McBride OW, Adesnik M, Nebert DW. Human dioxin-inducible cytosolic NAD(P)H:menadione oxidoreductase. cDNA sequence and localization of gene to chromosome 16. *J Biol Chem* 1988; 263: 13572-8.

[147] Traver RD, Horikoshi T, Danenberg KD, Stadlbauer TH, Danenberg PV, Ross D, Gibson NW. NAD(P)H:quinone oxidoreductase gene expression in human colon carcinoma cells: characterization of a mutation which modulates DT-diaphorase activity and mitomycin sensitivity. *Cancer Res* 1992; 52: 797-802.

[148] Ross D, Traver RD, Siegel D, Kuehl BL, Misra V, Rauth AM. A polymorphism in NAD(P)H:quinone oxidoreductase (NQO1): relationship of a homozygous mutation at position 609 of the NQO1 cDNA to NQO1 activity. *Br J Cancer* 1996; 74: 995-6.

[149] Siegel D, McGuinness SM, Winski SL, Ross D. Genotype-phenotype relationships in studies of a polymorphism in NAD(P)H:quinone oxidoreductase 1. *Pharmacogenetics* 1999; 9: 113-21.

[150] Rosvold EA, McGlynn KA, Lustbader ED, Buetow KH. Identification of an NAD(P)H:quinone oxidoreductase polymorphism and its association with lung cancer and smoking. *Pharmacogenetics* 1995; 5: 199-206.

[151] Lewis SJ, Cherry NM, Niven RM, Barber PV, Povey AC. Polymorphisms in the NAD(P)H: quinone oxidoreductase gene and small cell lung cancer risk in a UK population. *Lung Cancer* 2001; 34: 177-83.

[152] London SJ, Smart J, Daly AK. Lung cancer risk in relation to genetic polymorphisms of microsomal epoxide hydrolase among African-Americans and Caucasians in Los Angeles County. *Lung Cancer* 2000; 28: 147-55.

[153] Wiencke JK, Spitz MR, McMillan A, Kelsey KT. Lung cancer in Mexican-Americans and African-Americans is associated with the wild-type genotype of the NAD(P)H: quinone oxidoreductase polymorphism. *Cancer Epidemiol Biomarkers Prev* 1997; 6: 87-92.

[154] Chen H, Lum A, Seifried A, Wilkens LR, Le Marchand L. Association of the NAD(P)H:quinone oxidoreductase 609C-->T polymorphism with a decreased lung cancer risk. *Cancer Res* 1999; 59: 3045-58.

[155] Lin P, Wang HJ, Lee H, Lee HS, Wang SL, Hsueh YM, Tsai KJ, Chen CY. NAD(P)H: quinone oxidoreductase polymorphism and lung cancer in Taiwan. *J Toxicol Environ Health A* 1999; 58: 187-97.

[156] Xu LL, Wain JC, Miller DP, Thurston SW, Su L, Lynch TJ, Christiani DC.. The NAD(P)H:quinone oxidoreductase 1 gene polymorphism and lung cancer: differential susceptibility based on smoking behavior. *Cancer Epidemiol Biomarkers Prev* 2001; 10: 303-9.

[157] Kiyohara C, Otsu A, Shirakawa T, Fukuda S, Hopkin JM. Genetic polymorphisms and lung cancer susceptibility: a review. *Lung Cancer*. 2002; 37: 241-56.

[158] Hassett C, Robinson KB, Beck NB, Omiecinski CJ. The human microsomal epoxide hydrolase gene (EPHX1): complete nucleotide sequence and structural characterization. *Genomics* 1994; 23: 433-42.

[159] Seidegard J, Ekstrom G. The role of human glutathione transferases and epoxide hydrolases in the metabolism of xenobiotics. *Environ Health Perspect* 1997; 105: s791-9.

[160] Smith CA, Harrison DJ. Association between polymorphism in gene for microsomal epoxide hydrolase and susceptibility to emphysema. *Lancet* 1997; 350: 630-3.

[161] Harrison DJ, Hubbard AL, MacMillan J, Wyllie AH, Smith CA. Microsomal epoxide hydrolase gene polymorphism and susceptibility to colon cancer. *Br J Cancer* 1999; 79: 168-71.

[162] Oesch F. Mammalian epoxide hydrases: inducible enzymes catalysing the inactivation of carcinogenic and cytotoxic metabolites derived from aromatic and olefinic compounds. *Xenobiotica* 1973; 3: 305-40.

[163] Gelboin HV. Benzo[alpha]pyrene metabolism, activation and carcinogenesis: role and regulation of mixed-function oxidases and related enzymes. *Physiol Rev* 1980; 60: 1107-66.

[164] Pastorelli R, Guanci M, Cerri A, Negri E, La Vecchia C, Fumagalli F, Mezzetti M, Cappelli R, Panigalli T, Fanelli R, Airoldi L. Impact of inherited polymorphisms in glutathione S-transferase M1, microsomal epoxide hydrolase, cytochrome P450 enzymes on DNA, and blood protein adducts of benzo(a)pyrene-diolepoxide. *Cancer Epidemiol Biomarkers Prev* 1998; 7: 703-9.

[165] Miyata M, Kudo G, Lee YH, Yang TJ, Gelboin HV, Fernandez-Salguero P, Kimura S, Gonzalez FJ. Targeted disruption of the microsomal epoxide hydrolase gene. Microsomal epoxide hydrolase is required for the carcinogenic activity of 7,12-dimethylbenz[a]anthracene. *J Biol Chem* 1999; 274: 23963-8.

[166] Hassett C, Aicher L, Sidhu JS, Omiecinski CJ. Human microsomal epoxide hydrolase: genetic polymorphism and functional expression in vitro of amino acid variants. *Hum Mol Genet* 1994; 3: 421-8.

[167] Benhamou S, Reinikainen M, Bouchardy C, Dayer P, Hirvonen A. Association between lung cancer and microsomal epoxide hydrolase genotypes. *Cancer Res* 1998; 58: 5291-3.

[168] To-Figueras J, Gene M, Gomez-Catalan J, Pique E, Borrego N, Corbella J. Lung cancer susceptibility in relation to combined polymorphisms of microsomal epoxide hydrolase and glutathione S-transferase P1. *Cancer Lett* 2001; 173: 155-162

[169] Persson I, Johansson I, Lou YC, Yue QY, Duan LS, Bertilsson L, Ingelman-Sundberg M. Genetic polymorphism of xenobiotic metabolizing enzymes among Chinese lung cancer patients. *Int J Cancer* 1999; 81: 325-9.

[170] Yin L, Pu Y, Liu TY, Tung YH, Chen KW, Lin P. Genetic polymorphisms of NAD(P)H quinone oxidoreductase, CYP1A1 and microsomal epoxide hydrolase and lung cancer risk in Nanjing, China. *Lung Cancer* 2001; 33: 133-41.

[171] Wu X, Gwyn K, Amos CI, Makan N, Hong WK, Spitz MR. The association of microsomal epoxide hydrolase polymorphisms and lung cancer risk in African-Americans and Mexican-Americans. *Carcinogenesis* 2001; 22: 923-8.

[172] Lin P, Wang SL, Wang HJ, Chen KW, Lee HS, Tsai KJ, Chen CY, Lee H. Association of CYP1A1 and microsomal epoxide hydrolase polymorphisms with lung squamous cell carcinoma. *Br J Cancer* 2000; 82: 852-7.

[173] Zhou W, Thurston SW, Liu G, Xu LL, Miller DP, Wain JC, Lynch TJ, Su L, Christiani DC. The Interaction between Microsomal Epoxide Hydrolase Polymorphisms and Cumulative Cigarette Smoking in Different Histological Subtypes of Lung Cancer. *Cancer Epidemiol Biomarkers Prev* 2001; 10: 461-6.

[174] Hunninghake GW, Gadek JE, Kawanami O, Ferrans VJ, Crystal RG. Inflammatory and immune processes in the human lung in health and disease: evaluation by bronchoalveolar lavage. *Am J Pathol* 1979; 97: 149-206.

[175] Schmekel B, Hornblad Y, Linden M, Sundstrom C, Venge P. Myeloperoxidase in human lung lavage. II. Internalization of myeloperoxidase by alveolar macrophages. *Inflammation* 1990; 14: 455-61.

[176] Schmekel B, Karlsson SE, Linden M, Sundstrom C, Tegner H, Venge P. Myeloperoxidase in human lung lavage. I. A marker of local neutrophil activity. *Inflammation* 1990; 14: 447-54.

[177] Foote CS, Goyne TE, Lehrer RI. Assessment of chlorination by human neutrophils. *Nature* 1983; 301: 715-6.

[178] Prutz WA. Interactions of hypochlorous acid with pyrimidine nucleotides, and secondary reactions of chlorinated pyrimidines with GSH, NADH, and other substrates. *Arch Biochem Biophys* 1998; 349: 183-91.

[179] Tsuruta Y, Josephy PD, Rahimtula AD, O'Brien PJ. Peroxidase-catalyzed benzidine binding to DNA and other macromolecules. *Chem Biol Interact* 1985; 54: 143-58.

[180] Trush MA, Seed JL, Kensler TW. Oxidant-dependent metabolic activation of polycyclic aromatic hydrocarbons by phorbol ester-stimulated human polymorphonuclear leukocytes: possible link between inflammation and cancer. *Proc Natl Acad Sci (USA)* 1985; 82: 5194-8.

[181] Mallet WG, Mosebrook DR, Trush MA. Activation of (+/-)-trans-7,8-dihydroxy-7,8-dihydrobenzo[a]pyrene to diolepoxides by human polymorphonuclear leukocytes or myeloperoxidase. *Carcinogenesis* 1991; 12: 521-4.

[182] Petruska JM, Mosebrook DR, Jakab GJ, Trush MA. Myeloperoxidase-enhanced formation of (+/-)-trans-7,8-dihydroxy-7,8-dihydrobenzo[a]pyrene-DNA adducts in lung tissue in vitro: a role of pulmonary inflammation in the bioactivation of a procarcinogen. *Carcinogenesis* 1992; 13: 1075-81.

[183] Williams JA, Stone EM, Millar BC, Gusterson BA, Grover PL, Phillips DH. Determination of the enzymes responsible for activation of the heterocyclic amine 2-amino-3-methylimidazo[4,5-f]quinoline in the human breast. *Pharmacogenetics* 1998; 8: 519-28.

[184] Piedrafita FJ, Molander RB, Vansant G, Orlova EA, Pfahl M, Reynolds WF. An Alu element in the myeloperoxidase promoter contains a composite SP1-thyroid hormone-retinoic acid response element. *J Biol Chem* 1996; 271: 14412-20.

[185] Austin GE, Lam L, Zaki SR, Chan WC, Hodge T, Hou J, Swan D, Zhang W, Racine M, Whitsett C, Brown B. Sequence comparison of putative regulatory DNA of the 5' flanking region of the myeloperoxidase gene in normal and leukemic bone marrow cells. *Leukemia* 1993; 7: 1445-50.

[186] London SJ, Lehman TA, Taylor JA. Myeloperoxidase genetic polymorphism and lung cancer risk. *Cancer Res* 1997; 57: 5001-3.

[187] Le Marchand L, Seifried A, Lum A, Wilkens LR. Association of the myeloperoxidase -463G-->a polymorphism with lung cancer risk. *Cancer Epidemiol Biomarkers Prev* 2000; 9: 181-4.

[188] Cascorbi I, Henning S, Brockmoller J, Gephart J, Meisel C, Muller JM, Loddenkemper R, Roots I. Substantially reduced risk of cancer of the aerodigestive tract in subjects with variant--463A of the myeloperoxidase gene. *Cancer Res* 2000; 60: 644-9.

[189] Schabath MB, Spitz MR, Zhang X, Delclos GL, Wu X. Genetic variants of myeloperoxidase and lung cancer risk. *Carcinogenesis* 2000; 21: 1163-6.

[190] Misra RR, Tangrea JA, Virtamo J, Ratnasinghe D, Andersen MR, Barrett M, Taylor PR, Albanes D. Variation in the promoter region of the myeloperoxidase gene is not directly related to lung cancer risk among male smokers in Finland. *Cancer Lett* 2001; 164: 161-7.

[191] Cleaver JE. Defective repair replication of DNA in xeroderma pigmentosum. *Nature* 1968; 218: 652-6.

[192] Wood RD. DNA repair in eukaryotes. *Annu Rev Biochem* 1996; 65: 135-67.

[193] Asami S, Manabe H, Miyake J, Tsurudome Y, Hirano T, Yamaguchi R, Itoh H, Kasai H. Cigarette smoking induces an increase in oxidative DNA damage, 8-hydroxydeoxyguanosine, in a central site of the human lung. *Carcinogenesis* 1997; 18: 1763-6.

[194] Abrahams PJ, Houweling A, Cornelissen-Steijger PD, Jaspers NG, Darroudi F, Meijers CM, Mullenders LH, Filon R, Arwert F, Pinedo HM, Natarajan AP, Terleth C, Van Zeeland AA, van der Eb AJ. Impaired DNA repair capacity in skin fibroblasts from various hereditary cancer-prone syndromes. *Mutat Res* 1998; 407: 189-201.

[195] Bootsma d, Kraemer KH, Cleaver JE Hoeijmaker JH. Nucleotide excision repair syndromes: xeroderma pigmentosum, Cockayne Syndrome, and trichothiodystrophy. In: Vogelstein B, Kinzler KW, editors. *The Genetic Basis of Human Cancer*. New York: McGraw-Hill, 1998: 245-74.

[196] Van Duin M, Hoeijimakers JHL. Cloning of human repair genes by genomic DNA transfection. *Ann Inst Super Sanita* 1989; 25: 131-42.

[197] McWhir J, Selfridge J, Harrison DJ, Squires S, Melton DW. Mice with DNA repair gene (ERCC-1) deficiency have elevated levels of p53, liver nuclear abnormalities and die before weaning. *Nat Genet* 1993; 5: 217-24.

[198] Troelstra C, van Gool A, de Wit J, Vermeulen W, Bootsma D, Hoeijmakers JH. ERCC6, a member of a subfamily of putative helicases, is involved in Cockayne's syndrome and preferential repair of active genes. *Cell* 1992; 71: 939-53.

[199] Wei Q, Cheng L, Hong WK, Spitz MR. Reduced DNA repair capacity in lung cancer patients. *Cancer Res* 1996; 56: 4103-7.

[200] Wei Q, Cheng L, Amos CI, Wang LE, Guo Z, Hong WK, Spitz MR. Repair of tobacco carcinogen-induced DNA addcuts and lung cancer risk: a melecular epidemiologic study. *J Natl Cancer Inst* 2000; 92: 1764-72.

[201] Cheng L, Spitz MR, Hong WK, Wei Q. Reduced expression levels of nucleotide excision repair genes in lung cancer: a case-control analysis. *Carcinogenesis* 2000; 21: 1527-30.

[202] Ratnasinghe D, Yao SX, Tangrea JA, Qiao YL, Andersen MR, Barrett MJ, Giffen CA, Erozan Y, Tockman MS, Taylor PR. Polymorphisms of the DNA repair gene XRCC1 and lung cancer risk. *Cancer Epidemiol Biomarkers Prev* 2001; 10: 119-23.

[203] Divine KK, Gilliland FD, Crowell RE, Stidley CA, Bocklage TJ, Cook DL, Belinsky SA. The XRCC1 399 glutamine allele is a risk factor for adenocarcinoma of the lung. *Mutat Res* 2001; 461: 273-8.

[204] David-Beabes GL, London SJ. Genetic polymorphism of XRCC1 and lung cancer risk among African-Americans and Caucasians. *Lung Cancer* 2001; 34: 333-9.

[205] David-Beabes GL, Lunn RM, London SJ. No association between the XPD (Lys751G1n) polymorphism or the XRCC3 (Thr241Met) polymorphism and lung cancer risk. *Cancer Epidemiol Biomarkers Prev* 2001; 10: 911-912.

[206] Butkiewicz D, Rusin M, Enewold L, Shields PG, Chorazy M, Harris CC. Genetic polymorphisms in DNA repair genes and risk of lung cancer. *Carcinogenesis* 2001; 22: 593-7.

[207] Spitz MR, Wu X, Wang Y, Wang LE, Shete S, Amos CI, Guo Z, Lei L, Mohrenweiser H, Wei Q. Modulation of nucleotide excision repair capacity by XPD polymorphisms in lung cancer patients. *Cancer Res* 2001; 61: 1354-7.

[208] Kasai H, Nishimura S. Formation of 8-hydroxyguanosine in DNA by oxygen radicals and its biological significance. In: Sie H, editor. *Oxidative stress: oxidants and antioxidants*, London: Academic Press, 1991: 99-116.

[209] Wang D, Kreutzer DA, Essigmann JM. Mutagenicity and repair of oxidative DNA damage: insights from studies using defined lesions. *Mutat Res* 1998; 400: 99-115.

[210] Halliwell B. Free radicals, antioxidants, and human disease: curiosity, cause, or consequence? *Lancet* 1994; 344: 721-4.

[211] Moscow JA, Schmidt L, Ingram DT, Gnarra J, Johnson B, Cowan KH. Loss of heterozygosity of the human cytosolic glutathione peroxidase I gene in lung cancer. *Carcinogenesis* 1994; 15: 2769-73.

[212] Chu FF, Doroshow JH, Esworthy RS. Expression, characterization, and tissue distribution of a new cellular selenium-dependent glutathione peroxidase, GSHPx-GI. *J Biol Chem* 1993; 268: 2571-6.

[213] Takahashi K, Akasaka M, Yamamoto Y, Kobayashi C, Mizoguchi J, Koyama J. Primary structure of human plasma glutathione peroxidase deduced from cDNA sequences. *J Biochem (Tokyo)* 1990; 108: 145-8.

[214] Maiorino M, Chu FF, Ursini F, Davies KJ, Doroshow JH, Esworthy RS. Phospholipid hydroperoxide glutathione peroxidase is the 18-kDa selenoprotein expressed in human tumor cell lines. *J Biol Chem* 1991; 266: 7728-32.

[215] Forsberg L, de Faire U, Marklund SL, Andersson PM, Stegmayr B, Morgenstern R. Phenotype determination of a common Pro-Leu polymorphism in human glutathione peroxidase 1. *Blood Cells Mol Dis* 2000; 26: 423-6.

[216] Hardie LJ, Briggs JA, Davidson LA, Allan JM, King RF, Williams GI, Wild CP. The effect of hOGG1 and glutathione peroxidase I genotypes and 3p chromosomal loss on 8-hydroxydeoxyguanosine levels in lung cancer. *Carcinogenesis* 2000; 21: 167-72

[217] Cheng KC, Cahill DS, Kasai H, Nishimura S, Loeb LA. 8-Hydroxyguanine, an abundant form of oxidative DNA damage, causes G-T and A-C substitutions. *J Biol Chem* 1992; 267: 166-72.

[218] Shibutani S, Takeshita M, Grollman AP. Insertion of specific bases during DNA synthesis past the oxidation-damaged base 8-oxodG. *Nature* 1991; 349: 431-4.

[219] Aburatani H, Hippo Y, Ishida T, Takashima R, Matsuba C, Kodama T, Takao M, Yasui A, Yamamoto K, Asano M. Cloning and characterization of mammalian 8-hydroxyguanine-specific DNA glycosylase/apurinic, apyrimidinic lyase, a functional mutM homologue. *Cancer Res* 1997; 57: 2151-6.

[220] Kohno T, Shinmura K, Tosaka M, Tani M, Kim SR, Sugimura H, Nohmi T, Kasai H, Yokota J. Genetic polymorphisms and alternative splicing of the hOGG1 gene, that is involved in the repair of 8-hydroxyguanine in damaged DNA. *Oncogene* 1998; 16: 3219-25.

[221] Lu R, Nash HM, Verdine GL. A mammalian DNA repair enzyme that exicise oxidatively damaged quanines maps to a locus frequently lost in lung cancer. *Curr Biol* 1997; 7: 397-407.

[222] Hibi K, Takahashi T, Yamakawa K, Ueda R, Sekido Y, Ariyoshi Y, Suyama M, Takagi H, Nakamura Y, Takahashi T. Three distinct regions involved in 3p deletion in human lung cancer. *Oncogene* 1992; 7: 445-59.

[223] Ratnasinghe D, Tangrea JA, Andersen MR, Barrett MJ, Virtamo J, Taylor PR, Albanes D. Glutathione peroxidase codon 198 polymorphism variant increases lung cancer risk. *Cancer Res* 2000; 60: 6381-3.

[224] Sugimura H, Kohno T, Wakai K, Nagura K, Genka K, Igarashi H, Morris BJ, Baba S, Ohno Y, Gao C, Li Z, Wang J, Takezaki T, Tajima K, Varga T, Sawaguchi T, Lum JK, Martinson JJ, Tsugane S, Iwamasa T, Shinmura K, Yokota J. hOGG1 Ser326Cys polymorphism and lung cancer susceptibility. *Cancer Epidemiol Biomarkers Prev* 1999; 8: 669-74.

[225] Wikman H, Risch A, Klimek F, Schmezer P, Spiegelhalder B, Dienemann H, Kayser K, Schulz V, Drings P, Bartsch H. hOGG1 polymorphism and loss of heterozygosity (LOH): significance for lung cancer susceptibility in a caucasian population. *Int J Cancer* 2000; 88: 932-7.

[226] Ara S, Lee PS, Hansen MF, Saya H. Codon 72 polymorphism of the TP53 gene. *Nucleic Acids Res* 1990; 18: 4961.

[227] Hollstein M, Sidransky D, Vogelstein B, Harris CC. p53 mutations in human cancers. *Science* 1991; 253: 49-53.

[228] Marx J. Gene defect identified in common hereditary colon cancer. *Science* 1993; 262: 1645.

[229] Dulic V, Kaufmann WK, Wilson SJ, Tlsty TD, Lees E, Harper JW, Elledge SJ, Reed SI. p53-dependent inhibition of cyclin-dependent kinase activities in human fibroblasts during radiation-induced G1 arrest. *Cell* 1994; 76: 1013-23.

[230] Weinberg RA. Tumor suppressor genes. *Science* 1991; 254: 1138-46.

[231] Frebourg T, Friend SH. The importance of p53 gene alterations in human cancer: is there more than circumstantial evidence? *J Natl Cancer Inst* 1993; 85: 1554-7.

[232] Vogelstein B, Kinzler KW. p53 function and dysfunction. *Cell* 1992; 70: 523-6.

[233] Jensen RA, Page DL. p53: the promising story continues to unfold. *Hum Pathol* 1993; 24: 455-6.

[234] Harris CC. p53: at the crossroads of molecular Carcinogenesis and risk assessment. *Science* 1993; 262: 1980-1.

[235] Roy B, Beamon J, Balint E, Reisman D. Transactivation of the human p53 tumor suppressor gene by c-Myc/Max contributes to elevated mutant p53 expression in some tumors. *Mol Cell Biol* 1994; 14: 7805-15.

[236] Fujita T, Kiyama M, Tomizawa Y, Kohno T, Yokota J. Comprehensive analysis of p53 gene mutation characteristics in lung carcinoma with special reference to histological subtypes. *Int J Oncol* 1999; 15: 927-34.

[237] Oren M, Rotter V. Introduction: p53-the first twenty years. *Cell Mol Life Sci* 1999; 55: 9-11.

[238] Weston A, Perrin LS, Forrester K, Hoover RN, Trump BF, Harris CC, Caporaso NE. Allelic frequency of a p53 polymorphism in human lung cancer. *Cancer Epidemiol Biomarkers Prev* 1992; 1: 481-3.

[239] Weston A, Ling-Cawley HM, Caporaso NE, Bowman ED, Hoover RN, Trump BF, Harris CC. Determination of the allelic frequencies of an L-myc and a p53 polymorphism in human lung cancer. *Carcinogenesis* 1994; 15: 583-7.

[240] Kawajiri K, Nakachi K, Imai K, Watanabe J, Hayashi S. Germ line polymorphisms of p53 and CYP1A1 genes involved in human lung cancer. *Carcinogenesis* 1993; 14: 1085-9.

[241] Fan R, Wu MT, Miller D, Wain JC, Kelsey KT, Wiencke JK, Christiani DC. The p53 codon 72 polymorphism and lung cancer risk. *Cancer Epidemiol Biomarkers Prev* 2000; 9: 1037-42.

[242] Jin X, Wu X, Roth JA, Amos CI, King TM, Branch C, Honn SE, Spitz MR. Higher lung cancer risk for younger African-Americans with the Pro/Pro p53 genotype. *Carcinogenesis* 1995; 16: 2205-8.

[243] Birgander R, Sjalander A, Rannug A, Alexandrie AK, Sundberg MI, Seidegard J, Tornling G, Beckman G, Beckman L. P53 polymorphisms and haplotypes in lung cancer. *Carcinogenesis* 1995; 16: 2233-6.

[244] To-Figueras J, Gene M, Gomez-Catalan J, Galan C, Firvida J, Fuentes M, Rodamilans M, Huguet E, Estape J, Corbella J. Glutathione-S-Transferase M1 and codon 72 p53 polymorphisms in a northwestern Mediterranean population and their relation to lung cancer susceptibility. *Cancer Epidemiol Biomarkers Prev* 1996; 5: 337-42.

[245] Wang YC, Chen CY, Chen SK, Chang YY, Lin P. p53 codon 72 polymorphism in Taiwanese lung cancer patients: association with lung cancer susceptibility and prognosis. *Clin Cancer Res* 1999; 5: 129-34.

[246] Pierce LM, Sivaraman L, Chang W, Lum A, Donlon T, Seifried A, Wilkens LR, Lau AF, Le Marchand L. Relationships of TP53 codon 72 and HRAS1 polymorphisms with lung cancer risk in an ethnically diverse population. *Cancer Epidemiol Biomarkers Prev* 2000; 9: 1199-204.

[247] Murata M, Tagawa M, Kimura M, Kimura H, Watanabe S, Saisho H. Analysis of a germ line polymorphism of the p53 gene in lung cancer patients; discrete results with smoking history. *Carcinogenesis* 1996; 17: 261-4.

[248] Biros E, Kalina I, Kohut A, Stubna J, Salagovic J. Germ line polymorphisms of the tumor suppressor gene p53 and lung cancer. *Lung Cancer* 2001; 31: 157-62.
[249] Liu G, Miller DP, Zhou W, Thurston SW, Fan R, Xu LL, Lynch TJ, Wain JC, Su L, Christiani DC. Differential association of the codon 72 p53 and GSTM1 polymorphisms on histological subtype of non-small cell lung carcinoma. *Cancer Res* 2001; 61: 8718-22.
[250] Bergen AW, Caporaso N. Cigarette smoking. *J Natl Cancer Inst* 1999; 91: 1365-75.
[251] Yoshimasu K, Kiyohara C. Genetic influences on smoking behavior and nicotine dependence: a review. *J Epidemiol* 2003; 13: 183-192.
[252] Sibley DR, Monsma FJ Jr. Molecular biology of dopamine receptors. *Trends Pharmacol Sci* 1992; 13: 61-9.
[253] Gershanik O, Heikkila RE, Duvoisin RC. Behavioral correlations of dopamine receptor activation. *Neurology* 1983; 33: 1489-92.
[254] Walters JR, Bergstrom DA, Carlson JH, Chase TN, Braun AR. D1 dopamine receptor activation required for postsynaptic expression of D2 agonist effects. *Science* 1987; 236: 719-22.
[255] LaHoste GJ, Yu J, Marshall JF. Striatal Fos expression is indicative of dopamine D1/D2 synergism and receptor supersensitivity. *Proc Natl Acad Sci (USA)* 1993; 90: 7451-5.
[256] Civelli O, Bunzow JR, Grandy DK, Zhou OY, Van Tol HH. Molecular biology of the dopamine receptors. *Eur J Pharmacol* 1991; 207: 277-86.
[257] Seeman P. Dopamine receptors. In: Bloom FE, Kupfer DJ, editors. *Psychopharmacology: Fourth Generation of Progress*. Raven Press, Ltd., New York, 1995, 295-302.
[258] Bloom FE, Toth R. Dopamine. In: Cooper JR, Bloom FE, Roth RH, eds. *The Biochemical Basis of Neuropharmacology*. New York: Oxford University Press, 1996: 293-351.
[259] Van Tol HH, Bunzow JR, Guan HC, Sunahara RK, Seeman P, Niznik HB, Civelli O. Cloning of the gene for a human dopamine D4 receptor with high affinity for the antipsychotic clozapine. *Nature* 1991; 350: 610-4.
[260] Lahti RA, Evans DL, Stratman NC, Figur LM. Dopamine D4 versus D2 receptor selectivity of dopamine receptor antagonists: possible therapeutic implications. *Eur J Pharmacol* 1993; 236: 483-6.
[261] Crabbe JC, Belknap JK, Buck KJ. The D2 receptor gene. *Science* 1994; 266: 352-3.
[262] Stallings MC, Hewitt JK, Cloninger CR, Heath AC, Eaves LJ. Genetic and environmental structure of the Tridimensional Personality Questionnaire: three or four temperament dimensions? *J Pers Soc Psychol* 1996; 70: 127-40.
[263] Straub RE, Sullivan PF, Ma Y, Myakishev MV, Harris-Kerr C, Wormley B, Kadambi B, Sadek H, Silverman MA, Webb BT, Neale MC, Bulik CM, Joyce PR, Kendler KS. Susceptibility genes for nicotine dependence: a genome scan and followup in an independent sample suggest that regions on chromosomes 2, 4, 10, 16, 17 and 18 merit further study. *Mol Psychiatry* 1999; 4: 129-44.
[264] Bergen AW, Korczak JF, Weissbecker KA, Goldstein AM. A genome-wide search for loci contributing to smoking and alcoholism. *Genet Epidemiol* 1999; Suppl 1: S55-60.

[265] Rossing MA. Genetic influences on smoking: candidate genes. *Environ Health Perspect* 1998; 106: 231-8.
[266] Eubanks JH, Djabali M, Selleri L, Grandy DK, Civelli O, McElligott DL, Evans GA. Structure and linkage of the D2 dopamine receptor and neural cell adhesion molecule genes on human chromosome 11q23. *Genomics* 1992; 14: 1010-8.
[267] Grandy DK, Litt M, Allen L, Bunzow JR, Marchionni M, Makam H, Reed L, Magenis RE, Civelli O. The human dopamine D2 receptor gene is located on chromosome 11 at q22-q23 and identifies a TaqI RFLP. *Am J Hum Genet* 1989; 45: 778-85.
[268] Hauge XY, Grandy DK, Eubanks JH, Evans GA, Civelli O, Litt M. Detection and characterization of additional DNA polymorphisms in the dopamine D2 receptor gene. *Genomics* 1991; 10: 527-30.
[269] Noble EP, Blum K, Ritchie T, Montgomery A, Sheridan PJ. Allelic association of the D2 dopamine receptor gene with receptor-binding characteristics in alcoholism. *Arch Gen Psychiatry* 1991; 48: 648-54.
[270] Noble EP, St Jeor ST, Ritchie T, Syndulko K, St Jeor SC, Fitch RJ, Brunner RL, Sparkes RS. D2 dopamine receptor gene and cigarette smoking: a reward gene? *Med Hypotheses* 1994; 42: 257-60.
[271] Noble EP. Addiction and its reward process through polymorphisms of the D2 dopamine receptor gene: a review. *Eur Psychiatry* 2000; 15: 79-89.
[272] Blum K, Noble EP, Sheridan PJ, Montgomery A, Ritchie T, Jagadeeswaran P, Nogami H, Briggs AH, Cohn JB. Allelic association of human dopamine D2 receptor gene in alcoholism. *JAMA* 1990; 263: 2055-60.
[273] 1: Lawford BR, Young RM, Rowell JA, Qualichefski J, Fletcher BH, Syndulko K, Ritchie T, Noble EP. Bromocriptine in the treatment of alcoholics with the D2 dopamine receptor A1 allele. *Nat Med* 1995; 1: 337-41.
[274] Noble EP, Blum K, Khalsa ME, Ritchie T, Montgomery A, Wood RC, Fitch RJ, Ozkaragoz T, Sheridan PJ, Anglin MD, Paredes A, Treiman LJ, Sparkes RS. Allelic association of the D2 dopamine receptor gene with cocaine dependence. *Drug Alcohol Depend* 1993; 33: 271-85.
[275] Comings DE, Muhleman D, Ahn C, Gysin R, Flanagan SD. The dopamine D2 receptor gene: a genetic risk factor in substance abuse. *Drug Alcohol Depend* 1994; 34: 175-80.
[276] O'Hara BF, Smith SS, Bird G, Persico AM, Suarez BK, Cutting GR, Uhl GR. Dopamine D2 receptor RFLPs, haplotypes and their association with substance use in black and Caucasian research volunteers. *Hum Hered* 1993; 43: 209-18.
[277] 4: Noble EP, Noble RE, Ritchie T, Syndulko K, Bohlman MC, Noble LA, Zhang Y, Sparkes RS, Grandy DK. D2 dopamine receptor gene and obesity. *Int J Eat Disord* 1994; 15: 205-17.
[278] Wang GJ, Volkow ND, Logan J, Pappas NR, Wong CT, Zhu W, Netusil N, Fowler JS. Brain dopamine and obesity. *Lancet* 2001; 357: 354-7.
[279] Bierut LJ, Rice JP, Edenberg HJ, Goate A, Foroud T, Cloninger CR, Begleiter H, Conneally PM, Crowe RR, Hesselbrock V, Li TK, Nurnberger JI Jr, Porjesz B, Schuckit MA, Reich T. Family-based study of the association of the dopamine D2 receptor gene (DRD2) with habitual smoking. *Am J Med Genet* 2000; 90: 299-302.

[280] Spitz MR, Shi H, Yang F, Hudmon KS, Jiang H, Chamberlain RM, Amos CI, Wan Y, Cinciripini P, Hong WK, Wu X. Case-control study of the D2 dopamine receptor gene and smoking status in lung cancer patients. *J Natl Cancer Inst* 1998; 90: 358-63.

[281] Smith SS, O'Hara BF, Persico AM, Gorelick DA, Newlin DB, Vlahov D, Solomon L, Pickens R, Uhl GR. Genetic vulnerability to drug abuse. The D2 dopamine receptor Taq I B1 restriction fragment length polymorphism appears more frequently in polysubstance abusers. *Arch Gen Psychiatry* 1992; 49: 723-7.

[282] Yoshida K, Hamajima N, Kozaki Ki, Saito H, Maeno K, Sugiura T, Ookuma K, Takahashi T. Association between the dopamine D2 receptor A2/A2 genotype and smoking behavior in the Japanese. *Cancer Epidemiol Biomarkers Prev* 2001; 10: 403-5.

[283] Comings DE, Ferry L, Bradshaw-Robinson S, Burchette R, Chiu C, Muhleman D. The dopamine D2 receptor (DRD2) gene: a genetic risk factor in smoking. *Pharmacogenetics* 1996; 6: 73-9.

[284] Singleton AB, Thomson JH, Morris CM, Court JA, Lloyd S, Cholerton S. Lack of association between the dopamine D2 receptor gene allele DRD2*A1 and cigarette smoking in a United Kingdom population. *Pharmacogenetics* 1998; 8: 125-8.

[285] Barr CL, Kidd KK. Population frequencies of the A1 allele at the dopamine D2 receptor locus. *Biol Psychiatry* 1993; 34: 204-9.

[286] Wu X, Hudmon KS, Detry MA, Chamberlain RM, Spitz MR. D2 dopamine receptor gene polymorphisms among African-Americans and Mexican-Americans: a lung cancer case-control study. *Cancer Epidemiol Biomarkers Prev* 200; 9: 1021-6.

[287] George SR, Cheng R, Nguyen T, Israel Y, O'Dowd BF. Polymorphisms of the D4 dopamine receptor alleles in chronic alcoholism. *Biochem Biophys Res Commun* 1993; 196: 107-14.

[288] Shields PG, Lerman C, Audrain J, Bowman ED, Main D, Boyd NR, Caporaso NE. Dopamine D4 receptors and the risk of cigarette smoking in African-Americans and Caucasians. *Cancer Epidemiol Biomarkers Prev* 1998; 7: 453-8.

[289] Sunahara RK, Guan HC, O'Dowd BF, Seeman P, Laurier LG, Ng G, George SR, Torchia J, Van Tol HH, Niznik HB. Cloning of the gene for a human dopamine D5 receptor with higher affinity for dopamine than D1. *Nature* 1991; 350: 614-9.

[290] Vanyukov MM, Moss HB, Gioio AE, Hughes HB, Kaplan BB, Tarter RE. An association between a microsatellite polymorphism at the DRD5 gene and the liability to substance abuse: pilot study. *Behav Genet* 1998; 28: 75-82.

[291] Sullivan PF, Neale MC, Silverman MA, Harris-Kerr C, Myakishev MV, Wormley B, Webb BT, Ma Y, Kendler KS, Straub RE. An association study of DRD5 with smoking initiation and progression to nicotine dependence. *Am J Med Genet* 2001; 105: 259-65.

[292] Rose JE. Nicotine addiction and treatment. *Annu Rev Med* 1996; 47: 493-507

[293] Klink R, de Kerchove d'Exaerde A, Zoli M, Changeux JP. Molecular and physiological diversity of nicotinic acetylcholine receptors in the midbrain dopaminergic nuclei. *J Neurosci* 2001; 21: 1452-63.

[294] Phillips HA, Mulley JC.: SSCP variants within the alpha 4 subunit of the neuronal nicotinic acetylcholine receptor gene. *Clin Genet* 1997; 51: 135-6.

[295] : Steinlein OK, Deckert J, Nothen MM, Franke P, Maier W, Beckmann H, Propping P. Neuronal nicotinic acetylcholine receptor alpha 4 subunit (CHRNA4) and panic disorder: an association study. *Am J Med Genet* 1997; 74: 199-201.

[296] Weiland S, Steinlein O. Dinucleotide polymorphism in the first intron of the human neuronal nicotinic acetylcholine receptor alpha 4 subunit gene (CHRNA4). *Clin Genet* 1996; 50: 433-4.

[297] Lueders KK, Hu S, McHugh L, Myakishev MV, Sirota LA, Hamer DH. Genetic and functional analysis of single nucleotide polymorphisms in the beta2-neuronal nicotinic acetylcholine receptor gene (CHRNB2). *Nicotine Tob Res* 2002; 4: 115-25.

[298] Le Novere N, Zoli M, Lena C, Ferrari R, Picciotto MR, Merlo-Pich E, Changeux JP. Involvement of alpha6 nicotinic receptor subunit in nicotine-elicited locomotion, demonstrated by in vivo antisense oligonucleotide infusion. *Neuroreport* 1995; 10: 2497-501.

[299] Champtiaux N, Han ZY, Bessis A, Rossi FM, Zoli M, Marubio L, McIntosh JM, Changeux JP. Distribution and pharmacology of alpha 6-containing nicotinic acetylcholine receptors analyzed with mutant mice. *J Neurosci* 2002; 22: 1208-17.

[300] Ribeiro EB, Bettiker RL, Bogdanov M, Wurtman RJ. Effects of systemic nicotine on serotonin release in rat brain. *Brain Res* 1993; 621: 311-8.

[301] Mihailescu S, Palomero-Rivero M, Meade-Huerta P, Maza-Flores A, Drucker-Colin R. Effects of nicotine and mecamylamine on rat dorsal raphe neurons. *Eur J Pharmacol* 1998; 360: 31-6.

[302] Heils A, Teufel A, Petri S, Stober G, Riederer P, Bengel D, Lesch KP. Allelic variation of human serotonin transporter gene expression. *J Neurochem* 1996; 66: 2621-4.

[303] Lesch KP, Bengel D, Heils A, Sabol SZ, Greenberg BD, Petri S, Benjamin J, Muller CR, Hamer DH, Murphy DL. Association of anxiety-related traits with a polymorphism in the serotonin transporter gene regulatory region. *Science* 1996; 274: 1527-31.

[304] Hennings EC, Kiss JP, Vizi ES. Nicotinic acetylcholine receptor antagonist effect of fluoxetine in rat hippocampal slices. *Brain Res* 1997; 759: 292-4.

[305] Ishikawa H, Ohtsuki T, Ishiguro H, Yamakawa-Kobayashi K, Endo K, Lin YL, Yanagi H, Tsuchiya S, Kawata K, Hamaguchi H, Arinami T. Association between serotonin transporter gene polymorphism and smoking among Japanese males. *Cancer Epidemiol Biomarkers Prev* 1999; 8: 831-3.

[306] Lerman C, Caporaso NE, Audrain J, Main D, Boyd NR, Shields PG. Interacting effects of the serotonin transporter gene and neuroticism in smoking practices and nicotine dependence. *Mol Psychiatry* 2000; 5: 189-92.

[307] Hu S, Brody CL, Fisher C, Gunzerath L, Nelson ML, Sabol SZ, Sirota LA, Marcus SE, Greenberg BD, Murphy DL, Hamer DH. Interaction between the serotonin transporter gene and neuroticism in cigarette smoking behavior. *Mol Psychiatry* 2000; 5: 181-8.

[308] Kuikka JT, Tupala E, Bergstrom KA, Hiltunen J, Tiihonen J. Iodine-123 labelled PE2I for dopamine transporter imaging: influence of age in healthy subjects. *Eur J Nucl Med* 1999; 26: 1486-8.

[309] Seibyl JP, Laruelle M, van Dyck CH, Wallace E, Baldwin RM, Zoghbi S, Zea-Ponce Y, Neumeyer JL, Charney DS, Hoffer PB, Innis RB. Reproducibility of iodine-123-

beta-CIT SPECT brain measurement of dopamine transporters. *J Nucl Med* 1996; 37: 222-8.

[310] Lerman C, Caporaso NE, Audrain J, Main D, Bowman ED, Lockshin B, Boyd NR, Shields PG. Evidence suggesting the role of specific genetic factors in cigarette smoking. *Health Psychol* 1999; 18: 14-20.

[311] Sabol SZ, Nelson ML, Fisher C, Gunzerath L, Brody CL, Hu S, Sirota LA, Marcus SE, Greenberg BD, Lucas FR 4th, Benjamin J, Murphy DL, Hamer DH. A genetic association for cigarette smoking behavior. *Health Psychol* 1999; 18: 7-13.

[312] Jorm AF, Henderson AS, Jacomb PA, Christensen H, Korten AE, Rodgers B, Tan X, Easteal S. Association of smoking and personality with a polymorphism of the dopamine transporter gene: Results from a community survey. *Am J Med Genet* 2000; 96: 331-34.

[313] IARC. Application of biomarkers in cancer epidemiology. In: TonioloP, Boffetta P, Shuker D, Rothman N, Hulka B, Pearce N, editors. *IARC Sci Publ*, Vol. 142, 1997: 1-318.

[314] IARC. Metabolic polymorphisms and susceptibility to cancer. In: Vineis P, Maltas M, Lang M, d'Errico A, Caporaso N, Cuzick J, Boffetta P, editors. *IARC Sci Publ*, Vol. 148, 1999: 1-510.

[315] Todd JA. Interpretation of results from genetic studies of multifactorial diseases. *Lancet* 1999; 354 (Suppl. 1), S115-6.

[316] Fryer AA, Zhao L, Alldersea J, Boggild MD, Perrett CW, Clayton RN, Jones PW, Strange RC. The glutathione S-transferases: polymerase chain reaction studies on the frequency of the GSTM1 0 genotype in patients with pituitary adenomas. *Carcinogenesis* 1993; 14: 563-6.

[317] Kiyohara C, Shirakawa T, Hopkin JM. Genetic polymorphism of enzymes involved in xenobiotic metabolism and the risk of lung cancer. *Environ Health Prevent Med* 2002; 7: 47-59.

[318] Kaiser J. Environmental institute lays plans for gene hunt. *Science (Washington DC),* 1997; 278: 569-70.

In: Focus on Lung Cancer Research
Editor: Robert L. Carafaro, pp. 51-71

ISBN 1-59454-082-9

Chapter II

DNA METHYLATION IN THE PATHOGENESIS OF LUNG CANCER

***Sabine Zöchbauer-Müller*[1,*]*, Adi F. Gazdar*[2] *and John D. Minna*[2]

[1]Clinical Division of Oncology, Department of Medicine I, University Hospital, Währinger Gürtel 18-20, 1090 Vienna, Austria

[2]Hamon Center for Therapeutic Oncology Research, The University of Texas, Southwestern Medical Center at Dallas, 6000 Harry Hines Blvd., Dallas, TX 75390-8593, USA

ABSTRACT

Enormous progress recently has been made in understanding the molecular and cellular biology of lung cancer. Genetic abnormalities of proto-*Oncogene*s and tumor suppressor genes are well known changes which are frequently involved in lung cancer pathogenesis. However, a major finding which comes more and more into focus is that epigenetic inactivation of certain tumor suppressor genes by aberrant promoter methylation frequently occurs in lung carcinomas. Cytosine methylation at CpG dinucleotides is a post-replicative epigenetic modification of DNA that plays a crucial role in physiology and carcinogenesis. CpG islands which contain a high percentage of CpG dinucleotides are often located in the promoter region of tumor suppressor genes and it has been becoming increasingly apparent that aberrant cytosine methylation of CpG dinucleotides (referred to as methylation) in the promoter region of genes is the major mechanism of gene silencing in tumors. In addition, *in vitro* studies demonstrate that methylation can be reversed by methylation inhibitors resulting in gene re-expression. Moreover, DNA methylation has been linked to chromatin modifications recently suggesting a synergistic way to regulate gene transcription. These findings point to potential novel therapies to re-activate gene expression. So far, numerous genes have been identified which are frequently methylated in lung carcinomas demonstrating that

* Corresponding author: Sabine Zöchbauer-Müller, M.D., Clinical Division of Oncology, Department of Medicine I, University Hospital, Währinger Gürtel 18-20, 1090 Vienna, Austria, Phone: (+43) 1 40400-4429, Fax: (+43) 1 40400-4451, e-mail: sabine.zoechbauer-mueller@meduniwien.ac.at.

methylation plays an important role in the pathogenesis of this tumor type. These genes are involved in nearly all components of the "hallmarks of cancer" (Hanahan D and Weinberg RA, Cell. 2000;100:57-70). There are methylation patterns which distinguish small cell lung cancer (SCLC) from non-small cell lung cancer (NSCLC), which identify prior smoking behavior, and which give prognostic information on patient survival. Interestingly, methylation of certain genes can already be detected in smoking damaged bronchial epithelium from smokers suggesting that methylation may be a good biomarker for lung cancer risk assessment and early lung cancer detection. Translating these new findings into the clinic may help to prevent lung cancer and may hopefully result in new therapeutic strategies for patients suffering from this disease.

Key words: methylation, tumor suppressor gene, chromatin, lung cancer, preneoplastic lesion

Abbreviations

TSG	tumor suppressor gene
NSCLC	non-small cell lung cancer
SCLC	small cell lung cancer
DNMT	DNA methyltransferase
MSP	methylation-specific PCR
RASSF1	RAS association domain family 1 gene
TMS1	target of methylation-induced silencing gene
RARβ-2	retinoic acid receptor β-2 gene
FHIT	fragile histidine triad gene
TSLC1	tumor suppressor in lung cancer 1 gene
CDH1	E-cadherin gene
CDH13	H-cadherin gene
APC	adenomatous polyposis coli gene
p16	$p^{16INK4a}$ gene
DAPK	death-associated protein kinase gene
MGMT	O^6-methylguanine-DNA methyltransferase gene
SEMA 3B	Semaphorin 3B gene
TIMP-3	tissue inhibitor of metalloproteinase 3 gene
p14	$p14^{ARF}$ gene
GSTP1	glutathione-S-transferase P1 gene
COX2	cyclooxygenase 2 gene
CALCA	calcitonin gene
MTHFR	methylenetetrahydrofolate reductase gene
ESR1	estrogen receptor α gene
MYOD1	myogenic determinant 1 gene
MBD	methyl-CpG binding domain protein
BAL	bronchoalveolar lavage
5-aza-CR	5-aza-CR 5-azacytidine
5-aza-CdR	5-aza-2`-deoxycytidine
HDAC	histone deacetylase
TSA	trichostatin A

Introduction

Lung cancer is the leading cause of cancer deaths in the world causing over 1 million deaths worldwide each year [1]. The prognosis of lung cancer patients is still poor with 5-year survival rates of about 14% [2]. Thus, a better understanding of the pathogenesis of this disease is crucial for the development of new treatment strategies which could also be very helpful in detecting high risk individuals for lung cancer or patients at an early and therefore better treatable stage of disease. So far, enormous progress has been made in understanding the molecular and cellular biology of lung cancer including abnormalities of proto-*Oncogenes* and tumor suppressor genes (TSG), the role of angiogenesis and changes in growth factors and their receptors [3].

A topic which gains more and more interest is the inactivation of TSGs and other cancer-related genes by aberrant methylation of the promoter region of these genes [4]. TSGs involved in cancer pathogenesis require inactivation of both alleles. One allele is frequently inactivated by allelic loss, while the other one is inactivated by multiple mechanisms including point mutations, homozygous deletions or by aberrant methylation.

Methylation of DNA is essential for the development of mammals. The addition of methyl groups to the 5-position of cytosines alters the appearance of the major groove of DNA to which DNA binding proteins bind [4]. Methylation of CpG-rich promoters is used by mammals to prevent transcriptional initiation and to ensure the silencing of genes on the inactive X chromosome and imprinted genes [5].

Cancer can be caused and impacted by abnormal *de novo* methylation of CpG islands of TSGs and other cancer-related genes [5]. CpG dinucleotides are underrepresented in DNA. However, the distribution and methylation status of CpG sites are non-random. Clusters of CpG sites, called CpG islands, are often found in promoter regions and first exons of genes and are ~500-2000 bp in length. DNA methyltransferases (DNMT) play a crucial role in methylation of cytosine residues. DNMT1 is mainly responsible for maintenance of DNA methylation, whereas DNMT3a and DNMT3b have been shown to methylate hemimethylated and unmethylated DNA with equal efficiencies [6, 7]. It is becoming increasingly apparent that aberrant methylation (referred to as methylation) of the promoter region of genes is the major mechanism of gene silencing in tumors [4]. In various malignant diseases it has been demonstrated that methylation is tissue-specific resulting in different methylation patterns [8]. Besides other tumor entities, methylation plays a crucial role in the pathogenesis of lung carcinomas and in our review we want to focus on this tumor type.

Methods for Detecting Methylation

Several methods have been described for detecting methylation e.g. bisulfite genomic sequencing, methylation-specific PCR (MSP), real-time PCR-based assays and restriction enzyme digest. The principle of the MSP assay was described by Herman et al. [9]. Treatment of genomic DNA with sodium-bisulfite converts unmethylated but not methylated cytosines to uracil which are then converted to thymidine during the subsequent PCR step giving sequence differences between methylated and unmethylated DNA. These differences can be detected by DNA sequencing, the most specific way of detecting methylation. However, PCR primers which distinguish between methylated and unmethylated DNA sequences can also be used to establish a MSP assay. The authors reported that 0.1% of methylated DNA present in an otherwise unmethylated DNA sample can be detected with this method, a finding which was confirmed by other authors [10]. Thus, these results suggest that MSP is a very sensitive and fast method and is suitable to detect methylation in a large number of samples. However, a disadvantage of this method is that the results obtained have only qualitative but not quantitative character.

A quantitative PCR approach to detect methylation has been described recently [11-13]. By using fluorescence-based, real-time quantitative PCR the authors reported an even 10 fold higher sensitivity of this method compared to MSP. The use of different methods for detecting methylation may be a major reason for different frequencies of methylation of certain genes reported in the literature.

Frequently Methylated Tumor Suppressor Genes and Other Cancer-Related Genes in Lung Carcinomas which are Correlated with Clinicopathological Characteristics

Numerous studies investigating methylation in lung cancer have been published in the last few years. So far, more than 40 genes have been studied for methylation in lung cancer. However, the frequency of methylation of these genes varies in a broad range and we will focus here only on genes which were found frequently inactivated by methylation.

The RAS association domain family 1 (*RASSF1)* gene is a candidate TSG gene located at the chromosomal region 3p21.3, a region where frequent allelic loss and several homozygous deletions were found [14]. This gene has a predicted Ras association domain and homology to the Ras effector Nore 1 [15, 16]. The *RASSF1* gene encodes several major transcripts that are produced by alternative promoter selection and alternative mRNA splicing. Shivakumar et al. [17] reported that *RASSF1A* acts in the level of G_1/S-phase cell cycle progression and thus may be an important TSG. mRNA expression of one of the transcripts, *RASSF1A,* is frequently lost in various malignant tumors including lung carcinomas [15, 16, 18-20]. While only a few mutations have been detected methylation as the major mechanism for inactivating this gene has been identified [15]. The frequency of methylation of *RASSF1A* in primary non-small cell lung cancers (NSCLC) ranges between 30-40% [15, 16, 21-23]. The differences in the methylation frequencies may be due to different methods used to detect methylation. However, *RASSF1A* methylation was detected in an even higher percentage in primary small cell lung cancers (SCLC) [16, 24]. Interestingly, Burbee et al. [16] reported that *RASSF1A* methylation may be of prognostic impact in NSCLC patients. Patients whose tumor was *RASSF1A* methylated had a shorter overall survival compared to patients whose tumor was not *RASSF1A* methylated. Tomizawa et al. [25] investigated *RASSF1A* methylation and certain clinicopathological characteristics in stage I lung adenocarcinoma patients. The authors reported that *RASSF1A* methylation was predominantly detected in tumors with vascular invasion and was observed more frequently in poorly differentiated tumors. In addition, *RASSF1A* methylation correlated with adverse survival. Moreover, starting cigarette smoking at an early age is associated with *RASSF1A* methylation [23]. Young smokers who started smoking before the age of 19 were 4.23 times more likely to have *RASSF1A* methylated lung tumors than smokers who started smoking after the age of 19 [23]. In addition, also in this study *RASSF1A* methylation was associated with a poor prognosis in NSCLC patients [23].

The p16^{INK4a} (*p16*) gene is located at chromosome 9p21 a region which frequently undergoes allele loss [26]. *p16* functions in the pathway by binding to cyclin-dependent protein kinase 4 (CDK4) and inhibits the ability of CDK4 to interact with cyclin D1 [27]. Several authors reported that methylation of *p16* occurs frequently in NSCLCs [8, 22, 28, 29]. Belinsky et al. [30] even linked *p16* methylation to an early stage in the pathogenesis of lung cancer demonstrating that *p16* methylation was detected in 75% of carcinoma in situ lesions adjacent to squamous lung cancers harbouring this change. A higher prevalence of *p16* methylation in squamous cell carcinomas compared to adenocarcinomas was described [31]. Moreover, methylation of *p16* is significantly associated with pack-years smoked, duration of smoking and negatively with the time since quitting smoking [31].

The protein product of the adenomatous polyposis coli (*APC*) TSG at chromosome 5q21 is an important component of the Wnt signaling pathway which binds to and inactivates *β*-catenin [32]. Inactivation of *APC* is associated with both familial and sporadic colon cancer [32]. Virmani et al. [33] investigated *APC* methylation by MSP and reported that methylation of *APC* promoter 1A occurs frequently in primary NSCLCs (46%) and that *APC* methylation correlates with loss of *APC* expression by RT-PCR. Brabender et al. [13] used a real-time PCR assay to detect methylation and reported that 95% of primary NSCLC samples were *APC* methylated. A significantly longer survival for NSCLC patients with low *APC* methylation status compared to patients with high *APC* methylation status was seen [13].

The retinoic acid receptor β-2 (*RARβ-2*) gene located at 3p24 functions as a key retinoid receptor mediating growth control responses [34-37]. Frequent loss of *RARβ-2* mRNA expression has been described in both primary NSCLCs and bronchial biopsy specimens from heavy smokers [37-39]. Moreover, diminished or absent RARβ-2 protein expression was seen in ~50% of resected NSCLCs [40]. Virmani et al [41] identified methylation as the underlying mechanism for this frequent loss of *RARβ-2* expression. 43% of primary resected NSCLCs were *RARβ-2* methylated. In addition, the authors demonstrated that *RARβ-2* methylation is also important in the pathogenesis of SCLCs finding 62% of primary SCLCs methylated for *RARβ-2*. Finally, a close correlation between methylation of *RARβ-2* and loss of *RARβ-2* expression was found.

Recently, a myosin family gene, *MYO18B*, located at the chromosomal region 22q12.1 has been cloned [42]. This gene is located in a region where frequent allelic loss occurs in NSCLCs and SCLCs and frequent loss of expression was observed. Expression of *MYO18B* was restored by treatment with 5-aza-2`-deoxycytidine (5-aza-CdR) in several lung cancer cell lines with reduced expression. The authors reported that 35% of primary lung cancers were *MYO18B* methylated while 13% of primary lung carcinomas were found to be mutated. In conclusion, these results suggest that *MYO18B* is a strong candidate for a TSG.

Table 1: Selected genes which are frequently methylated in lung carcinomas

Gene	Location	Function	NSCLCs	SCLCs
LAMC2	1q25-31	Laminin-5-encoding gene	22%	58%
LAMB3	1q32	Laminin-5-encoding gene	25%	77%
FHIT	3p14	Pro-apoptotic	37%	64%*
RASSF1A	3p21.3	Cell cycle regulation	30-40%	72-85%
BLU	3p21.3	Putative TSG	19%	14%
SEMA3B	3p21.3	Putative TSG	41%	ND
RARβ-2	3p24	Growth regulation	40-43%	45%
SLIT2	4p15.2	Ligand for ROBO receptors	53%	36%
APC	5q21	Inhibitor of β-catenin	46-96%	15%
p16	9p21	Cyclin-dependent kinase inhibitor	25-41%	5%
DAPK	9q34.1	Pro-apoptotic	16-44%	33%
MGMT	10q26	DNA repair	16-38%	16%
TSLC1	11q23.2	Cell adhesion	79%§	ND
TMS1	16p11	Pro-apoptotic	40%	41%
CDH1	16q22.1	Cell adhesion	18-33%	60%
CDH13	16q24.2-3	Cell adhesion	43-45%	15%
LAMA3	18q11.2	Laminin-5-encoding gene	42%	65%
TIMP-3	22q12-q13	Pro-apoptotic	19-26%	ND
MYO18B	22q12.1	Putative TSG	31%	45%

* Data are from tumor cell lines; § Tumors with allelic loss at chromosomal region 11q23.2; ND, not done; Data extracted from references [8, 13, 15, 16, 21-25, 28, 29, 33, 41-43, 48, 50, 51, 53-55, 57-59, 62-64]

The tumor suppressor in lung cancer 1 (*TSLC1*) gene was cloned from the chromosomal region 11q23.2, a region where frequent allelic loss was observed in lung carcinomas [43]. Expression of *TSLC1* is frequently lost in lung carcinomas and Kuramochi et al. [43] found this gene methylated in 79% of primary NSCLC samples which showed allelic loss at the *TSLC1* locus.

The fragile histidine triad (*FHIT*) gene, a candidate TSG that spans the FRA3B common fragile site at 3p14.2, was found to be frequently abnormal in lung cancer [44, 45]. Aberrant *FHIT* transcripts were detected in 80% of SCLC and 40% of NSCLC specimens [44, 45] and absent Fhit protein expression was found in ~50% of all lung cancers [46, 47]. We found *FHIT* frequently methylated in NSCLC (64%) and SCLC (64%) cell lines as well as in primary NSCLCs (37%) [48]. In addition, a significant correlation between *FHIT* methylation and loss of Fhit protein expression by immunostaining was observed.

CDH1 (E-cadherin) and *CDH13* (H-cadherin) belong to the cadherin-family which are cell surface glycoproteins responsible for homophilic cell recognition and adhesion [49]. *CDH1* is frequently methylated in lung carcinomas [50]. *CDH13* expression is frequently absent in lung cancers and Toyooka et al. [51] found 43% of primary NSCLCs *CDH13* methylated.

The death-associated protein kinase (*DAPK*) gene is a pro-apoptotic serine/threonine kinase involved in apoptosis [52]. *DAPK* methylation was reported in NSCLCs in up to 44%

by MSP [28, 53, 54]. Toyooka et al. [55] investigated *DAPK* methylation by combined bisulfite restriction analysis and bisulfite DNA sequencing and obtained a similar frequency of methylation as reported by MSP. Tang et al. [54] who studied *DAPK* methylation in stage I NSCLC observed a statistically significant poorer probability of overall survival at 5 years in patients whose tumors exhibited *DAPK* methylation than in those without *DAPK* methylation. Moreover, the groups with and without *DAPK* methylation showed a striking difference in the probability of disease-specific survival [54].

The target of methylation-induced silencing gene (*TMS1*) is a CpG island-associated gene that functions in the regulation of apoptosis and encodes a caspase recruitment domain, a recently described motif in apoptotic signalling molecules [56]. Virmani et al. [57] investigated methylation of *TMS1* in lung carcinomas and found 41% of primary SCLCs and 40% of primary NSCLCs and an even higher percentage of lung cancer cell lines methylated suggesting that methylation of *TMS1* plays a role in the pathogenesis of lung cancer.

Another gene which is frequently silenced by promoter methylation is the DNA repair gene O^6-methylguanine-DNA-methyltransferase (*MGMT*). Brabender et al. [58] detected *MGMT* methylation in 38% of primary NSCLCs and in 18% of matching normal lung tissues by real-time PCR. However, the mean *MGMT* methylation level was significantly higher in tumors than in matching normal tissues. Patients without *MGMT* methylation showed a significantly better survival than patients with *MGMT* methylation.

Sathyanarayana et al. [59] investigated loss of expression of 3 laminin-5 (LN5)-encoding genes (*LAMA3*, *LAMB3*, *LAMC2*) in lung cancer cell lines and primary lung carcinomas and the underlying mechanism for loss of expression. Laminins are the major component of the basement membrane and thus play a major role in anchorage dependence [60]. In breast cancer, a downregulation of LN5 mRNA has been observed and a role for LN5 in controlling tumor growth has been proposed [61]. The authors observed frequent loss of expression in NSCLC (20-60%) and SCLC (65-85%) cell lines [59]. Methylation was identified as the major mechanism for gene silencing and was found more frequently in SCLC (60-80%) compared to NSCLC (15-60%) cell lines [59]. The results were similar in primary lung carcinomas demonstrating a higher frequency of methylation in primary SCLCs (58-77%) compared to primary NSCLCs (22-42%).

It has also been reported that the *SLIT2* gene, located at the chromosomal region 4p15.2, and the genes *BLU* and Semaphorin 3B (*SEMA3B*), both located at 3p21.3, are frequently methylated in lung carcinomas [62-64].

While the majority of authors investigated only a single gene some authors studied the occurrence of methylation of several genes in the same group of samples. We investigated the frequency of methylation of 8 different genes [*RARβ*, tissue inhibitor of metalloproteinase-3 (*TIMP-3*), *p16*, *MGMT*, *DAPK*, *CDH1*, $p14^{ARF}$ (*p14*), and glutathione S-transferase P1 (*GSTP1*)] in more than 100 primary NSCLCs and in the corresponding non-malignant lung tissues [28]. While methylation of *RARβ*, *TIMP-3*, *p16*, *MGMT*, *DAPK* and *CDH1* occurred frequently in tumors methylation of these genes was not seen in the vast majority of corresponding non-malignant lung tissues. A total of 82% of the NSCLCs showed methylation of at least one of these genes. We found lymph node involvement more frequently in samples with any gene methylated than in samples where no genes showed methylation [28]. Moreover, similar to the results of Kim et al. [31] *p16* methylation was more frequently detected in squamous compared to adenocarcinomas, and was only seen in smokers [28].

Toyooka et al. [22] performed a comprehensive study about smoke exposure, histologic type and geography-related differences in the methylation profiles of NSCLC patients. The authors investigated over 500 NSCLC samples from 4 countries (USA, Australia, Japan, Taiwan) for the methylation status of 7 genes (*p16*, *RASSF1A*, *APC*, *RARβ-2, CDH13, MGMT, GSTP1*). The rates of methylation of *p16* and *APC* and the mean methylation index were significantly higher in ever smokers than in never smokers and the mean methylation index of tumors arising in former smokers was significantly lower than in current smokers. Moreover, the methylation rates of *APC*, *CDH13* and *RARβ-2* were significantly higher in adenocarcinomas than in squamous cell carcinomas and the methylation rates of *MGMT* and *GSTP1* were significantly higher in USA and Australian cases than in those from Japan and Taiwan. However, no significant gender-related differences in methylation patterns were noted.

In conclusion, these results from several studies demonstrate that methylation is a major mechanism for the inactivation of certain TSGs in lung cancers.

Methylation Differences between NSCLC and SCLC Samples

A comparison of the frequencies of methylation of certain genes between lung carcinomas of different histologies was performed in the following 2 studies: The pattern of methylation of 7 different genes (*APC*, *CDH13*, *GSTP1*, *MGMT*, *RARβ-2*, *CDH1*, *RASSF1A*) was analyzed in 198 lung tumors consisting of SCLCs, NSCLCs and bronchial carcinoids by Toyooka et al. [50]. The profile of methylated genes in the neuroendocrine tumors (SCLC and carcinoids) were very different from that of NSCLCs. While the overall pattern of methylation of carcinoids was similar to that of SCLCs, carcinoids had lower frequencies of methylation for some of the genes tested. There were also significant differences in the methylation profiles between the major types of NSCLC, adenocarcinomas and squamous cell carcinomas. The authors concluded that SCLCs, carcinoids, squamous cell carcinomas and adenocarcinomas of the lung have unique profiles of methylation. These findings may be helpful in understanding differences in the pathogenetic mechanisms of lung carcinomas.

Virmani et al. [65] investigated if the pattern of methylation could be used to distinguish between different histological subtypes of lung cancer. The methylation status of 23 loci in 91 lung cancer cell lines using quantitative real-time PCR was performed. The genes *COX2*, *CALCA*, *MTHFR*, *ESR1*, *MGMT*, *MYOD1* and *APC* showed statistically significant differences in the level of methylation between SCLC and NSCLC cell lines. Hierachial clustering using a panel consisting of these 7 loci yielded 2 major groups, one which contained 78% of the SCLC cell lines. The authors concluded that similar to the study by Toyooka et al. [22] the methylation pattern differs between NSCLC and SCLC cell lines and suggest that the pattern may be helpful to achieve accurate diagnosis of lung cancer. Taken together, these studies indicate that while most genes can be methylated in either SCLC or

NSCLC, there are distinct methylation signatures which distinguish these major histologic types.

DNA Methylation, Chromatin and Transcription

After detecting that methylation leads to gene silencing the question was: How does DNA methylation modulate gene expression? Bird and his colleagues defined a family of proteins, the methyl-CpG binding domain proteins (MBDs), which bind to methyl-cytosines and which can inhibit gene transcription [66, 67]. Two of these MBDs, MeCP2 and MBD2, have shown to also participate in protein complexes that recruit transcriptional co-repressors, chromatin remodeling complexes and histone deacetylases (HDAC) [68-70]. Through these complexes sites of methylated DNA can target the formation of chromatin including the deacetylated state of histones which is typical for transcriptionally repressive domains [66-70]. Thus, these results suggest that DNA methylation and histone deacetylation work together in gene silencing and may also explain the synergistic effect of methylation inhibitors and HDAC inhibitors on re-expression of silenced genes in tumors [71]. Moreover, it has been reported that DNMT1 can directly bind HDACs and that, in addition, DNMT1 can also bind transcriptional co-repressors and directly suppress, in a partially HDAC-dependent manner, gene transcription [72-74].

Methylation in Serum DNA and Exfoliative Material of the Aerodigestive Tract from Lung Cancer Patients

Esteller et al. [53] investigated if methylation can be detected in serum DNA from lung cancer patients by MSP. The authors analyzed primary NSCLCs and matched serum samples from 22 patients for the methylation pattern of 4 TSGs (*DAPK*, *GSTP1*, *p16*, *MGMT*). Methylation of at least 1 of these genes was detected in 68% of NSCLCs. Comparing primary tumors with methylation and matched serum samples 73% of the matched serum samples were found to be methylated. In addition, none of the sera from patients with tumors not demonstrating methylation was positive.

Usadel et al. [75] investigated the frequency of *APC* methylation in primary NSCLCs and paired preoperative serum or plasma samples of these patients by semiquantitative methylation-specific fluorogenic real-time PCR. 47% of serum and/or plasma samples from patients with *APC* methylated tumors carried detectable amounts of methylated *APC* promoter DNA. In contrast, no methylated *APC* promoter DNA was detected in serum samples from 50 healthy controls.

The methylation status of *p16* was investigated besides some other molecular changes in tumors and bronchoalveolar lavage (BAL) samples from 50 NSCLC patients [76]. *p16* methylation was observed in 19 out of 50 tumors and in the corresponding BALs from 12 out of 19 patients.

Table 2: Frequencies of methylation in the aerodigestive tract epithelium from smokers

Material	Number of samples	Gene	Frequency of methylation	Reference number
Sputum	32	p16	19%	78
	66	p16	35%	81
	25	p16	16%	77
	73	p16	5%	84
	15	*RASSF1A*	33%	83
	66	*RASSF1A*	3%	81
	73	*RASSF1A*	4%	84
	32	*MGMT*	16%	78
	66	*MGMT*	14%	81
	66	*DAPK*	23%	81
	73	*CDH13*	10%	84
	73	*RARβ-2*	27%	84
	39	*FHIT*	15%	84
Bronchial brush	25	p16	8%	77
	100	p16	17%	80
	87	p16	7%	84
	87	*RASSF1A*	6%	84
	100	DAPK	17%	80
	87	*CDH13*	7%	84
	100	GSTP1	6%	80
	87	*RARβ-2*	20%	84
	35	*FHIT*	17%	48
Bronchial biopsy	70	p16	19%	82
BAL fluid	25	p16	12%	77
	43	p16	0%	84
	43	*RASSF1A*	5%	84
	43	*CDH13*	5%	84
	43	*RARβ-2*	9%	84
Oropharyngeal brush	42	p16	0%	84
	42	*RASSF1A*	2%	84
	42	*CDH13*	0%	84
	42	*RARβ-2*	10%	84

Kersting et al. [77] analyzed the frequency of *p16* methylation in exfoliative material from lung cancer patients. *p16* methylation was detected in 35% in sputum samples, in 22% in bronchial lavage samples and in 16% in bronchial brushings from patients with lung cancer.

Sputum samples and matched squamous cell cancer specimens were studied for the occurrence of methylation of *p16* and *MGMT* [78]. All of the 10 patients investigated had a history of smoking and about 50% were exposed to radon. One or both of the genes were methylated in all of the sputum samples. *p16* methylation was present in sputum from all 8 patients whose tumors were also positive for this marker, but not in sputum from the 2 patients whose tumors were negative for this change. Four of 6 patients with *MGMT* methylation in their tumors were also tested positive in the sputum samples.

Methylation of *hMLH1* was detected in 56% of primary NSCLCs and in 38% in the corresponding sputum samples [79]. The concordance of methylation between sputum samples and matched resected tumors was 72%.

Methylation in Cancer-Free Smokers

Since methylation of certain genes is frequent in lung carcinomas researchers started to investigate if methylation occurs already in aerodigestive tract samples from cancer-free smokers. So far, only a few genes have already been investigated. *p16* methylation was found in 16% of sputum samples, in 12% of bronchial lavage samples and in 8% of bronchial brushings from cancer-free chronic smokers [77].

Palmisano et al. [78] investigated if lung cancer can be predicted by detection of methylation in sputum samples. By using a highly sensitive PCR approach to detect methylation the authors detected methylation of *p16* and /or *MGMT* in DNA from sputum in 100% of patients with squamous cell lung carcinomas up to 3 years before clinical diagnosis.

Soria et al. [80] reported methylation of *p16*, *DAPK* and *GSTP1* in bronchial brush samples from former cigarette smokers in 17%, 17% and 6% of the samples, respectively [80]. However, no correlation was found between methylation of any of these genes and the smoking characteristics of the individuals analyzed.

A comparison of methylation in bronchial epithelium between current and former smokers was performed by Belinsky et al. [81]. Methylation of *p16* and *DAPK* was seen as frequently in bronchial epithelium from current smokers as from former smokers. This suggests that methylation changes persist.

In another study 70 biopsies from precancerous bronchial lesions from 37 high-risk individuals without invasive cancer were investigated for *p16* methylation and p16 protein expression was studied by immunohistochemistry on contiguous parallel biopsies [82]. Methylation of *p16* was found in 19% of the samples. However, no association between methylation and tobacco and asbestos exposure was observed.

Honorio et al. [83] investigated *RASSF1A* methylation in sputum samples from current and former smokers. *RASSF1A* methylation was detected in 1 of 2 former and 4 of 13 current smokers.

Recently, we performed a study investigating methylation of the genes *p16*, *RASSF1A*, *RARβ-2* and *CDH13* in different types of specimens (oropharyngeal brushes, sputum samples, bronchial brushes and bronchioloalveolar lavage [BAL] samples) of the upper aerodigestive tract epithelium from heavy smokers without evidence of cancer but with morphometric evidence of sputum atypia [84]. At least one gene was methylated in one or more specimens from 48% of the smokers. Methylation occurred more frequently in samples from the central airways (sputum, bronchial brushes) compared to the peripheral airways

(BAL), and only occasionally in the oropharynx. *RARβ-2* was the most frequently methylated gene while the frequency of methylation for the other genes was lower. In addition, an important fact was that data from sputum samples and bronchial brushes were comparable.

Another gene which was found frequently methylated in heavy smokers is the *FHIT* gene. We detected methylation of *FHIT* in 17% in bronchial brushes and in 15% in sputum samples suggesting that *FHIT* methylation already occurs in preneoplastic lesions in the smoking damaged bronchial epithelium from heavy smokers [48, 84].

In conclusion, the results demonstrate that methylation of certain genes can be an early event in the pathogenesis of lung cancer and a panel of such methylated genes might be an useful biomarker for lung cancer risk assessment and for monitoring the response to chemopreventive agents.

Inhibitors of DNA Methylation

5-aza-2`-cytidine (5-aza-CR) and 5-aza-2`-deoxycytidine (5-aza-CdR) are potent inhibitors of DNA methylation and inducer of cellular differentiation [85]. While 5-aza-CR is incorporated into both DNA and RNA 5-aza-CdR is incorporated only in DNA. Incorporation of one of these agents into DNA of cultured cells leads to rapid loss of DNMT1 activity because the enzyme becomes irreversibly bound to the 5-aza nucleotide [86]. A large number of studies demonstrated that genes which have been silenced by methylation can be re-expressed after treatment with these agents *in vitro* [16, 41, 48, 51]. *In vivo*, 5-aza-CR has been used in patients with leukemias or certain solid tumors and the greatest successes were seen in patients with myelodysplastic syndrome, chronic and acute myeloid leukemia [87]. The number of clinical trials of 5-aza-CR and 5-aza-CdR in patients with solid tumors is small and responses are low compared to conventional therapy. However, interesting results were obtained by Momparler et al. [88]. The authors performed a pilot clinical trial on 5-aza-CdR in patients with stage IV NSCLC. Patients were administered an 8 hour i.v. infusion of 5-aza-CdR for one or more cycles at intervals of 5 to 7 weeks depending on recovery of the granulocyte count. The patients did not receive any prior chemotherapy. Seven patients were included and for all but one the survival time increased with the number of cycles of 5-aza-CdR administered. Interestingly, 1 patient survived more than 6 years. In this study the authors observed a delayed action of 5-aza-CdR on tumor growth which begins to occur after one or more cell divisions suggesting that patients require several treatment cycles before antitumor activity becomes evident.

Because side effects of 5-aza-CR and 5-aza-CdR such as nausea, vomiting, diarrhea, myelosuppression and the ability to form mutagenic lesions are common the search for new methylation inhibitors with less toxic side effects is underway. Recently, alternative inhibitors of DNMT1 have been described [89, 90]. These include antisense oligonucleotides directed against DNMT1 mRNA and hairpin-structured oligonucleotide substrate mimics. However, clinical trials about the toxicity and efficacy of these drugs are necessary.

Recent studies demonstrated a synergy in reactivating gene expression between 5-aza-CdR and the HDAC inhibitor trichostatin A (TSA) [71]. The combination of these agents has shown promising results on both cell kill and cancer-related gene reactivation in cancer cell lines [71, 91]. These data suggest that the dose of 5-aza-CdR used in clinical studies could be reduced when used in combination with HDAC inhibitors resulting in potentially less side effects associated with 5-aza-CdR. However, clinical trials are necessary to prove this concept.

How May Methylation Fit into the Clinic?

So far, several authors reported a prognostic impact of methylation of certain genes detected in primary tumors from lung cancer patients (e.g. *RASSF1A, APC, CDH1, MGMT*) [13, 16, 25, 54, 58]. This finding may influence future treatment strategies for lung cancer patients. Finding genes of prognostic impact methylated in tumors could allow one to "individualize" therapy for those lung cancer patients. These patients potentially might benefit from a more aggressive treatment strategy or the use of methylation inhibitors. The combination of methylation inhibitors and HDAC inhibitors needs to be tested in cancer patients in clinical trials.

Because methylation is tissue-specific the methylation pattern of several genes can also be used to distinguish between different tumor histologies [8]. A different methylation pattern is not only found between various tumor entities but also between histologic subtypes of lung carcinomas [50, 65]. Thus, it might be helpful to use the detection of certain methylation patterns to distinguish between NSCLC and SCLC.

However, methylation could also be used in lung cancer risk assessment and early lung cancer detection. Methylation can be detected in the bronchial epithelium from cancer-free smokers and was already observed up to 3 years prior to the diagnosis of lung cancer [78]. However, the frequencies of methylation of genes in the bronchial epithelium are different and it will take some time to identify genes with the most predictive value for an increased lung cancer risk. By this way it would be possible to assess the "individual" risk for a subject. The current data suggest that it will be necessary to test a panel of genes for methylation to identify individuals at high risk of developing lung cancer. This subgroup of people could then undergo other, more costly, procedures for early detection of lung cancer such as spiral computer tomography scan and would also be ideal candidates for chemoprevention trials. These methylated genes could then be followed as surrogate biomarkers of the efficacy of chemoprevention. Another important issue is that the material which will be tested for methylation in smokers has to be available in an easy, non-invasive and cheap way. We reported that the frequencies of methylation of certain gene were comparable between bronchial brushes and sputum samples obtained from heavy smokers suggesting that sputum samples are ideal for this kind of studies [84].

Hypomethylation and Gene Overexpression

While numerous studies have shown the association between hypermethylation of the promoter region of TSGs and loss of expression of these genes in tumors the biological significance of DNA hypomethylation in cancer is less understood. Genome-wide hypomethylation has been described in various human cancers and has been associated with genetic instability characterized by chromosomal aberrations or elevated mutation rates [92, 93]. The genome-wide DNA hypomethylation found in cancers is prevalent in nomally methylated repeat sequences [94]. Interestingly, DNA hypomethylation at unique sequences can increase expression of cancer-promoting genes and the extent of hypomethylation appears to correlate with tumor grade and with prognosis in certain cancers suggesting an important role of DNA hypomethylation in the overexpression of genes in tumors [94, 95]. Sato et al. [96] recently investigated the methylation status of several genes which are frequently overexpressed in pancreatic cancer and found a high prevalence of hypomethylation. However, similar studies have not been reported yet in lung cancer and thus need to be done in the future.

Summary

In recent years it has become increasingly apparent that epigenetic changes play a critical role in gene silencing. So far, multiple genes were found to be frequently methylated in lung carcinomas and methylation of certain genes has been linked to early preneoplastic changes in the multistage pathogenesis of lung cancer. Detection of these methylation changes represents a new method for risk assessment, screening, and chemoprevention studies. Re-expression of silenced genes by methylation inhibitors in combination with HDAC inhibitors has been successfully performed *in vitro* suggesting these as new therapeutic modalities. However, all of these concepts needs to be tested in clinical trials. If these work in the clinic then important steps towards prevention and improved treatment of cancer patients can be taken.

Acknowledgments

This work was supported by the Medical-Scientific Fund of the Mayor of the Federal Capital Vienna, a grant from the Austrian Federal Ministry of Education, Science and Culture (GZ 200.062/2-VI/1/2002) and a National Cancer Institute Lung Cancer SPORE grant (P50 CA70907).

References

[1] Parkin DM, Bray FI, Devesa SS. Cancer burden in the year 2000. The global picture. *Eur J Cancer* 2001;37:S4-66.

[2] Travis WD, Travis LB, Devesa SS. Lung cancer. *Cancer* 1995;75:191-202.

[3] Zöchbauer-Müller S, Gazdar AF, Minna JD. Molecular pathogenesis of lung cancer. *Annu Rev Physiol* 2002;64:681-708.

[4] Baylin SB, Esteller M, Rountree MR, Bachman KE, Schuebel K, Herman JG. Aberrant patterns of DNA methylation, chromatin formation and gene expression in cancer. *Hum Mol Genet* 2001;10:687-92.

[5] Jones PA, Baylin SB. The fundamental role of epigenetic events in cancer. *Nat Rev Genet* 2002;3:415-28.

[6] Okano M, Bell DW, Haber DA, Li E. DNA methyltransferases Dnmt3a and Dnmt3b are essential for de novo methylation and mammalian development. *Cell* 1999;99:247-57.

[7] Rhee I, Bachman KE, Park BH, Jair KW, Yen RW, Schuebel KE, Cui H, Feinberg AP, Lengauer C, Kinzler KW, Baylin SB, Vogelstein B. DNMT1 and DNMT3b cooperate to silence genes in human cancer cells. *Nature* 2002;416:552-6.

[8] Esteller M, Corn PG, Baylin SB, Herman JG. A gene hypermethylation profile of human cancer. *Cancer Res* 2001;61:3225-9.

[9] Herman JG, Graff JR, Myöhänen S, Nelkin BD, Baylin SB. Methylation-specific PCR: a novel PCR assay for methylation status of CpG islands. *Proc Natl Acad Sci U S A* 1996;93:9821-6.

[10] Virmani AK, Muller C, Rathi A, Zöchbauer-Müller S, Mathis M, Gazdar AF. Aberrant methylation during cervical carcinogenesis. *Clin Cancer Res* 2001;7:584-9.

[11] Eads CA, Danenberg KD, Kawakami K, Saltz LB, Danenberg PV, Laird PW. CpG island hypermethylation in human colorectal tumors is not associated with DNA methyltransferase overexpression. *Cancer Res* 1999;59:2302-6.

[12] Eads CA, Danenberg KD, Kawakami K, Saltz LB, Blake C, Shibata D, Danenberg PV, Laird PW. MethyLight: a high-throughput assay to measure DNA methylation. *Nucleic Acids Res* 2000;28.

[13] Brabender J, Usadel H, Danenberg KD, Metzger R, Schneider PM, Lord RV, Wickramasinghe K, Lum CE, Park J, Salonga D, Singer J, Sidransky D, Holscher AH, Meltzer SJ, Danenberg PV. Adenomatous polyposis coli gene promoter hypermethylation in non-small cell lung cancer is associated with survival. *Oncogene* 2001;20:3528-32.

[14] Lerman MI, Minna JD. The 630-kb lung cancer homozygous deletion region on human chromosome 3p21.3: identification and evaluation of the resident candidate tumor suppressor genes. The International Lung Cancer Chromosome 3p21.3 Tumor Suppressor Gene Consortium. *Cancer Res* 2000;60:6116-33.

[15] Dammann R, Li C, Yoon JH, Chin PL, Bates S, Pfeifer GP. Epigenetic inactivation of a RAS association domain family protein from the lung tumour suppressor locus 3p21.3. *Nat Genet* 2000;25:315-9.

[16] Burbee DG, Forgacs E, Zöchbauer-Müller S, Shivakumar L, Fong KM, Gao B, Randle D, Kondo M, Virmani A, Bader S, Sekido Y, Latif F, Milchgrub S, Toyooka S, Gazdar AF, Lerman MI, Zabarovsky E, White M, Minna JD. Epigenetic inactivation of RASSF1A in lung and breast cancers and malignant phenotype suppression. *J Natl Cancer Inst* 2001;93:691-699.

[17] Shivakumar L, Minna J, Sakamaki T, Pestell R, White MA. The RASSF1A tumor suppressor blocks cell cycle progression and inhibits cyclin D1 accumulation. *Mol Cell Biol* 2002;22:4309-18.

[18] Dammann R, Yang G, Pfeifer GP. Hypermethylation of the cpG island of Ras association domain family 1A (RASSF1A), a putative tumor suppressor gene from the

3p21.3 locus, occurs in a large percentage of human breast cancers. *Cancer Res* 2001;61:3105-9.

[19] Dreijerink K, Braga E, Kuzmin I, Geil L, Duh FM, Angeloni D, Zbar B, Lerman MI, Stanbridge EJ, Minna JD, Protopopov A, Li J, Kashuba V, Klein G, Zabarovsky ER. The candidate tumor suppressor gene, RASSF1A, from human chromosome 3p21.3 is involved in kidney tumorigenesis. *Proc Natl Acad Sci U S A* 2001;98:7504-9.

[20] Kuzmin I, Gillespie JW, Protopopov A, Geil L, Dreijerink K, Yang Y, Vocke CD, Duh FM, Zabarovsky E, Minna JD, Rhim JS, Emmert-Buck MR, Linehan WM, Lerman MI. The RASSF1A tumor suppressor gene is inactivated in prostate tumors and suppresses growth of prostate carcinoma cells. *Cancer Res* 2002;62:3498-502.

[21] Agathanggelou A, Honorio S, Macartney DP, Martinez A, Dallol A, Rader J, Fullwood P, Chauhan A, Walker R, Shaw JA, Hosoe S, Lerman MI, Minna JD, Maher ER, Latif F. Methylation associated inactivation of RASSF1A from region 3p21.3 in lung, breast and ovarian tumours. *Oncogene* 2001;20:1509-18.

[22] Toyooka S, Maruyama R, Toyooka KO, McLerran D, Feng Z, Fukuyama Y, Virmani AK, Zöchbauer-Müller S, Tsukuda K, Sugio K, Shimizu N, Shimizu K, Lee H, Chen CY, Fong KM, Gilcrease M, Roth JA, Minna JD, Gazdar AF. Smoke exposure, histologic type and geography-related differences in the methylation profiles of non-small cell lung cancer. *Int J Cancer* 2003;103:153-60.

[23] Kim DH, Kim JS, Ji YI, Shim YM, Kim H, Han J, Park J. Hypermethylation of RASSF1A promoter is associated with the age at starting smoking and a poor prognosis in primary non-small cell lung cancer. *Cancer Res* 2003;63:3743-6.

[24] Dammann R, Takahashi T, Pfeifer GP. The CpG island of the novel tumor suppressor gene RASSF1A is intensely methylated in primary small cell lung carcinomas. *Oncogene* 2001;20:3563-7.

[25] Tomizawa Y, Kohno T, Kondo H, Otsuka A, Nishioka M, Niki T, Yamada T, Maeshima A, Yoshimura K, Saito R, Minna JD, Yokota J. Clinicopathological significance of epigenetic inactivation of RASSF1A at 3p21.3 in stage I lung adenocarcinoma. *Clin Cancer Res* 2002;8:2362-8.

[26] Serrano M, Lee H, Chin L, Cordon-Cardo C, Beach D, DePinho RA. Role of the INK4a locus in tumor suppression and cell mortality. *Cell* 1996;85:27-37.

[27] Sherr CJ. Cancer cell cycles. *Science* 1996;274:1672-7.

[28] Zöchbauer-Müller S, Fong KM, Virmani AK, Geradts J, Gazdar AF, Minna JD. Aberrant promoter methylation of multiple genes in non-small cell lung cancers. *Cancer Res* 2001;61:249-55.

[29] Kashiwabara K, Oyama T, Sano T, Fukuda T, Nakajima T. Correlation between methylation status of the p16/CDKN2 gene and the expression of p16 and Rb proteins in primary non-small cell lung cancers. *Int J Cancer* 1998;79:215-20.

[30] Belinsky SA, Nikula KJ, Palmisano WA, Michels R, Saccomanno G, Gabrielson E, Baylin SB, Herman JG. Aberrant methylation of p16 (INK4a) is an early event in lung cancer and a potential biomarker for early diagnosis. *Proc Natl Acad Sci U S A* 1998;95:11891-6.

[31] Kim DH, Nelson HH, Wiencke JK, Zheng S, Christiani DC, Wain JC, Mark EJ, Kelsey KT. p16(INK4a) and histology-specific methylation of CpG islands by exposure to tobacco smoke in non-small cell lung cancer. *Cancer Res* 2001;61:3419-24.

[32] Polakis P. The adenomatous polyposis coli (APC) tumor suppressor. *Biochim Biophys Acta* 1997;7:F127-47.

[33] Virmani AK, Rathi A, Sathyanarayana UG, Padar A, Huang CX, Cunnigham HT, Farinas AJ, Milchgrub S, Euhus DM, Gilcrease M, Herman J, Minna JD, Gazdar AF. Aberrant methylation of the adenomatous polyposis coli (APC) gene promoter 1A in breast and lung carcinomas. *Clin Cancer Res* 2001;7:1998-2004.

[34] Gebert JF, Moghal N, Frangioni JV, Sugarbaker DJ, Neel BG. High frequency of retinoic acid receptor beta abnormalities in human lung cancer. *Oncogene* 1991;6:1859-68.

[35] Geradts J, Chen JY, Russell EK, Yankaskas JR, Nieves L, Minna JD. Human lung cancer cell lines exhibit resistance to retinoic acid treatment. *Cell Growth Differ* 1993;4:799-809.

[36] Lu XP, Fanjul A, Picard N, Pfahl M, Rungta D, Nared-Hood K, Carter B, Piedrafita J, Tang S, Fabbrizio E. Novel retinoid-related molecules as apoptosis inducers and effective inhibitors of human lung cancer cells in vivo. *Nat Med* 1997;3:686-90.

[37] Xu XC, Sozzi G, Lee JS, Lee JJ, Pastorino U, Pilotti S, Kurie JM, Hong WK, Lotan R. Suppression of retinoic acid receptor beta in non-small-cell lung cancer in vivo: implications for lung cancer development. *J Natl Cancer Inst* 1997;89:624-9.

[38] Xu XC, Lee JS, Lee JJ, Morice RC, Liu X, Lippman SM, Hong WK, Lotan R. Nuclear retinoid acid receptor beta in bronchial epithelium of smokers before and during chemoprevention. *J Natl Cancer Inst* 1999;91:1317-21.

[39] Ayoub J, Jean-Francois R, Cormier Y, Meyer D, Ying Y, Major P, Desjardins C, Bradley WE. Placebo-controlled trial of 13-cis-retinoic acid activity on retinoic acid receptor-beta expression in a population at high risk: implications for chemoprevention of lung cancer. *J Clin Oncol* 1999;17:3546-52.

[40] Picard E, Seguin C, Monhoven N, Rochette-Egly C, Siat J, Borrelly J, Martinet Y, Martinet N, Vignaud JM. Expression of retinoid receptor genes and proteins in non-small-cell lung cancer [see comments]. *J Natl Cancer Inst* 1999;91:1059-66.

[41] Virmani AK, Rathi A, Zöchbauer-Müller S, Sacchi N, Fukuyama Y, Bryant D, Maitra A, Heda S, Fong KM, Thunnissen F, Minna JD, Gazdar AF. Promoter methylation and silencing of the retinoic acid receptor-beta gene in lung carcinomas. *J Natl Cancer Inst* 2000;92:1303-7.

[42] Nishioka M, Kohno T, Tani M, Yanaihara N, Tomizawa Y, Otsuka A, Sasaki S, Kobayashi K, Niki T, Maeshima A, Sekido Y, Minna JD, Sone S, Yokota J. MYO18B, a candidate tumor suppressor gene at chromosome 22q12.1, deleted, mutated, and methylated in human lung cancer. *Proc Natl Acad Sci U S A* 2002;99:12269-74.

[43] Kuramochi M, Fukuhara H, Nobukuni T, Kanbe T, Maruyama T, Ghosh HP, Pletcher M, Isomura M, Onizuka M, Kitamura T, Sekiya T, Reeves RH, Murakami Y. TSLC1 is a tumor-suppressor gene in human non-small-cell lung cancer. *Nat Genet* 2001;27:427-30.

[44] Sozzi G, Veronese ML, Negrini M, Baffa R, Cotticelli MG, Inoue H, Tornielli S, Pilotti S, De Gregorio L, Pastorino U, Pierotti MA, Ohta M, Huebner K, Croce CM. The FHIT gene 3p14.2 is abnormal in lung cancer. *Cell* 1996;85:17-26.

[45] Fong KM, Biesterveld EJ, Virmani A, Wistuba I, Sekido Y, Bader SA, Ahmadian M, Ong ST, Rassool FV, Zimmerman PV, Giaccone G, Gazdar AF, Minna JD. FHIT and FRA3B 3p14.2 allele loss are common in lung cancer and preneoplastic bronchial lesions and are associated with cancer-related FHIT cDNA splicing aberrations. *Cancer Res* 1997;57:2256-67.

[46] Sozzi G, Sard L, De Gregorio L, Marchetti A, Musso K, Buttitta F, Tornielli S, Pellegrini S, Veronese ML, Manenti G, Incarbone M, Chella A, Angeletti CA, Pastorino U, Huebner K, Bevilaqua G, Pilotti S, Croce CM, Pierotti MA. Association between cigarette smoking and FHIT gene alterations in lung cancer. *Cancer Res* 1997;57:2121-3.

[47] Geradts J, Fong KM, Zimmerman PV, Minna JD. Loss of Fhit expression in non-small-cell lung cancer: correlation with molecular genetic abnormalities and clinicopathological features. *Br J Cancer* 2000;82:1191-7.

[48] Zöchbauer-Müller S, Fong KM, Maitra A, Lam S, Geradts J, Ashfaq R, Virmani AK, Milchgrub S, Gazdar AF, Minna JD. 5' CpG island methylation of the FHIT gene is correlated with loss of gene expression in lung and breast cancer. *Cancer Res* 2001;61:3581-5.

[49] Takeichi M. Cadherin cell adhesion receptors as a morphogenetic regulator. *Science* 1991;251:1451-5.

[50] Toyooka S, Toyooka KO, Maruyama R, Virmani AK, Girard L, Miyajima K, Harada K, Ariyoshi Y, Takahashi T, Sugio K, Brambilla E, Gilcrease M, Minna JD, Gazdar AF. DNA methylation profiles of lung tumors. *Mol Cancer Therapeutics* 2001;1:61-7.

[51] Toyooka KO, Toyooka S, Virmani AK, Sathyanarayana UG, Euhus DM, Gilcrease M, Minna JD, Gazdar AF. Loss of expression and aberrant methylation of the CDH13 (H-cadherin) gene in breast and lung carcinomas. *Cancer Res* 2001;61:4556-60.

[52] Kogel D, Prehn JH, Scheidtmann KH. The DAP kinase family of pro-apoptotic proteins: novel players in the apoptotic game. *Bioessays* 2001;23:352-8.

[53] Esteller M, Sanchez-Cespedes M, Rosell R, Sidransky D, Baylin SB, Herman JG. Detection of aberrant promoter hypermethylation of tumor suppressor genes in serum DNA from non-small cell lung cancer patients. *Cancer Res* 1999;59:67-70.

[54] Tang X, Khuri FR, Lee JJ, Kemp BL, Liu D, Hong WK, Mao L. Hypermethylation of the death-associated protein (DAP) kinase promoter and aggressiveness in stage I non-small-cell lung cancer. *J Natl Cancer Inst* 2000;92:1511-6.

[55] Toyooka S, Toyooka KO, Miyajima K, Reddy JL, Toyota M, Sathyanarayana UG, Padar A, Tockman MS, Lam S, Shivapurkar N, Gazdar AF. Epigenetic down-regulation of death-associated protein kinase in lung cancers. *Clin Cancer Res* 2003;9:3034-41.

[56] Conway KE, McConnell BB, Bowring CE, Donald CD, Warren ST, Vertino PM. TMS1, a novel proapoptotic caspase recruitment domain protein, is a target of methylation-induced gene silencing in human breast cancers. *Cancer Res* 2000;60:6236-42.

[57] Virmani A, Rathi A, Sugio K, Sathyanarayana UG, Toyooka S, Kischel FC, Tonk V, Padar A, Takahashi T, Roth JA, Euhus DM, Minna JD, Gazdar AF. Aberrant methylation of TMS1 in small cell, non small cell lung cancer and breast cancer. *Int J Cancer* 2003;106:198-204.

[58] Brabender J, Usadel H, Metzger R, Schneider PM, Park J, Salonga D, Tsao-Wei DD, Groshen S, Lord RV, Takebe N, Schneider S, Holscher AH, Danenberg KD, Danenberg PV. Quantitative O(6)-methylguanine DNA methyltransferase methylation analysis in curatively resected non-small cell lung cancer: associations with clinical outcome. *Clin Cancer Res* 2003;9:223-7.

[59] Sathyanarayana UG, Toyooka S, Padar A, Takahashi T, Brambilla E, Minna JD, Gazdar AF. Epigenetic inactivation of laminin-5-encoding genes in lung cancers. *Clin Cancer Res* 2003;9:2665-72.

[60] Colognato H, Yurchenco PD. Form and function: the laminin family of heterotrimers. *Dev Dyn* 2000;218:213-34.

[61] Martin KJ, Kwan CP, Nagasaki K, Zhang X, O'Hare MJ, Kaelin CM, Burgeson RE, Pardee AB, Sager R. Down-regulation of laminin-5 in breast carcinoma cells. *Mol Med* 1998;4:602-13.

[62] Dallol A, Da Silva NF, Viacava P, Minna JD, Bieche I, Maher ER, Latif F. SLIT2, a human homologue of the Drosophila Slit2 gene, has tumor suppressor activity and is frequently inactivated in lung and breast cancers. *Cancer Res* 2002;62:5874-80.

[63] Agathanggelou A, Dallol A, Zöchbauer-Müller S, Morrissey C, Honorio S, Hesson L, Martinsson T, Fong KM, Kuo MJ, Yuen PW, Maher ER, Minna JD, Latif F. Epigenetic inactivation of the candidate 3p21.3 suppressor gene BLU in human cancers. *Oncogene* 2003;22:1580-8.

[64] Kuroki T, Trapasso F, Yendamuri S, Matsuyama A, Alder H, Williams NN, Kaiser LR, Croce CM. Allelic loss on chromosome 3p21.3 and promoter hypermethylation of semaphorin 3B in non-small cell lung cancer. *Cancer Res* 2003;63:3352-5.

[65] Virmani AK, Tsou JA, Siegmund KD, Shen LY, Long TI, Laird PW, Gazdar AF, Laird-Offringa IA. Hierarchical clustering of lung cancer cell lines using DNA methylation markers. *Cancer Epidemiol Biomarkers Prev* 2002;11:291-7.

[66] Bird AP, Wolffe AP. Methylation-induced repression--belts, braces, and chromatin. *Cell* 1999;99:451-4.

[67] Ng HH, Bird A. DNA methylation and chromatin modification. *Curr Opin Genet Dev* 1999;9:158-63.

[68] Jones PL, Veenstra GJ, Wade PA, Vermaak D, Kass SU, Landsberger N, Strouboulis J, Wolffe AP. Methylated DNA and MeCP2 recruit histone deacetylase to repress transcription. *Nat Genet* 1998;19:187-91.

[69] Nan X, Ng HH, Johnson CA, Laherty CD, Turner BM, Eisenman RN, Bird A. Transcriptional repression by the methyl-CpG-binding protein MeCP2 involves a histone deacetylase complex. *Nature* 1998;393:386-9.

[70] Wade PA, Gegonne A, Jones PL, Ballestar E, Aubry F, Wolffe AP. Mi-2 complex couples DNA methylation to chromatin remodelling and histone deacetylation. *Nat Genet* 1999;23:62-6.

[71] Cameron EE, Bachman KE, Myohanen S, Herman JG, Baylin SB. Synergy of demethylation and histone deacetylase inhibition in the re-expression of genes silenced in cancer. *Nat Genet* 1999;21:103-7.

[72] Fuks F, Burgers WA, Brehm A, Hughes-Davies L, Kouzarides T. DNA methyltransferase Dnmt1 associates with histone deacetylase activity. *Nat Genet* 2000;24:88-91.

[73] Robertson KD, Ait-Si-Ali S, Yokochi T, Wade PA, Jones PL, Wolffe AP. DNMT1 forms a complex with Rb, E2F1 and HDAC1 and represses transcription from E2F-responsive promoters. *Nat Genet* 2000;25:338-42.

[74] Rountree MR, Bachman KE, Baylin SB. DNMT1 binds HDAC2 and a new co-repressor, DMAP1, to form a complex at replication foci. *Nat Genet* 2000;25:269-77.

[75] Usadel H, Brabender J, Danenberg KD, Jeronimo C, Harden S, Engles J, Danenberg PV, Yang S, Sidransky D. Quantitative adenomatous polyposis coli promoter methylation analysis in tumor tissue, serum, and plasma DNA of patients with lung cancer. *Cancer Res* 2002;62:371-5.

[76] Ahrendt SA, Chow JT, Xu LH, Yang SC, Eisenberger CF, Esteller M, Herman JG, Wu L, Decker PA, Jen J, Sidransky D. Molecular detection of tumor cells in bronchoalveolar lavage fluid from patients with early stage lung cancer. *J Natl Cancer Inst* 1999;91:332-9.

[77] Kersting M, Friedl C, Kraus A, Behn M, Pankow W, Schuermann M. Differential frequencies of p16(INK4a) promoter hypermethylation, p53 mutation, and K-ras mutation in exfoliative material mark the development of lung cancer in symptomatic chronic smokers. *J Clin Oncol* 2000;18:3221-9.

[78] Palmisano WA, Divine KK, Saccomanno G, Gilliland FD, Baylin SB, Herman JG, Belinsky SA. Predicting lung cancer by detecting aberrant promoter methylation in sputum. *Cancer Res* 2000;60:5954-8.

[79] Wang YC, Lu YP, Tseng RC, Lin RK, Chang JW, Chen JT, Shih CM, Chen CY. Inactivation of hMLH1 and hMSH2 by promoter methylation in primary non-small cell lung tumors and matched sputum samples. *J Clin Invest* 2003;111:887-95.

[80] Soria JC, Rodriguez M, Liu DD, Lee JJ, Hong WK, Mao L. Aberrant promoter methylation of multiple genes in bronchial brush samples from former cigarette smokers. *Cancer Res* 2002;62:351-5.

[81] Belinsky SA, Palmisano WA, Gilliland FD, Crooks LA, Divine KK, Winters SA, Grimes MJ, Harms HJ, Tellez CS, Smith TM, Moots PP, Lechner JF, Stidley CA, Crowell RE. Aberrant promoter methylation in bronchial epithelium and sputum from current and former smokers. *Cancer Res* 2002;62:2370-7.

[82] Lamy A, Sesboue R, Bourguignon J, Dautreaux B, Metayer J, Frebourg T, Thiberville L. Aberrant methylation of the CDKN2a/p16INK4a gene promoter region in preinvasive bronchial lesions: a prospective study in high-risk patients without invasive cancer. *Int J Cancer* 2002;100:189-93.

[83] Honorio S, Agathanggelou A, Schuermann M, Pankow W, Viacava P, Maher ER, Latif F. Detection of RASSF1A aberrant promoter hypermethylation in sputum from chronic smokers and ductal carcinoma in situ from breast cancer patients. *Oncogene* 2003;22:147-50.

[84] Zöchbauer-Müller S, Lam S, Toyooka S, Virmani AK, Toyooka KO, Seidl S, Minna JD, Gazdar AF. Aberrant methylation of multiple genes in the upper aerodigestive tract epithelium of heavy smokers. *Internatl J Cancer* 2003;107:612-6.

[85] Momparler RL, Bouffard DY, F. ML, Dionne J, Belanger K, Ayoub J. Pilot phase I-II study on 5-Aza-2`deoxycytidine (Decitabine) in patients with metastatic lung cancer. *Anti-Cancer Drugs* 1997;8:358-68.

[86] Ferguson AT, Vertino PM, Spitzner JR, Baylin SB, Muller MT, Davidson NE. Role of estrogen receptor gene demethylation and DNA methyltransferase.DNA adduct formation in 5-aza-2'deoxycytidine-induced cytotoxicity in human breast cancer cells. *J Biol Chem* 1997;272:32260-6.

[87] Santini V, Kantarjian HM, Issa JP. Changes in DNA methylation in neoplasia: pathophysiology and therapeutic implications. *Ann Intern Med* 2001;134:573-86.

[88] Momparler RL, Eliopoulos N, Ayoub J. Evaluation of an inhibitor of DNA methylation, 5-aza-2'-deoxycytidine, for the treatment of lung cancer and the future role of gene therapy. *Adv Exp Med Biol* 2000;465:433-46.

[89] Fournel M, Sapieha P, Beaulieu N, Besterman JM, MacLeod AR. Down-regulation of human DNA-(cytosine-5) methyltransferase induces cell cycle regulators p16(ink4A) and p21(WAF/Cip1) by distinct mechanisms. *J Biol Chem* 1999;274:24250-6.

[90] Bigey P, Knox JD, Croteau S, Bhattacharya SK, Theberge J, Szyf M. Modified oligonucleotides as bona fide antagonists of proteins interacting with DNA. Hairpin antagonists of the human DNA methyltransferase. *J Biol Chem* 1999;274:4594-606.

[91] Bovenzi V, Momparler RL. Antineoplastic action of 5-aza-2'-deoxycytidine and histone deacetylase inhibitor and their effect on the expression of retinoic acid receptor beta and estrogen receptor alpha genes in breast carcinoma cells. *Cancer Chemother Pharmacol* 2001;48:71-6.

[92] Gama-Sosa MA, Slagel VA, Trewyn RW, Oxenhandler R, Kuo KC, Gehrke CW, Ehrlich M. The 5-methylcytosine content of DNA from human tumors. *Nucleic Acids Res* 1983;11:6883-94.

[93] Goelz SE, Vogelstein B, Hamilton SR, Feinberg AP. Hypomethylation of DNA from benign and malignant human colon neoplasms. *Science* 1985;228:187-90.

[94] Ehrlich M. DNA methylation in cancer: too much, but also too little. *Oncogene* 2002;21:5400-13.

[95] Lin CH, Hsieh SY, Sheen IS, Lee WC, Chen TC, Shyu WC, Liaw YF. Genome-wide hypomethylation in hepatocellular carcinogenesis. *Cancer Res* 2001;61:4238-43.

[96] Sato N, Maitra A, Fukushima N, van Heek NT, Matsubayashi H, Iacobuzio-Donahue CA, Rosty C, Goggins M. Frequent hypomethylation of multiple genes overexpressed in pancreatic ductal adenocarcinoma. *Cancer Res* 2003;63:4158-66.

In: Focus on Lung Cancer Research
Editor: Robert L. Carafaro, pp. 73-120
ISBN 1-59454-082-9

Chapter III

THE PATHOGENIC CONTRIBUTION OF MATRIX METALLOPROTEINASES TO LUNG CANCER

Hiroyuki Ohbayashi*
Department of Internal Medicine,
Nagoya University School of Medicine, Japan.

ABSTRACT

The extracellular matrix (ECM) is a complex network of interstitial connective tissue filling the extracellular space of the submucosa, which functions by mechanically supporting the three dimensional structure of the cell body, maintaining tissue homeostasis, and it also affects various biologic cell functions. The matrix metalloproteinases (MMPs), a growing family of zinc-dependent neutral endopeptidases, are the key enzymes in the degradation of the ECM, which belong to the metzincin superfamily. The expression of MMPs if strictly regulated to maintain proper homeostasis in the normal stomal environment. On the other hand, during cancer progression, it is well recognized that MMPs promote tumor invasion and metastasis via ECM degradation. Furthermore, abundant evidence has recently accumulated showing that MMPs also play a pivotal role in the early stage of carcinogenesis, tumor growth, migration, angiogenesis, and apoptosis. This chapter reports on the findings of research on the pathogenic contribution of MMPs to lung cancer.

For at least 30 years, researchers have continued to develop synthetic MMP inhibitors have been continued to develop as the next generation of anti-cancer drugs. Although the results of human clinical trials of these inhibitors have been disappointing, the accumulated ideas and knowledge will surely lead to the next promising drug. This chapter focuses upon the major synthetic MMP inhibitors with some prospects for future therapy.

* Correspondence: Hiroyuki Ohbayashi, Internal Medicine, JA Gifu Tohno Kousei Hospital, 76-1, Toki-cho, Mizunami City, Gifu Pref. 509-6101, Japan, TEL:+81-572-68-4111, FAX:+81-572-68-8934, E-mail: ohbayasi@nn.iij4u.or.jp.

Key words: matrix metalloproteinases (MMPs), lung cancer, MMP inhibitor, extracellular matrix (ECM), tissue inhibitor of metalloproteinases (TIMP), extracellular matrix metalloproteinase inducer (EMMPRIN)

1. Introduction

The occurrence of cancer invasion and metastases is the hallmark of tumors including those of lung cancer, severely affecting a good prognosis and survival. Only a few and limited effective therapeutic methods have been found to prevent cancer invasion and metastases at present. However, considering that cancer cells have to penetrate through the epithelial basement membrane and remove a complex network of extracellular matrix (ECM) tissue in order to invade and for metastasis to occur, the prevention of ECM degradation by tumor cells may possibly become a key method to block cancer invasion and metastases.

2. The Extracellular Matrix (ECM)

The extracellular matrix (ECM) is a complex network of interstitial connective tissue filling the extracellular space of the submucosa. The ECM contains collagens, many other non-collagenous glycoproteins such as laminins and fibronectins, and proteoglycans. ECM not only functions in mechanically supporting the three dimensional structure of a cell body, but also affects various biologic cell functions such as cell growth and differentiation, migration, tissue repair, proliferation and apoptosis, which maintains tissue homeostasis [1, 2, 3]. The ECM proteins also directly interact with cell surface receptors to initiate signal transduction pathways and to modulate those triggered by differentiation and growth factors, and they can control the activity and presentation of a wide range of growth factors [4].

The key enzymes responsible for ECM degradation are matrix metalloproteinases (MMPs). MMPs can collectively degrade all of the components of the ECM including collagens, proteoglycans, laminins, fibronectins and many other glycoproteins. The expression of MMPs is strictly regulated to maintain proper homeostasis in the normal stromal environment.

Furthermore, cleavage of ECM proteins by MMPs often exposes and activates their putative cryptic sites [4]. The proteolytic cleavage of collagen type IV by MMP-2, a major component of the vascular basement membrane, exposes a functionally important angiogenesis-associated cryptic site HUIV26 hidden within its triple helical structure [5]. The HUIV26 cryptic site contributes to angiogenesis in part by regulating endothelial cell–integrin interactions. The denaturation of the triple helical structure of collagen IV can shift integrin binding specificity from that of a beta 1 dependency to both beta 1 and alpha v beta 3 integrin. As a result, alpha v beta 3 integrin may function as a receptor for the HUIV26 cryptic epitope [5]. MMP-2 can also directly bind to integrin alpha v beta 3 on the surface of angiogenic blood vessels, facilitating cell-mediated ECM degradation [6]. In contrast, a fragment of MMP-2, which comprises the C-terminal hemopexin-like domain, termed PEX, prevents MMP-2 binding to alpha v beta 3 and blocks cell surface collagenolytic activity [7]. A naturally occurring form of PEX, as a natural inhibitor of MMP-2 activity, could be detected in vivo in conjunction with alpha v beta 3 expression in tumors and during developmental retinal neovascularization [7].

Additionally, Laminin-5, an ECM protein predominantly expressed in many epithelial basement membranes, normally functions to promote cell adhesion and hemidesmosome formation. The Laminin-5 molecule, in particular its gamma2 chain, has recently been considered as an important player in the tumor cascade and progression to metastatic disease [8]. Giannelli G et al first showed that specific cleavage of laminin-5 gamma2 subunit by MMP-2, exposed and activated the putative cryptic promigratory site on Laminin-5, which resulted in the induction of breast epithelial cell migration [9]. Later, they also reported the primary role of MT1-MMP is to trigger cell migration via Laminin-5 in colon and breast cancer tissue specimens [10]. On the other hand, the alpha-chain of Laminin-5 is the most prominent laminin heterotrimer in normal adult tissues. The laminin alpha5 peptide AQARSAASKVKVSMKF markedly increased the expression of MMP-9 mRNA and gelatinolytic activity in conditioned media [11]. AQARSAASKVKVSMKF was also chemotactic for neutrophils and macrophages in vitro, and induced expression of membrane-type-1 MMP (MT1-MMP), while MMP-2, MMP-3, MMP-7, MMP-12, and MMP-13 were not induced. [11].

3. Matrix Metalloproteinases

Matrix metalloproteinases (MMPs), a growing family of zinc-dependent neutral endopeptidases, belong to the metzincin superfamily [12]. According to sequence and structural similarities, the metzincins superfamily is grouped in four distinct categories: MMPs (also called the matrixins), the adamalysins (reprolysins, or snake venom metalloproteinases (SVMPs) [13, 14] and disintegrin-like and metalloprotease-containing proteins (ADAMs) [15]), the astacins, and the serralysins (large bacterial proteinases) **(Table 1)**. MMPs are characterized by their consensus sequence and structural features including a HEXXHXXGXXH zinc-binding segment and a methionine-containing turn (the 'Met-turn') [12]. The three histidine (H) residues in the zinc-binding motif HEXXHXXGXXH are ligands of the catalytic zinc atom. MMPs share a basic structural organization composed of propeptide, catalytic, hinge and hemopexin-like domain, with a few exceptions [16] **(Figure 1)**. To date, at least 23 kinds of MMPs in human (28 kinds of whole MMPs are presently identified) have been detected **(Table 2)**. They can be classified into the following groups according to their structure and substrate specificity: soluble type MMPs including gelatinases, collagenases, stromelysins and others, and the membrane-type MMPs. However, as the MMP family is a growing one, MMPs are also generally called according to a sequential numbering system. As shown in Table 2, MMPs have various cellular sources including stromal cells. The gene expression and protein secretion of MMPs are tightly regulated by growth factors and their receptors, cytokines and chemokines, adhesion receptors and cell surface proteoglycans and a variety of enzymes at several different levels including transcription and protein activation [17, 18]. MMPs are synthesized as prepro-enzymes and secreted outside the cell as latent proenzymes in most cases [16]. The interaction between a cysteine-sulphydryl group in the propeptide domain and the zinc ion bound to the catalytic domain keeps the proenzymes of MMPs inactive, requiring the proteolytic removal of the propeptide prodomain by other activated MMPs or serine proteinases in order to exert the MMPs potentialities [19]. It is also well-known that MT1-MMP can induce activation of proMMP-2 on the cell surface [20]. MT1-MMP also activates proMMP-13 (procollagenase 3) [21]. In contrast, MMP-11, MMP-28 and the membrane-type MMPs can also be activated by intracellular furin-like serine proteinases before they reach the cell surface [19].

Table 1. Families of proteinases

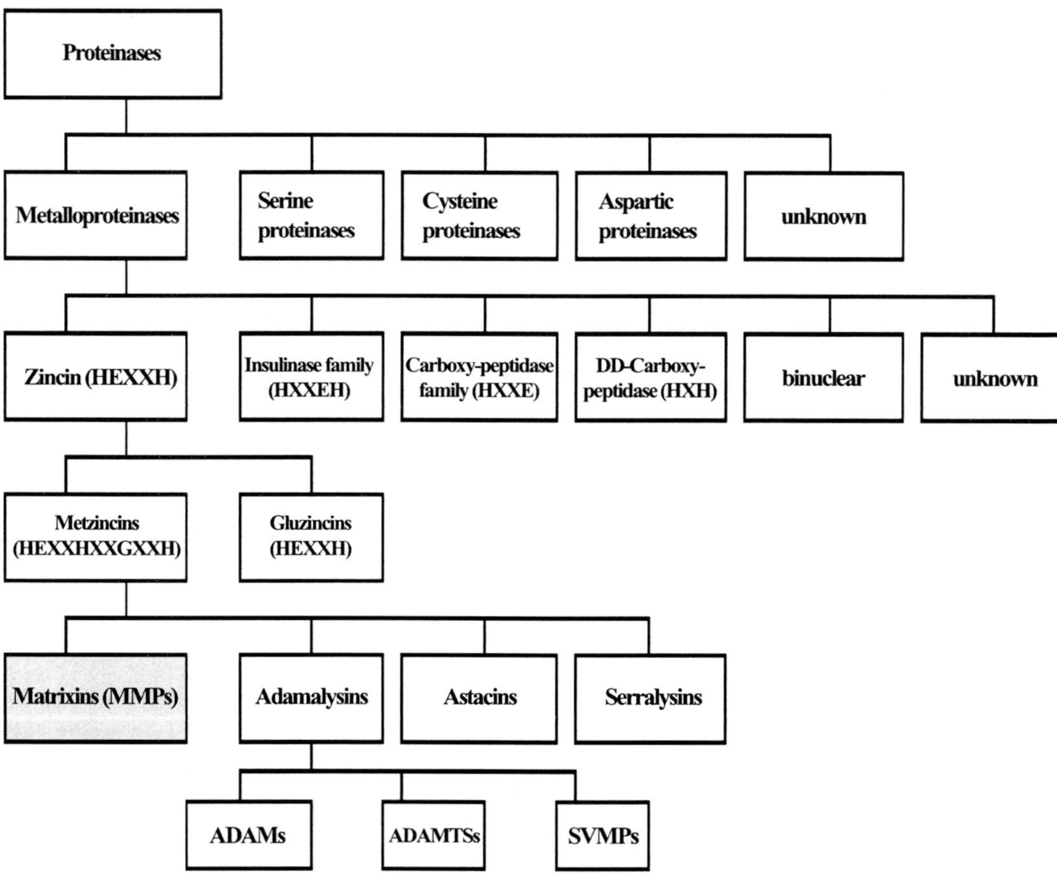

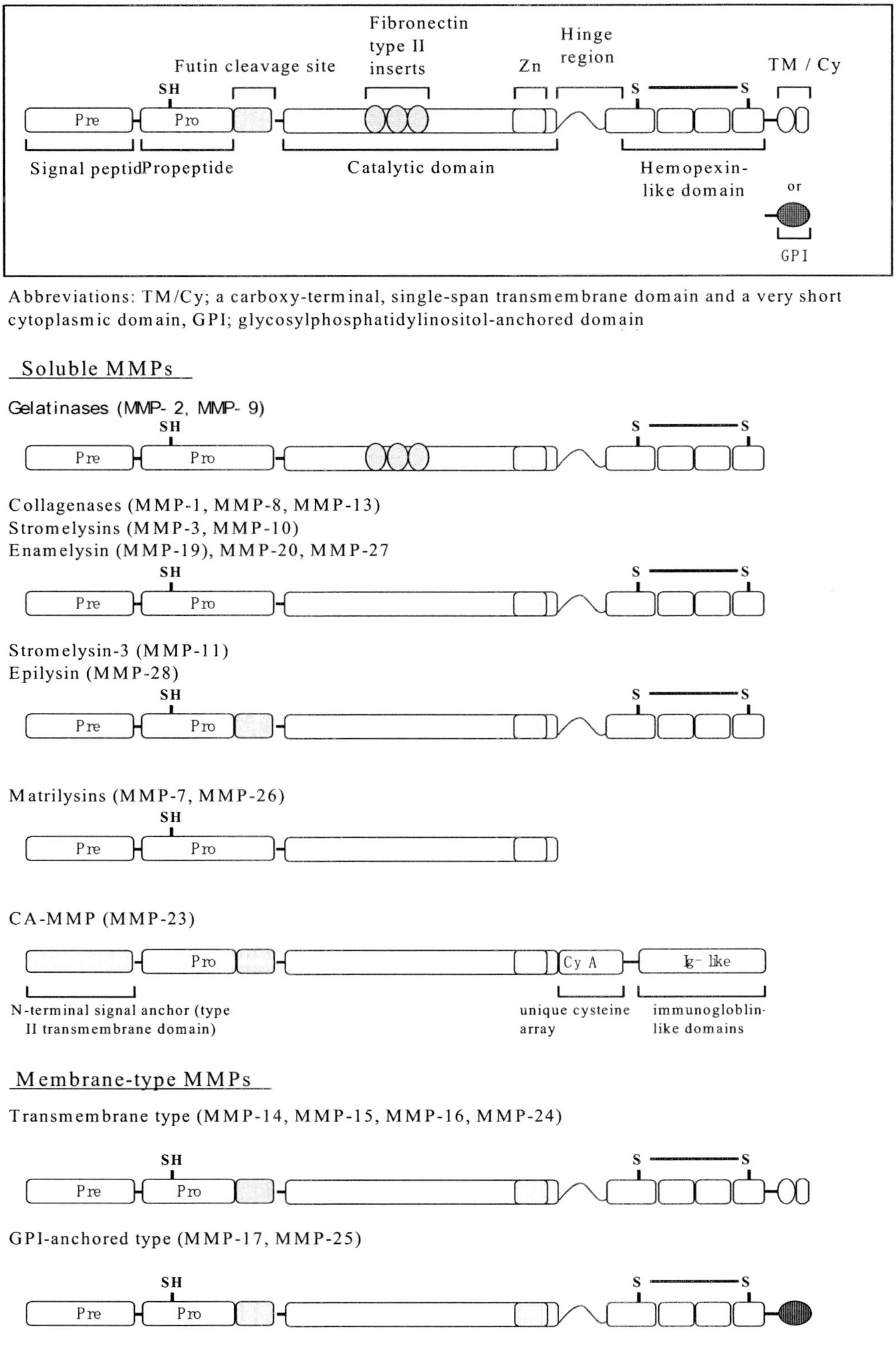

Figure 1. The domain structure of MMPs

Table 2. Human MMP family at present detected.

Soluble MMPs

MMP subfamily	MMP No.	Other names	Chromosomal location	Molecular weight (kDa) (latent/active)	ECM Substrates	Cellular source
Gelatinases	MMP-2	Gelatinase-A, 72 kDa Gelatinase, 72kDa type IV Collagenase, neutrophil gelatinase	16q13	72 / 66	C-I, II, III, IV, V, VII, X, XI, XIV, gelatin, elastin, fibronectin, aggrecan	Fibro, Endo, Neu, Mac, T lymphocytes
	MMP-9	Gelatinase-B, 92 kDa Gelatinase, 92kDa type IV Collagenase	20q12-13	92 / 82, 65	C-IV, V, VII, X, XIV, gelatin, fibronectin, elastin, aggrecan	Epi, Neu, Mac, Eo, Fibro, Endo, T lymphocytes, dendritic cells, keratinocytes, osteoblasts, trophoblasts
Collagenases	MMP-1	Collagenase-1, Interstitial Collagenase, Fibroblast collagenase, Tissue collagenase	11q22.2-22.3	52 / 41	C-I, II, III, VII, VIII, X, aggrecan, gelatin	Epi, Endo, Mac, Fibro, keratinocytes, osteoblasts, hepatocytes
	MMP-8	Neutrophil collagenase, Collagenase-2, PMN collagenase, granurocyte collagenase	11q22.2-22.3	85 / 64	C-I, II, III, VII, VIII, X, aggrecan, gelatin	Neu, Fibro, Endo
	MMP-13	Collagenase-3	11q22.2-22.3	65 / 55	C-I, II, III, aggrecan, gelatin	Fibro, bone
Stromelysins	MMP-3	Stromelysin-1, Transin-1, Procollagenaseactivating protein, Proteoglycanase	11q22.2-22.3	57 / 45, 28	C-II, III, IV, IX, X, XI, fibronectin, laminin, elastin, gelatin, aggrecan	Fibro, Epi, Endo, Mac, vascular smooth muscle, keratinocytes, chondrocytes
	MMP-10	Stromelysin-2, Transin-2	11q22.2-3	56 / 47, 24	C-III, IV, V, fibronectin, laminin, elastin, gelatin	Fibro, Epi, T lymphocytes, keratinocytes
	MMP-11	Stromelysin-3	22q11.2	58 / 28	fibronectin, laminin, gelatin	Fibro, Epi, Mac, mesenchymal cells
Others	MMP-7	Matrilysin, Pump-1, Matrin, Small uterine metalloproteinase	11q22.2-22.3	28 / 19	fibronectin, laminin, elastin, vecronectin, tenascin	Epi, Mac, mesangial cells
	MMP-12	Macrophage metalloelastase, Macrophage elastase	11q22.2-22.3	54 / 45, 22	fibronectin, elastin, vecronectin	Fibro, Epi, Mac, mesenchymal cells
	MMP-19	rheumatoid arthritis synovium inflamed (RASI)-1	12q14	57 / 45	C-I, IX, fibronectin, gelatin, tenascin	T lymphocytes
	MMP-20	Enamelysin	11q22	54 / 22	enamel matrix, gelatin	dental enamel
	MMP-21	Homologue of Xenopus XMMP	not applicable	70 / 53	unknown	unknown
	MMP-23	Cysteine array MMP, CA-MMP, Femalsin, MIFR	1p36	unknown	unknown	ovary, testis, prostate
	MMP-26	Matrilysin-2, Endometase	11q22.2	28 / 19	C-IV, gelatin, fibronectin	placenta, uterus
	MMP-27	No trivial name	not applicable	unknown	unknown	unknown
	MMP-28	Epilysin	17q11.2	unknown / 58, 55	unknown	testis, keratinocyte

Membrane-type MMPs

MMP subfamily	MMP No.	Other names	Chromosomal location	Molecular weight (kDa) (latent/active)	ECM Substrates	Cellular source
Transmembrane-type	MMP-14	Membrane-type-1 MMP (MT1-MMP)	14q12.2	66 / 60	C-I, II, III, fibronectin, laminin, gelatin, elastin, vecronectin, tenascin	Fibro, Epi, Mac, osteoblasts, vascular smooth muscle
	MMP-15	Membrane-type-2 MMP (MT2-MMP)	16q12.2	68 / 62	fibronectin, laminin, gelatin	Fibro, Mac
	MMP-16	Membrane-type-3 MMP (MT3-MMP)	8q21	64 / 55	C-III, fibronectin	vascular smooth muscle, brain, placenta
	MMP-17	Membrane-type-4 MMP (MT4-MMP)	12q24	57 / 53	unknown	lymphocytes, brain
GPI-anchored type	MMP-24	Membrane-type-5 MMP (MT5-MMP)	20q11.2	63 / 45	unknown	brain
	MMP-25	Membrane-type-6 MMP (MT6-MMP), leukolysin	16q13.3	73 / 64	C-IV, gelatin, fibronectin	Neu

Abbreviations: C: collagen, ECM: extracellular matrix, Epi: epithelial cells, Endo:endothelial cells, Eo: eosinophils, Epi: epithelial cells, Fibro: fibroblasts, Mac; macrophages, Mo: monocytes, Neu; neutrophils

4. A Disintegrin-Like and Metalloprotease-Containing Proteins (ADAMs)

The metzincins superfamily contains other important zinc-dependent proteinases, a disintegrin-like and metalloprotease-containing proteins (ADAMs) and ADAMs with one or more thrombospondin (TS) domains (ADAMTSs) **(Table 1)**. As the term "ADAM" suggests, there are two key structural domains, containing a disintegrin and a metalloproteinase, in these molecules. At least 31 kinds of ADAMs [22] and 10 ADAMTSs have been detected at present [23]. ADAMs is a family of membrane-associated multidomain zinc-dependent metalloproteinases [24]. 19 of the 31 presently known ADAMs are regarded as the active ones based upon their characteristics of the zinc-binding motif HEXXHXXGXXH. Although their exact functions are unknown, ADAMs are widely distributed in many tissues including lung tissue [15]. ADAMs share all or some of the following domain structure: a signal peptide, a propeptide, a metalloproteinase, a disintegrin, a cysteine-rich and an epidermal growth factor (EGF)-like domains, a transmembrane region, and a cytoplasmic tail, suggesting a possible role for ADAMs in cell to cell and cell to matrix interactions [15]. In addition to the similarity of the active sites of ADAMs/ADAMTSs with those of MMPs, ADAMs were reported to exhibit high sensitivity to competitive inhibitors of MMPs [25]. TNF-alpha converting enzyme (TACE; ADAM-17) is a membrane-bound disintegrin metalloproteinase that processes the membrane-associated cytokine proTNF-alpha to the soluble form. As TACE is elevated in several inflammatory diseases, TACE often becomes a significant target in drug discovery. A recent genetic linkage study confirmed that polymorphisms in ADAM33 are associated with asthma and bronchial hyperresponsiveness, suggesting important pathogenic linkages of MMPs to asthma [26]. Further investigation concerning these important metzincins, ADAMs/ADAMTSs, is anticipated.

5. Extracellular Matrix Metalloproteinase Inducer (EMMPRIN)

Extracellular matrix metalloproteinase inducer (EMMPRIN) is a member of the IgG superfamily [27]. EMMPRIN was isolated from human non small cell lung carcinoma (NSCLC) cell membrane [28], and its human gene was determined by Biswas et al [29]. The protein core of EMMPRIN is approximately 27 kDa and varies from 43 to 66 kDa in the glycosylate forms [27]. EMMPRIN is also known by other names: CD147 and M6 in human, basigin and gp42 in mouse [30], OX47 and CE9 in rat, and HT7, meurothelin and 5A11 in chicken. EMMPRIN normally increases in the lung during development, while little is expressed in normal adult lung [31]. However, this protein is enriched on the surface of several types of human tumor cells in vitro and in vivo and stimulates nearby human fibroblasts to synthesize MMPs [32]. The EMMPRIN protein was detected by immunohistochemistry prominently in malignant proliferations of the lung and the breast cells, being present in particular at the surface of both tumor epithelial and peritumor stromal cells [31]. Tumor cells can induce adjacent stromal cells to synthesize MMPs using EMMPRIN and cytokine stimulatory mechanisms [33]. Most MMPs in tumors are made by stromal cells including fibroblasts and inflammatory cells, not by the carcinoma cells themselves. The fact that peritumoral stromal cells synthesize MMPs by EMMPRIN on the surface of the cancer cell is interesting and important to know the role of EMMPRIN in tumor dissemination.

Previous study demonstrated that EMMPRIN stimulated in vitro the fibroblast production of various MMPs such as MMP-1, MMP-2 and MMP-3 [34]. Another study showed that the upregulation of MMP-1 mRNA expression in human lung fibroblast caused by EMMPRIN required the activation of the p38 signal transduction pathway [35]. EMMPRIN not only stimulates the production of MMP-1 but also forms a complex with MMP-1 at the tumor cell surface [36]. MMP-2, MT1-MMP, and EMMPRIN mRNA were concurrently expressed in invasive breast carcinoma, suggesting that these proteins interact and are important for the invasive phenotype in breast carcinoma [37]. Using in situ hybridization and gelatin substrate zymography, increased MMP-2 and MMP-9 expression were also detected accompanied by enhanced EMMPRIN in human MDA-MB-436 breast cancer cells [38]. A very recent study using immunofluorescence staining detected the increased expression of EMMPRIN and overexpression of MMP-1, MMP-2, and MMP-9 in multidrug resistant cancer cells [39]. The expression and activities of these MMPs in the multidrug resistant cell lines were inhibited with an anti-EMMPRIN antibody [39]. Another very recent study showed that EMMPRIN was increased in bronchoalveolar lavage fluid of smokers [40], suggesting that EMMPRIN is involved in smoking-induced lung pathology such as lung cancer and COPD.

Very recent studies demonstrated the wide participation of EMMPRIN in various cancers. EMMPRIN can induce MMP-9 in skin pigment cells of malignant melanomas [41]. EMMPRIN is also expressed in laryngeal squamous cell carcinoma [42], and is associated with the biological progression and aggressiveness of bone giant cell tumor [43]. EMMPRIN is a pivotal factor in tumor progression, causing tumor-associated stromal cells to increase their MMP production, thus facilitating tumor invasion and neoangiogenesis. These facts suggest that inhibition of EMMPRIN could be a promising therapeutic target for treating lung cancer.

6. Endogenous MMP Inhibitors

The activities of MMPs are normally regulated by binding of endogenous inhibitors such as tissue inhibitor of metalloproteinases (TIMP) and alpha2-macroglobulin. TIMPs are well-known and the most relevant endogenous MMP inhibitors. Four kinds of TIMPs have been detected in human: TIMP-1, TIMP-2, TIMP-3, and TIMP-4 [44, 45]. TIMP-1,-2, and -4 are found in a soluble form, while TIMP-3 is anchored to the ECM [46]. TIMP-1 and TIMP-2 are major endogenous MMP inhibitors. They can bind the active or the latent form of MMPs and form 1:1 complexes, specifically inhibiting the activities of MMPs. A latent form MMP-9 (Pro-MMP-9) binds to TIMP-1 [47], while pro-MMP-2 binds to TIMP-2 [48, 49] and to TIMP-4 [50]. TIMP-1, -2 and -4 are specific MMP inhibitors, while TIMP-3 can inhibit some of members of the ADAMs including TNF-alpha convertase (TACE, ADAM-17) [51, 52], ADAM-12S [53], aggrecanase-1 (ADAM-TS4), and aggrecanase-2 (ADAM-TS5) [54]. After changing the activated form of MMPs, any TIMPs can bind to the catalytic domain of the MMPs and inhibit their enzymatic activities [47, 55]. TIMPs play a key regulatory role not only in the homeostasis of the ECM by controlling the activity of MMPs, but they can also affect various phases of cancer progression including tumor growth, invasion, metastasis and angiogenesis [56]. Current knowledge concerning TIMPs has been reviewed in detail by Jiang Y et al [57].

As well, an abundant plasma protein alpha2-macroglobulin can function as a "molecular trap", and nonspecifically inhibit most proteinases including MMPs. The alpha2-macrogloblin and MMP complex binds to a scavenger receptor, and then is irreversibly cleared by endocytosis. This has been reviewed in detail by Sottrup-Jensen L [58]. As well as alpha2-macroglobulin, thrombospondin-1 and thrombospondin-2 can nonspecifically bind to some MMPs and act as agents for their removal from the extracellular environment [59]. Thrombospondin-1 can directly inhibit the activation of pro-MMP-2 and -9 through binding to them [60, 61]. However, it has recently been reported that thrombospondin-1 activates MMP-2 and MMP-9 [62, 63]. On the other hand, thrombospondin-2 forms the complex with MMP-2, which binds to a scavenger receptor and then irreversibly clears MMP-2 by endocytosis [64].

In addition, reversion-including cysteine-rich protein with Kazal motifs (RECK), a membrane-anchored glycoprotein recently described, can negatively regulate the secretion and enzymatic activities of MMPs such as MMP-9, MMP-2 and MT1-MMP, resulting in the inhibition of tumor metastasis and angiogenesis [65, 66]. Furthermore, although their physiological significance is unclear, other proteins such as domains of netrins, the procollagen C-terminal proteinase enhancer (PCPE) and tissue factor pathway inhibitor (TFPI-2) show modest inhibitory activity against some of the MMPs [59].

7. MMPs and Cancer Progression

It has been long been thought that MMPs are produced by tumor cells alone and that MMPs play a pivotal role only in tumor invasion and metastasis. However, as mentioned the following section, a lot of accumulated evidence has recently shown that most MMPs are produced and secreted by adjacent stromal cells, and furthermore MMPs can act in various important pathogenic functions other than tumor invasion and metastasis [66, 67, 68]. In addition, MMPs can degrade substrates other than components of the ECM. Although the accurate mechanism as to how MMPs pathogenically contribute to cancer progression is still unclear, our knowledge in this field is rapidly expanding.

7.1. MMPs in Tumor Invasion and Metastasis

In order to promote tumor invasion, tumor cells have to traverse the following two types of ECM. Basement membrane, a thin layer of specialized ECM beneath the (airway) epithelium, is the first physical barrier. The details of concerning the contribution of the basement membrane matrix to cancer has been reviewed by Engbring JA et al [70]. ECM in the interstitial stroma, a matrix of a dense meshwork composed by collagen, proteoglycans, elastin and other glycoproteins, is the second barrier for the tumor cells [71]. Staining for type IV collagen disclosed discontinuities in basement membranes from basal cell hyperplasia to dysplasia, progressing to destruction in carcinoma in situ and invasive carcinoma [72].

The following traditional three-step theory of tumor invasion has been considered as correct for a long time. (I) Tumor cells attach to the ECM via specific ECM receptors on the cell surface, (II) tumor cells express and secret MMPs to focally degrade ECM at the attachment site, and (III) they migrate to the area where the ECM is degraded. And then, with the cyclic repetition of these three steps, tumor cells can further invade the surrounding tissues [68, 71]. Abundant expression of MMPs in tumor tissues has long been considered to be due to production by tumor cells themselves. However, a lot of evidence has shown that most MMPs are expressed and secreted from adjacent stromal cells, including fibroblasts and inflammatory cells, rather than from the carcinoma cells themselves [73]. Tumor cells induce adjacent stromal cells to produce and secret MMPs via stimulation by cytokines, growth factors and EMMPRIN [4]. MMPs secreted by stromal cells recruit around tumor cells in a paracrine manner and degrade ECM at the tumor attachment site. The Akt/protein kinase B (PKB) a serine/threonine kinase, is a pivotal mediator in the phosphoinositide-3 kinase (PI3K)-Akt kinase pathway, which is correlated with many cell survival and proliferation signaling pathways. Recent studies showed that Akt/PKB contributed to promote tumor invasion by activating the productions of MMP-9 [74], MMP-2 [75] and MT1-MMP [76].

The occurrence of metastases is another hallmark of cancer progression, severely affecting prognosis and survival. In order to metastasize from the primary organ to secondary remote ones, tumor cells have to overcome several steps, with avoiding the host immune attacks. After leaving from the primary site, tumor cells intravasate into the blood or lymphatic circulation and must survive transportation in the circulation before extravasating at a distant site. And then they need to establish themselves at the new site before forming a metastatic colony.

Degradation of collagenous matrix causes the extending specialized cell surface protrusions called "invadopodia" at sites of cell invasion into the ECM [77]. Invasive cancer cells make contact with the ECM via the specialized plasma membrane protrusions invadopodia. Invadopodia promotes proteolysis of a wide variety of ECM proteins and is thought to be necessary for cancer cell invasion [77]. On the other hand, Chen WT et al reported that there are other surface protrusions called lamellipodia, analogous invadopodia, which also make contact with the underlying ECM at the leading edge of an invasive cell [78]. Although they exhibit similar structure and mobility to invadopodia, lamellipodia, by virtue of their location at the cellular periphery, are readily accessible to the soluble TIMP-2 and blood-borne inhibitors. TIMP-2 co-localizes with MT1-MMP and MMP-2 at lamellipodia [78].

Many previous studies demonstrated that proteolysis of ECM by MMPs at invadopodia facilitates cancer cell invasion in human breast cancer [79, 80] and human malignant melanoma cells [81]. In particular MT1-MMP, MMP-2 and 170-kD gelatinase (seprase) degrade ECM at invadopodia. The overexpressed MT1-MMP in RPMI7951 human melanoma cells activated soluble and ECM-bound MMP-2 and degraded ECM [81]. The MT-MMP transmembrane /cytoplasmic domain mediates the spatial organization of MT-

MMP into invadopodia and the subsequent degradation of the ECM [81]. Seprase also called fibroblast activation protein alpha (FAPalpha), a large gelatin-degrading membrane-protease complex, is localized in invadopodia and plays a prominent role in locally degrading ECM, resulting in cancer cell invasion during tumor invasion, angiogenesis and metastasis [82]. Both seprase and active MMP-2 are coexpressed at the invasive front of malignant melanoma cells [83]. Formation of seprase and the urokinase plasminogen activator receptor (uPAR) membrane complex can be found in the plasma membrane of LOX malignant melanoma cells which are dependent upon the involvement of beta 1-integrins [84]. Alpha 3 beta 1 integrin is a docking protein for seprase to form functional invadopodia [85]. In addition, alpha 5 beta 1 integrin may participate in the adhesion process necessary for invadopodial formation [85]. As well, a complex of cortactin, paxillin and protein kinase C mu were also detected in the invadopodia-enriched membranes of invasive breast cancer cells, while they were not detected in lysates from non-invasive cells that did not form invadopodia, suggesting a relationship between this complex of molecules and the formation and function of invadopodia during cellular invasion [86].

The Cell-ECM interaction is essential for cancer cell invasion [87]. A transmembrane glycoprotein CD44, primarily known as a cell surface receptor for hyaluronate, is one of the ECM receptors which can mediate cell migration [88, 89]. CD44 is a ubiquitous multistructural and multifunctional cell surface adhesion molecule involved in cell-cell and cell-ECM interactions [89]. Although at least 20 different CD44 transcripts have been described at present, the most abundant form is the standard hematopoietic type CD44H [89]. CD44 is abundantly present in a wide variety of tissues including lung [89]. On the other hand, a high expression of CD44 is found on the surfaces of invasive tumor as well as their metastases, CD44H is also abundantly expressed in human cancer cells [89]. CD44 is shed from the cell surface by proteolytic processing [89, 90], and higher levels of soluble CD44 have been detected in serum from the patients with advanced gastric or colon cancer [91], colorectal cancer [92, 93], and non-Hodgkin's lymphoma [94]. CD44 cleavage is induced by MT-MMPs during tumor cell migration and consequently promotes CD44-mediated cancer cell migration [90]. Among the MT-MMPs, MT1-MMP is frequently expressed in invasive cancer cells [95]. MT1-MMP acts as a processing enzyme for CD44H, releasing it into the medium as a soluble 70-kD fragment which may stimulate cell motility in an autocrine and paracrine manner [96]. Another previous study also showed that CD44 served to anchor MMP-9 on the cell surface and was involved in CD44-mediated tumor invasion [97]. In addition, as referred to in the above section, specific cleavage of laminin-5 by MT1-MMT as well as MMP2 exposed and activated the putative cryptic promigratory site on Laminin-5, inducing cancer cell migration [9, 10]. Thus, these facts suggest that MT1-MMP is a powerful tool for tumor invasion by triggering direct as well as indirect ECM proteolysis on the cell surface.

On the other hand, E-cadherin is a calcium-dependent cell-cell adhesion molecule and is associated with intracellular molecules catenins. The E-cadherin-catenin complex proteins function in cell-cell adhesion and are critical for intercellular adhesiveness and maintenance of normal and malignant tissue architecture [98]. Reduced expression of this complex in malignant disease including lung cancer is thought to happen early in cancer development, which is also associated with tumor invasion, metastasis, and poor prognosis [98]. As well in lung cancer, the reduced expression of E-cadherin also developed malignant phenotype in NSCLC, even though the genetic mutation of E-cadherin gene was not involved in the pathogenesis of NSCLC [99]. Another study reported that tumor cell dedifferentiation correlated with reduced expression for E-cadherin, beta-catenin, gamma-catenin, and p120 in squamous cell carcinomas but not in adenocarcinomas [100]. There was an inverse correlation between nodal metastasis and expression of E-cadherin and gamma-catenin [100]. Very recently research by Ohira T et al showed that WNT7a, encoded on 3p25, activated E-cadherin expression via a beta-catenin specific mechanism in lung cancer cells [101]. The expression of WNT7a was frequently downregulated in lung cancer, which was involved in loss of E-cadherin or beta-catenin, inducing a poor prognosis [101]. The epidermal growth factor-receptor (EGF-R) modulation also regulates the E-cadherin/catenin complex and cell motility in human lung epithelial carcinoma cells [102]. The expressions of E-cadherin and beta-catenin can become prognostic markers in pathological stage I NSCLC [103]. Another study demonstrated that E-cadherin alone can become an independent prognostic factor for NSCLC survival [100]. A recent study also reported that the 5-year survival rate of patients with E-cadherin-negative NSCLC was significantly lower than that of patients with E-cadherin-positive NSCLC [104]. Reduced expression of E-cadherin and beta-catenin indicated tumor cell dedifferentiation, while reduced expression of beta-catenin had poor recurrence free survival in adenocarcinoma of the resected stage I NSCLC, but not in squamous cell carcinoma. [103]. Other studies showed that beta-catenin expression loss was associated with advanced tumor stage and was an independent predictor of shortened patient survival in NSCLC [105] and in SCLC [106]. However, in contrast, another study showed that, although the expression of alpha-catenin, beta-catenin, and gamma-catenin is related to histological type and differentiation in NSCLC, catenins had no independent prognostic value [107]. Both MMP-3 and MMP-7 cleave E-cadherin at the cell surface and release an invasion promoter E-cadherin fragment soluble E-cadherin (sE-CAD) [108]. A very recent in vitro study by Nawrocki-Raby B et al showed that sE-CAD induced the expression of MMP-2, -9 and MT1-MMP, but not MMP-1, -3 and -7, resulting in tumor invasion in human lung cancer cells [109].

7.2. MMPs and Tumorigenisis

MMPs can also affect tumorigenicity in various cancer cells during early stages of tumor progression [110, 111]. Recent studies in transgenic and knock-out animals suggested that MMPs can promote very early stages of various tumor progressions. The expression of MMP-1 in the skin of transgenic mice increased the susceptibility to chemical tumorigenisis [112]. MMP-9 also triggered the angiogenic switch during *Carcinogenesis* of pancreatic islets in transgenic mice [113].

The absence of MMP-7 resulted in reduced mean multiplicity and the diameter of early-stage human colorectal tumors in MMP-7 deficient mice [114]. Chemical mutagenesis resulted in decreased tumorigenisis in MMP-11 deficient mice [115]. Tumor progression also reduced in MMP-2-deficient mice [116]. There is plenty of evidence concerning the close relationship between MMPs and mammary carcinogenesis. The expression of MMP-7 in the mammary epithelium enhanced the early-stage mammary tumorigenisis and produced hyperplastic nodules [117]. The expression of MMP-3 [118] and MT1-MMP [119] also remarkably induced hyperplasias and dysplasias in mammary gland of transgenic mice, which could have the ability to progress to aggressive adenocarcinoma. A recent study showed the spontaneous development of premalignant and malignant lesions in the mammary glands of transgenic mice expressing MMP-3 under the control of the whey acidic protein gene promoter [120].

On the other hand, TIMPs have been reported to suppress oncogenicity. The downregulation of TIMP-1 by antisense mRNA in murine fibroblasts imposed tumorigenic and metastatic behavior [121]. The overexpression of TIMP-1 in transgenic mice also inhibited intradermal tumor growth and spontaneous metastasis of ESbL-lacZ T-lymphoma cells, leading to the prolonged survival of the mice, while the opposite effects occurred in low TIMP-1expression [122]. Previous studies also showed that overexpression of TIMP-1 [123] and TIMP-2 [124] reduced tumor growth in human melanoma cells.

7.3. MMPs and Tumor Neoangiogenesis

Tumor cells can facilitate the formation of a blood supply through new blood vessel formation, known as neoangiogenesis (also called neovascularization). The process of tumor neoangiogenesis also has three steps similar to those involved in tumor invasion: proliferation of endothelial cells, ECM degradation and endothelial cell migration. During these steps, MMPs degrade the ECM, which allows the budding endothelial cells to invade into stromal tissue in both normal angiogenesis and tumor vascularization. There have been many previous studies which have indicated the direct contribution of MMPs to tumor angiogenesis [125, 126, 127]. Furthermore, both synthetic and endogenous MMP inhibitors have been reported to prevent angiogensis both in vitro and in vivo [128, 129, 130]. Among MMP family, in particular MMP-2, -9, and -14 (MT1-MMP) can directly regulate tumor angiogenesis [73]. A previous study demonstrated that tumor-induced angiogenesis was suppressed in MMP-2-deficient mice, suggesting that host-derived MMP-2 plays an important role in angiogenesis [116]. Suppression of MMP-2 activity resulted in decreased angiogesis both in vitro and in vivo in the chick chorioallantoic membrane model, suggesting that the activity of MMP-2 is required for the switch to the angiogenic phenotype [131]. As mentioned in above section, cleavage of type IV collagen by MMP-2 exposes the HUIV26 cryptic site which facilitates angiogenesis in vivo [5]. Exposure of the HUIV26 epitope was associated with a loss of alpha 1 beta 1 integrin binding and the gain of alpha v beta 3 binding, and the alpha v beta 3 integrin may function as a receptor for the HUIV26 cryptic epitope. Brooks et al showed that in melanoma cells in vivo expression of integrin alpha v beta 3 on the surface of cancer cells enabled them to bind directly to MMP-2 in a proteolytically active form on the surface of invasive cells, and co-localization of MMP-2 and alpha v beta 3 on angiogenic blood vessels and melanoma cells in vivo, facilitated cell-mediated collagen degradation [6]. A monoclonal antibody (mAb HUIV26) directed to this site blocked integrin-dependent endothelial cell interactions and potently inhibited angiogenesis and tumor growth, suggesting the important role of interaction between MMP-2 and v beta 3 integrin in neoangiogenesis [5].

In addition, recent study showed that MMP-9 triggered the angiogenic switch during *Carcinogenesis* in the RIPI-Tag2 transgenic insulinoma model [132]. In a mouse model of skin cancer, transgenic mice lacking MMP-9 showed the reduced *Carcinogenesis* which could be completely restored by bone-marrow transplantation of MMP-9-expressing cells [133]. MT1-MMP-deficient mice were found to have severe defects in angiogenesis, indicating an essential role for MT1-MMP in the processes of angiogenesis [134]. MT1-MMP regulates angiogenesis by acting as pericellular fibrinolysins during the neovascularization process [135]. Another recent study also showed that MT1-MMP played an important role in endothelial cell migration, and its activity could modulate endothelial migration, invasion, and formation of capillary tubes during the angiogenic response [136]. MT1-MMP is related to the cleavage of CD44, and CD44 expressed on the endothelial cell surface is also involved in the angiogenesis process [137]. In contrast, MMP-12 is reported to inhibit tumor angiogenesis. The formation of capillary structures by human foreskin microvascular endothelial cells (hMVECs) in a 3-dimensional fibrin matrix requires a functional urokinase-type plasminogen activator receptor (u-PAR). The endothelial cell-derived MMP-12 inhibits tumor angiogenesis by cleaving and shedding angiogenesis-related u-PAR [138]. Furthermore, the cleavage of collagen by MMPs also generates functional fragments which can inhibit angiogenesis. Angiostatin is generated from plasminogen via cleaving by MMP-12 [139, 140], -2, -3, and -9 [141]. Angiostatin inhibits endothelial-cell proliferation [140, 141] and has been reported to inhibit growth and metastasis in Lewis lung carcinoma in mice [139, 142]. A very recent study showed that human angiostatin(4.5) may function in vivo to block blood vessel formation by specifically inducing vascular endothelial cells to apoptosis [143]. On the other hand, Endostatin, a 20 kDa C-terminal fragment of collagen XVIII, is generated by MMP-3, -9, -12, -13, and -20 and specifically inhibits endothelial proliferation and potently inhibits angiogenesis and tumor growth [144, 145, 146]. Endostatin inhibits the activities of MMP-2 and MT1-MMP, resulting in inhibition of endothelial cell proliferation [147] and migration [148], and also inducing endothelial cell apoptosis [149].

Angiogenesis is a recently described prognostic factor in NSCLC [150]. Distinct differences in the role of angiogenic molecules between NSCLC and SCLC [150]. A reduced expression of both vascular endothelial growth factor (VEGF) and its receptor (Flt) correlated with less tumor angiogenesis and a better prognosis in patients with a pulmonary adenocarcinoma [151]. Coexpression of VEGF and basic fibroblast growth factor (bFGF) was associated with significantly increased vessel density in human epidermoid lung carcinoma, suggesting that VEGF and bFGF might act cooperatively in the neovascularization of lung carcinomas [152]. Recent study also showed that combined overexpression of VEGF and MMP-2 revealed poor prognosis in NSCLC [153]. Platelet-derived endothelial cell growth factor (PD-ECGF), shown to be the enzyme thymidine phosphorylase (TP), also induces angiogenesis in NSCLC and is related to a worse prognosis [154]. Anti-apoptotic gene bcl-2-positive NSCLC may be related to low tumor vascularization and a strong inverse relationship between bcl-2 and angiogenesis has also been found in NSCLC [155]. Normal lung epithelium expresses bcl-2, while loss of bcl-2 may be involved in tumor progression. In addition, N(neural)-cadherin expression is associated with tumor angiogenesis, and its expression is a prognostic factor of patients with large cell carcinomas [104].

7.4. MMPs and Apoptosis

Apoptosis, also thought of as cell suicide, is an active physiological cell death which fundamentally regulates tissue homeostasis by keeping an appropriate balance between cell proliferation and cell death, thereby avoiding aberrant cellular accumulation and increased tumor incidence [156]. The Fas antigen (CD95/Apo-1) is a member of the tumor necrosis factor receptor superfamily [157, 158]. Cross-linking of Fas and Fas ligand (FasL) are complementary receptor-ligand proteins that lead to apoptosis in Fas-bearing cells. Both Fas and FasL are widely expressed in normal human tissues including bronchial epithelium [159]. Although the expressions of both Fas and FasL are also found on the surface of many tumor cells including lung cancer cells [160, 161], they can often escape against spontaneous apoptosis, with the expression of Fas pathway inhibitors including soluble Fas (sFas), Fas-associated phosphatase-1 (FAP-1) [162] and bcl-2 [163]. The expression of sFas and FAP-1 and, in part, loss of Fas expression, rather than Fas gene alteration or bcl-2 expression, may be involved in the Fas resistance of human hepatocellular carcinoma in vivo [164]

The relationship between some MMPs and apoptosis or anti-apoptosis has been reported. Previous study showed that MMP-7 proteolytically generated active soluble Fas ligand (sFasL) in epithelial tissue and potentiated epithelial cell apoptosis [165]. A 67% reduction in the apoptotic index in the involuting prostate was shown in MMP-7 deficient mice compared with wild-type animals, thereby implicating MMP-7 in this FasL-mediated process [165]. In contrast, another study demonstrated that MMP-7 efficiently cleaved recombinant FasL in vitro and reduced cell surface FasL expression, decreasing cancer cell apoptosis [166]. In addition, MMP-7 prevented apoptosis by forming a complex with heparin-binding epidermal growth factor precursor (pro-HB-EGF) and cleaving it to generate mature HB-EGF, which resulted in the activation of ErbB4 receptor tyrosine kinase leading to cell survival [167]. As well, MMP-3, MMP-9 and MMP-11 have been reported to inhibit cell apoptosis. MMP-3 induced mammary epithelial cell apoptosis in mice [168, 169]. MMP-9 was also reported to prevent apoptosis of hypertrophic chondrocytes [170]. MMP-11 suppressed tumor cell apoptosis in a murine model [171]. High cancer cell death in syngeneic tumors developed in MMP-11 deficient mice [172]. The insulin-like growth factor-I (IGF-I) plays a very important role in promoting survival of cells against a variety of apoptotic agents [173]. MMP-11 also increased IGF-I by cleaving insulin-like growth factor-binding protein-1 (IGFBP-1), thereby promoting the survival of cells and inhibiting apoptosis [174]. MMP-11 mRNA was highly upregulated and required during apoptotic tissue remodeling in Xenopus laevis metamorphosis [175]. These facts suggested that MMP expression by stromal cells surrounding cancer cells contributes to tumorigenesis in a paracrine manner. This party results from decreased cancer cell death through apoptosis.

There have been several reports showing that high levels of TIMP-3 inhibited apoptosis in cancer cell lines [176, 177]. A very recent study demonstrated the accelerated epithelial apoptosis in TIMP-3-deficient mice during mammary gland involution [178]. Furthermore, Ahonen M et al recently reported that TIMP-3 induced apoptosis through stabilization of three distinct death receptors in melanoma cells: tumor necrosis factor receptor-1 (TNF-RI), Fas, and TNF-related apoptosis inducing ligand receptor-1 (TRAIL-RI) [179]. Stabilization of death receptors by TIMP-3 results in activation of caspase-8 and caspase-3, and subsequent apoptosis is blocked by specific caspase-8 inhibitor (Z-IETD-FMK) and by pan-caspase inhibitor (Z-DEVD-FMK) [179].

In addition, tumor necrosis is a consequence of chronic cellular hypoxia, which correlates with poor prognosis in solid tumors. A recent retrospective study demonstrated that the extent of tumor necrosis reflected an aggressive tumor phenotype in NSCLC, which was correlated with the expression of epidermal growth factor receptor (EGFR), Bcl-2, p53 and MMP-9 [180].

8. MMPs and Lung Cancer

Small cell carcinoma (SCLC) has a differenct clinical response to chemotherapy from other types of lung cancers including adenocarcinoma, squamous cell carcinoma, and large cell carcinoma. These latter three lung cancers are collectively called non-small cell lung carcinoma (NSCLC), and are often discussed together. In this section, the author discusses the accumulated knowledge about the association of MMPs to NSCLC and SCLC.

8.1. MMPs and Non-Small Cell Lung Carcinoma (NSCLC)

There is a lot of evidence reported that MMPs and TIMPs, in particular MMP-2 and MMP-9, are closely associated with NSCLC. Previous study detected the increased mRNA expressions of MMP-2 and MMP-9, together with TIMP-1 and TIMP-2 mRNA, in both lung cancer cell lines and NSCLC tumor samples [181]. A recent study also showed high coexpression of MMP1, MMP2, MMP9, TIMP1 and TIMP2 in stage II NSCLC [182].

As for MMP-2, its close relationship with the pathogenesis of NSCLC has previously been reported [183, 184]. A recent study demonstrated that the inactive precursor of MMP-2 was specifically expressed in adenocarcinoma or lung metastases of extrapulmonary tumors [185]. A high level of the active form of MMP-2 in lung carcinomas and the near lack of its activation in normal lung parenchyma showed that MMP-2 activation was also associated with the malignant phenotype and may serve as a good marker of malignancy [186]. The incidence of MMP-2 immunoreactivity was higher in poorly differentiated lung adenocarcinoma than in well differentiated ones, and lower in bronchioloalveolar carcinoma compared with other subtypes of adenocarcinoma [187]. Hyaluronan (HA), a nonsulfated high-molecular mass glycoaminoglycan, strongly activates MMP-2 secretion and the mitogen-activated protein kinase in a human cancer cell line QG90 in a time- and dose-dependent manner, which is strongly inhibited by treatment with anti-CD44, a mitogen-activated protein/extracellular signal-regulated kinase kinase 1 inhibitor, PD98059, or by the phosphatidylinositol 3'-kinase inhibitors, wortmannin and LY294002 [188]. These results suggest that HA-CD44s signaling plays a key role in the HA-dependent secretion of MMP-2 and, hence, in the invasiveness of QG90 cells.

As well shown in other immunohistochemical studies of breast cancer [189] and skin melanoma [190], the overexpression of MMP-2 is also closely associated with a poor prognosis in NSCLC. The prognosis for patients with MMP-2 positive immunoreactivities was significantly poorer than for those with a MMP-negative tumor [187]. MMP-2 expression itself was reported to become an independent risk factor for poor prognosis in NSCLC [191]. Another study showed that the degradation of tenascin-C by MMP-2 in lung cancer is a reliable marker for the potential recurrence of stage-1 NSCLC [192]. The combined overexpression of VEGF and MMP-2 also revealed significant poor prognosis in NSCLC [153]. However, another recent study showed that the correlation between MMP2 protein-staining status and the overall survival rate reached significance in the univariate analysis, but not in the multivariate analysis, suggesting that the detection of MMP2 may be of limited value in informing a prognosis in NSCLC [193].

Furthermore, the positive correlation between MMP-2 and cycloxygenase-2 (COX-2) expression has been recently often mentioned. The expression of COX-2 was related to lymphatic invasion in gastric and colon cancer [194, 195]. The COX-1 or COX-2, derived from human breast cancer cell line Hs578T, could mediate the processing of MMP-2 through induction of MTI-MMP [196]. Expression of COX-2 also promoted the release of MMP-2 and MMP-9 in fetal rat hepatocytes [197]. The constitutive expression of COX-2 could lead to phenotypic changes accompanied by activation of MMP-2 and increased RNA levels for the MT1-MMP, resulting in the enhanced metastatic potential of colorectal cancer cells [198]. As well, in lung cancer, a COX-2 selective inhibitor NS398 also prevented the mRNA expression and enzymatic activity of MMP-2, not MMP-9, in human lung cancer cells, suggesting that the inhibition of COX-2 may possibly become a useful target to prevent lung metastasis [199]. There are various agents contained in cigarette smoke that activate nuclear factor-kappa B (NF-kappaB), leading to lung carcinogenesis. A very recent study by Dohadwala M et al indicated that prostaglandin E2, a COX-2 product, can regulate COX-2-dependent, CD44- and MMP-2-mediated NSCLC invasiveness in an autocrine/paracrine manner through EP4 receptor signaling [200]. Another very recent study showed that curcumin (diferuloylmethane) could down-regulate cigarette smoke-induced NF-kappaB activation through inhibition of IkappaBalpha kinase in human lung epithelial cells, which correlated with suppression of cigarette smoke-induced NF-kappaB-dependent cyclin D1, COX-2 and MMP-9 expression [201].

A lot of evidence has been reported concerning the contribution of MMP-9 to NSCLC. Experimental metastasis was suppressed in MMP-9-deficient mice, suggesting that host-derived MMP-9 may be an important factor in the process of metastasis [202]. Reactivity for MMP-9 was mild in basal cell hyperplasia and squamous metaplasia, while it increased in carcinoma in situ and invasive carcinoma. In contrast, reactivity for MMP-1 was strong in basal cell hyperplasia and squamous metaplasia, decreasing in carcinoma in situ and invasive carcinoma [72]. Confocal microscopy also showed MMP-9-positive cells could pass through fragmented basement membranes [72]. Elevated levels of circulating plasma MMP-9 was also shown in patients with NSCLC [203], especially for types of squamous cell carcinoma and large cell carcinoma [204]. The pretreatment serum level of MMP-9 was identified as an independent prognostic factor in patients with NSCLC [205]. The prognosis for patients with MMP-9 positive immunoreactivities was significantly poorer than for those with a MMP-9 negative tumor [184]. Higher levels of MMP-9 mRNA have been detected in stage III NSCLC compared to stage I and II [205]. The incidence of MMP-9 immunoreactivity was also higher in poorly differentiated adenocarcinomas than in well-differentiated ones, and lower in bronchioloalveolar carcinoma compared with other subtypes of adenocarcinoma [187]. Another immunohistochemical study also indicated that MMP-9 was an independent prognostic factor in post-operative patients with resected stage I-IIIa NSCLC [206]. However, a recent study using quantitative zymography and computer-assisted image analysis demonstrated that, in spite of the significant elevation of mean serum MMP-9 levels in cancer samples compared with normal sera, there was no significant correlation between serum MMP-9 activity and the histological type and stage of lung cancer [207]. Another study also showed that there was no significant correlation between MMP-9 expression and the prognosis of patients with NSCLC [208].

The importance of the contribution of MMP-1 to a poor prognosis has also been reported in colorectal carcinomas [209] and oesophageal cancer [210]. As well, the overexpression of MMP-1 was reported to correlate with an overall poor prognosis in T1 adenocarcinoma of the lung [187]. Another immunohistochemical study demonstrated that MMP-1 was strongly expressed in adenocarcinoma compared with squamous cell carcinoma, together with the overexpressions of MMP-11, MMP-13, MMP-14, TIMP-1 and/or TIMP-2 [211]. another immunohistochemical study by Galateau-Salle et al reported that the reactivity of MMP-1 strongly expressed the basal cell hyperplasia and squamous metaplasia, but in contrast decreased in carcinoma in situ and invasive carcinoma, which was interestingly the inverse of the relationship between MMP-1 and the progression of cancer [72]. Zhu et al recently reported a significant association between the 2G/2G genotype and lung cancer susceptibility, especially in current smokers, suggesting that molecular epidemiological evidence of the MMP-1 promoter polymorphism may be associated with the development of lung cancer [212].

As for other MMPs, there has been some relationship reported. The overexpression of MMP-11 showed significant linkage with the lymphnode involvement in NSCLC [213]. MMP-11 expression was also reported to correlate with the prognosis of NSCLC [211]. MMP-14 (MT1-MMP), a tumor-specific activator of pro-MMP-2, was also correlated with the invasion of lung carcinoma and with lymph node metastasis [20]. Neoplastic cells in carcinoma in situ and invasive carcinoma were positive to MMP-3 [72].

The association of TIMPs with NSCLC has also been often reported. TIMP-1 was expressed in all bronchial washings of NSCLC and pulmonary metastases of extrapulmonary tumors, while TIMP-2 was not detectable [185]. As well, both TIMP-1 and MMP-9 levels were found to be higher in lung cancer than in controls, whereas TIMP-2 and MMP-2/TIMP-2 complex levels were lower in lung cancer than in the sera of the control subjects [203]. High serum levels of TIMP-1 indicated a poor prognosis, especially in squamous cell cancer and in NSCLC patients with stage III [203]. In contrast, another study showed that TIMP1 mRNA expression levels were heterogeneous in NSCLC, but was significantly higher in adenocarcinoma compared to squamous cell carcinoma [214]. Adenocarcinoma, which expressed TIMP-1 and/or TIMP-2 more potently, was positively associated with a more advanced cancer stage and poorer prognosis, compared with squamous cell carcinoma [211].

Furthermore, another previous study reported a significant correlation between TIMP-2 immunoreactivity and cancer stage in NSCLC [181].

8.2. MMPs and Small Cell Lung Carcinoma (SCLC)

There were more positive immunohistochemical expressions of MMP-11, MMP-13, MMP-14, TIMP-2 and TIMP-3 (shown in 70 to 100% of SCLC patients) in SCLC, compared to those of MMP-1 and MMP-9 (shown in 60 to 70% of them), suggesting different contributions of MMPs in SCLC from those in NSCLC [215]. Zhang et al recently demonstrated that Hyaluronan stimulates QG90, a cell line derived from human SCLC, to activate the secretion of MMP-2 in a focal adhesion kinase (FAK)-dependent manner [216]. It is expected that there will be further research concerning the pathogenic contribution of MMPs to SCLC.

9. Synthetic MMP Inhibitors for Treatment of Lung Cancer

The standard treatment for early-stage NSCLC is surgery. However, considering the 5-year survival rates were only 50–60% even though still in stages I and II [217, 218], it requires a more effective clinical strategy other than the present therapeutic methods. MMP inhibitors may be that strategy. The most extensively studied class of MMP inhibitors includes peptidomimetics and nonpeptidomimetic inhibitors of the MMP active site, tetracycline derivatives, and bisphosphonates [219]. A number of synthetic MMP inhibitors have had their development terminated because of adverse effects and insufficient anti-cancer effect to cause tumor shrinkage. At present, several MMP inhibitors are under intensive investigation. The chemical structures of each MMP inhibitor are shown in **Figure 2**.

9.1 Peptidomimetic MMP Inhibitors

Mimicking the structure of MMPs substrates, peptidomimetic MMP inhibitors can act as their substrates, and reversibly and competitively inhibit the activities of MMPs via interacting with the zinc ion of the catalytic site of MMPs. This section focuses upon the major peptidomimetic MMP inhibitors: Batimastat (BB-94), Marimastat (BB-2516), BMS-275291, FKY-1388, Ilomastat (Galardin), PKF-242-484 and PKF-242-466.

Batimastat (BB-94)

Batimastat (BB-94), a low-molecular-weight broad-spectrum hydroxamate-based compound, was the first MMP inhibitor to enter clinical trials. The intraperitonealy administered BB-94 was well tolerated with no serious adverse events and no specific toxicities observed in patients with malignant ascites [220]. In a phase I trial of malignant pleural effusions, intrapleural administration of BB-94 could significantly reduce symptoms and the frequency of therapeutic pleural aspirations [221]. Nevertheless, the development of batimastat has been terminated because of insufficient clinical effect and poor water solubility. There was a recent surprising study which reported that batimastat caused liver-specific overexpression of MMPs-2, -9, and mRNA up-regulation of angiogenesis factors and promoted liver metastasis in the experimental mouse model [222].

Marimastat (BB-2516)

Marimastat (BB-2516), an orally bioavailable analogue of batimastat, is also a low-molecular-weight broad-spectrum hydroxamate-based compound.

Having a collagen-mimicking hydroxamate structure, BB-2516 can also facilitate chelation of the zinc ion in the active site of the MMPs. Marimastat inhibits the activities of MMP-1, -2, -3, -7, -9 and -12 [223]. In a phase I clinical study with patients with advanced lung cancer, the highest dose of marimastat (100 mg orally twice daily) was well tolerated and the most significant toxicity was a symptomatic inflammatory polyarthritis that persisted for up to 8 weeks after discontinuation of the study drug and was dose-limiting [224]. In another phase I trial with advanced inoperable gastric or gastro-oesophageal tumors, marimastat starting dose of 50 mg twice daily or 25 mg once daily for 28 days was generally well tolerated with the principal treatment-related toxicity being pain and stiffness of the musculoskeletal system, and favorable changes in endoscopic findings and improvement of the survival of stable gastric cancer patients were obtained [224]. This compound provided clinical benefits in clinical trials with patients with recurrent colorectal cancer [226] and advanced pancreatic cancer [227]. In these studies, serum levels of tumor markers carcinoembryonic antigen (CEA) [226] and CA19-9 [227] decreased in response to the treatment with marimastat. However, in above these trials, musculoskeletal adverse events caused by the principal drug-related toxicity of marimastat, occurred in a dose- and time-dependent fashion. In a randomized phase II pilot trial of adjuvant marimastat in patients with early-stage breast cancer, marimastat caused the same musculoskeletal adverse events [228]. In the prospective, randomized, double-blind, placebo-controlled trial of marimastat after response to first-line chemotherapy in patients with SCLC, treatment with marimastat after induction therapy for SCLC did not result in improved survival, while significant musculoskeletal toxicity required approximately 20% of patients to discontinue the therapy and caused a significant worsening of their quality of life [229]. There have been other clinical randomized trials in patients with SCLC and stage III NSCLC supported by Brithsh Biotech, but they have not been published yet [230]. Furthermore, marimastat has been studied in other several phase III clinical trials for treatment of patients with unresectable pancreatic cancer [231], advanced ovarian cancer [232] and gliosarcoma [233], but favorable clinical improvements could not obtained. On the other hand, 369 patients with histological proof of advanced gastric adenocarcinoma, who had received no more than a single regimen of 5-fluorouracil-based chemotherapy, were randomised to receive either marimastat (10 mg b.d.) or placebo [234]. As a result over a further 2 years of follow-up, the median survival was 138 days for the placebo and 160 days for marimastat, with 2-year survival rates of 3% and 9% respectively, suggesting a survival benefit of marimastat in advanced gastric cancer. Further clinical trials with marimastat will be continued in the treatment of gastric cancer [235].

BMS-275291

BMS-275291 is a water-soluble and an orally bioavailable broad spectrum MMP inhibitor. The compound can inhibit the activities of MMP-1, -2, -7, -9, and MMP-14. In an experimental a B16BL6 murine metastatic model, BMS-275291 inhibited tumor growth and dose-dependently reduced the number of lung metastases reduction compared with vehicle controls [236]. BMS-275291 also inhibited angiogenesis in a murine angiogenesis model, where once-daily treatment with BMS-275291 resulted in a dose-dependent inhibition of endothelial cell migration [236]. In a randomized phase II study in patients with stage IIIB or IV NSCLC, BMS-275291 has been clinically evaluated in combination with an eight cycle of paclitaxel plus carboplatin every other days for 3 weeks [237]. It was concluded that BMS-275291 was well tolerated in combination with paclitaxel plus carboplatin, with no dose-limiting arthrotoxicity and no adverse impact on early tumor shrinkage [238]. The study has progressed to phase III and the clinical efficacy of BMS-275291 in combination with paclitaxel and carboplatin is being further investigated. Detailed information concerning BMS-275291 has been reviewed by Poulaki V et al [238].

peptidomimetic MMP inhibitors

Batimastat (BB-94)

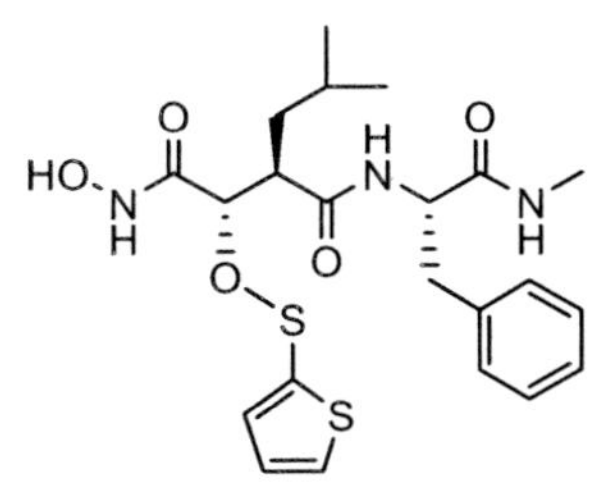

Marimastat (BB-2516)

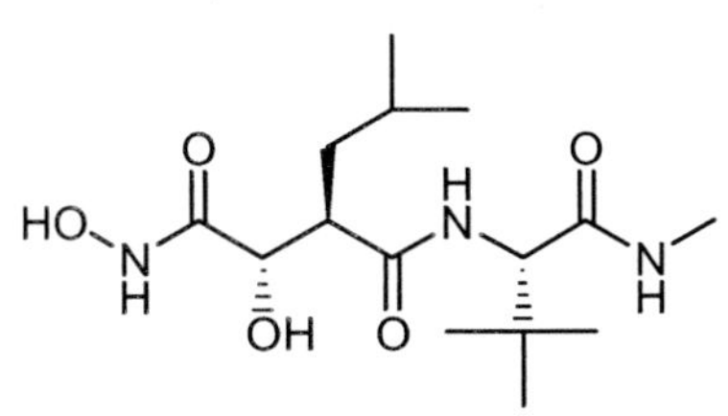

BMS-275291

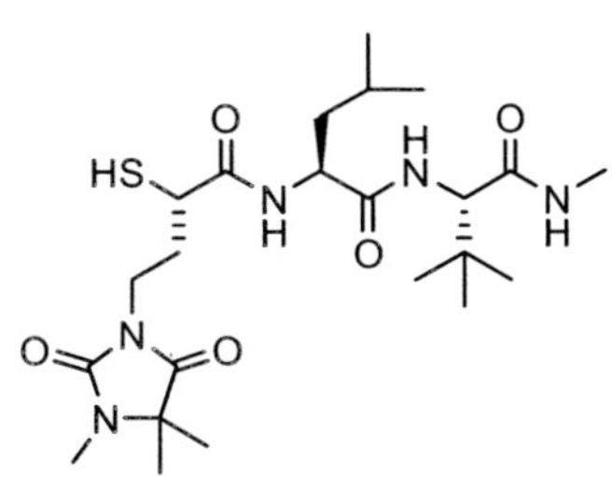

FYK-1388

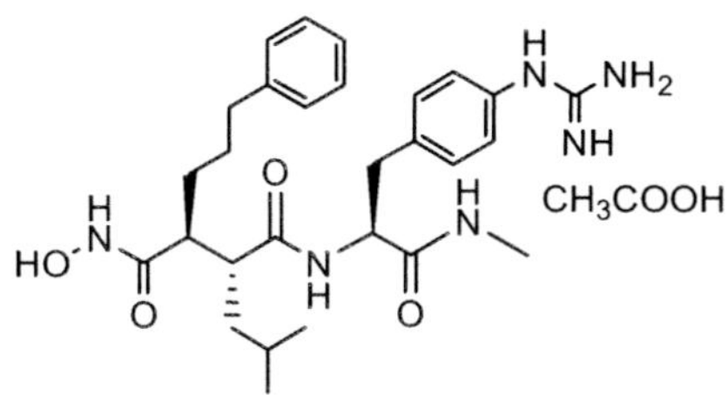

Ilomastat

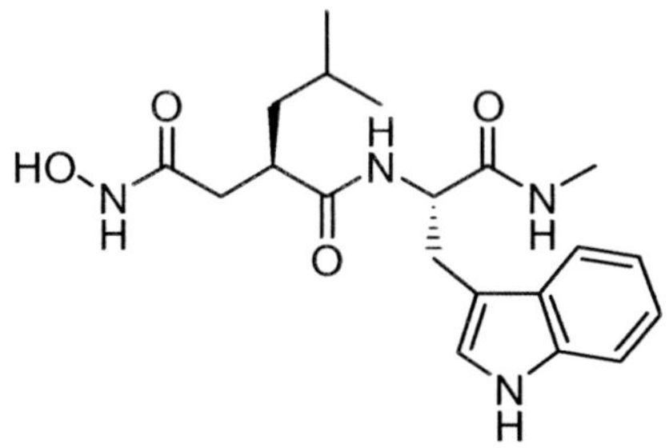

PKF-242-484

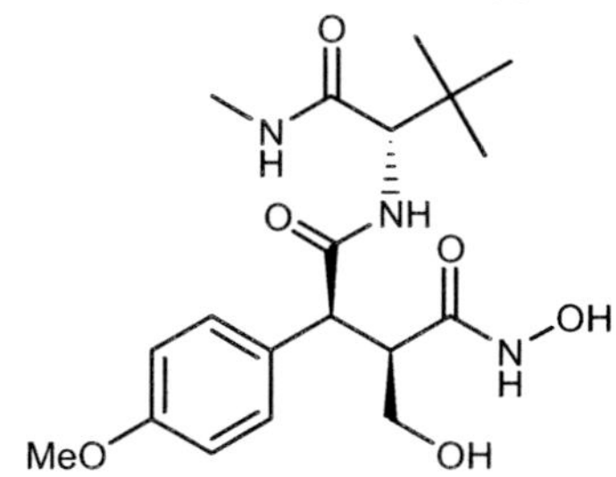

Non-peptidic MMP inhibitors

Prinomastat (AG-3340)

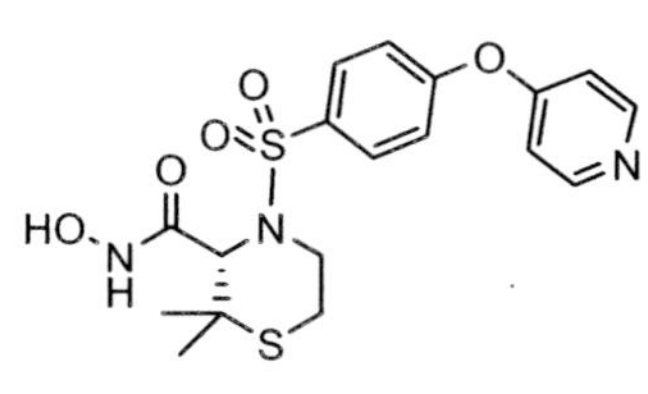

BAY-12-9566

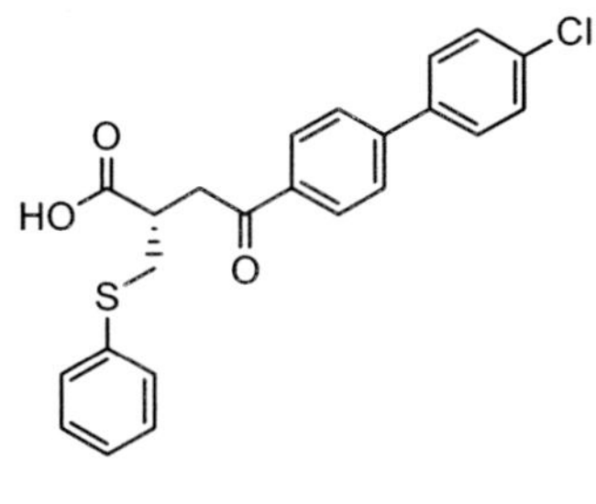

ONO-4817

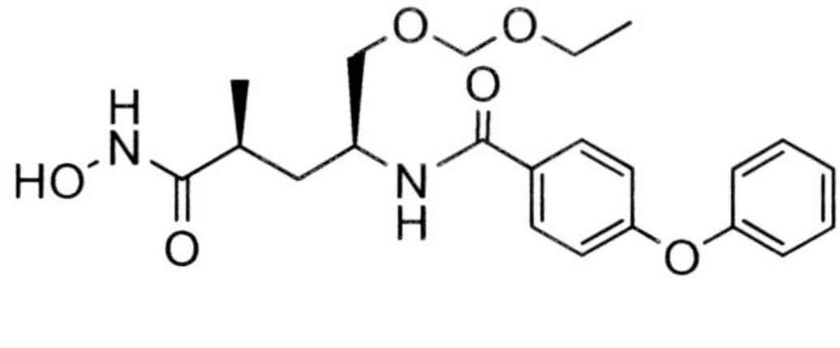

OJ-R11793

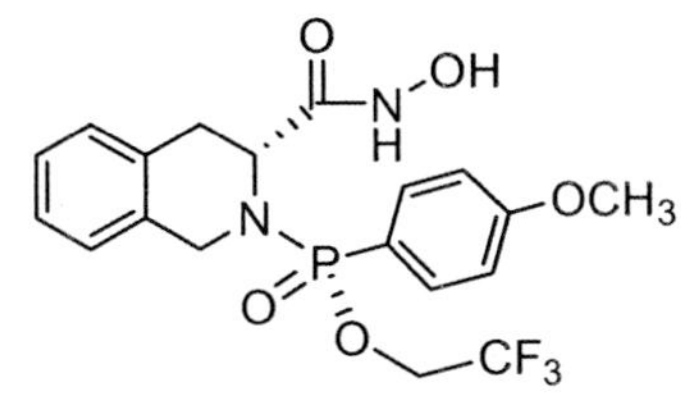

SC-77964

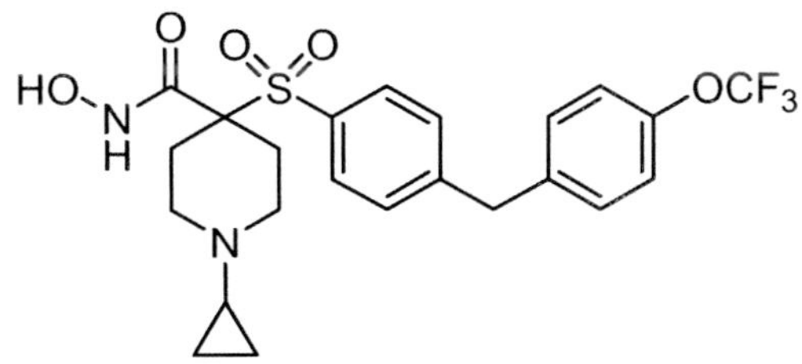

S-3304

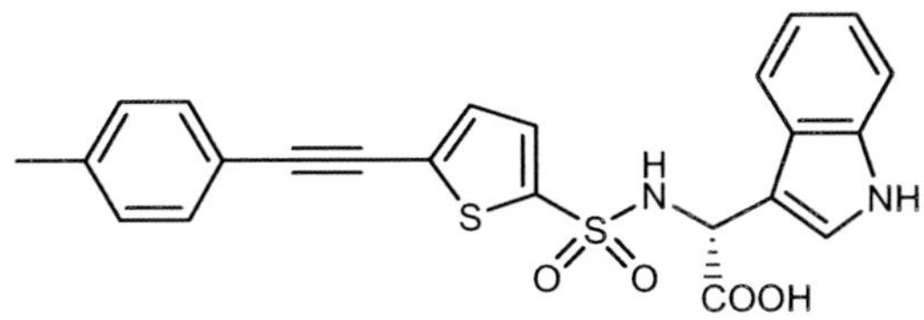

Others

Neovastat: Extract from natural source (shark cartilage)

Metastat (Col-3, CMT-3)

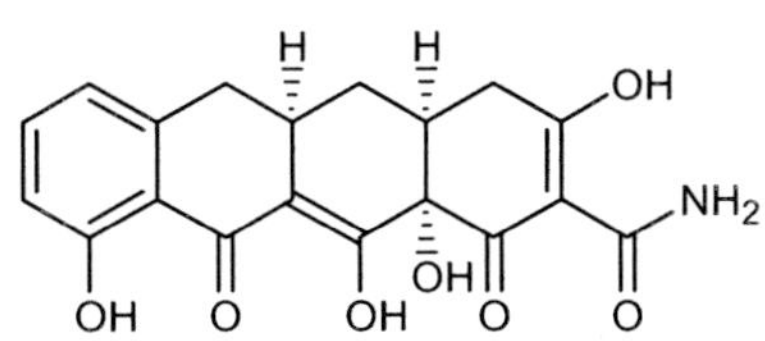

Figure 2 SyntheticMMP inhibitors

FKY-1388

FKY-1388 is a novel broad MMP inhibitor which blocks the activity of MMP-1, -2 ,-3, -7, -9, -13 and -14, in particular it effectively inhibits MMP-2 and -9 [239]. FKY-1388 inhibited the production of MMP-2 and -9 in the human fibrosarcoma cell line HT-1080 at a dose of 10^{-8}M. FYK-1388 also significantly inhibited in vivo tumor growth, experimental lung metastasis and tumor-induced angiogenesis in mouse [239]. These results suggest that FYK-1388 possesses anti-tumor efficacy as a result of inhibiting angiogenesis via the suppression of MMP-2 and -9 activities.

Ilomastat

Ilomastat (Galardin) is a broad spectrum, small-molecule matrix metalloprotease inhibitor, under development by Arriva for the treatment of inflammatory respiratory diseases such as smoking-related emphysema and COPD [240].

PKF242-484 and PKF241-466

PKF242-484 and PKF241-466 are potent dual inhibitors of TNF-alpha converting enzyme (TACE) and MMPs, which are under development by Novartis for the treatment of respiratory inflammation disorders. PKF242-484 and PKF241-466 inhibited purified MMP-1, -2, -3, -9, -13 and rat collagenase at a low nanomolar range [241]. Both compounds inhibited the TNF-alpha release from activated human peripheral blood mononuclear cells with IC(50) values of 56+/-28 and 141+/-100 nM, respectively. In a mouse inflammation model, intranasal administration of PKF-242-484 or PKF241-466 (3-30mg/kg) inhibited LPS-induced airway neutrophil and lymphocyte influx and TNF-alpha release from activated human monocytes [241]. In sensitised C57BL/6 mice, intranasal PKF-242-484 (1-10mg/kg) inhibited ovalbumin-induced airway leucocyte influx [241]. Although no detailed data concerning lung cancer have been published yet, further investigation of these inhibitors is expected.

9.2. Non-Peptidic Inhibitors

The nonpeptidic MMP inhibitors were synthesized in an attempt to improve oral bioavailability and enhance pharmaceutical properties compared with the peptidomimetic inhibitors. These inhibitors have also been synthesized to bind on the base of the 3-dimensional conformation of the zinc ion catalytic site of MMPs, resulting in increased specificity. Some compounds of this class are undergoing evaluation in phase III clinical trials. This section picks up the major nonpeptidic MMP inhibitors, Prinomastat (AG-3340), BAY 12-9566 and ONO-4817. A new approach against the adverse effects observed in conventional MMP inhibitors will be reported. A novel phosphonamide-based MMP-inhibitor OJ-R11793 developed by Nippon Organon, which is quite different from other MMP inhibitors, may allow new applications for MMP inhibitors in general.

Prinomastat (AG-3340)

Prinomastat (AG-3340) is a low-molecular-weight and lipophilic MMP synthetic inhibitor, which inhibits the activity of MMP-3, -9, -13 and MT1-MMP, in particular MMP-2 and MMP-9 more specifically. Prinomastat can inhibit tumor growth and angiogenesis in several xenograft models [219]. There have been two phase III trials of prinomastat in NSCLC. In spite of promising preclinical data, the randomized Phase III trials of prinomastat in patients with advanced NSCLC showed no beneficial clinical effect [242]. Furthermore, another phase III study in combination with gemcitibine and cisplatin in NSCLC also failed to result in any survival advantage [243].

BAY 12-9566

BAY 12-9566, an orally bioavailable biphenyl compound, inhibits the activity of MMP-2, -3, -9 and -13, but not of MMP-1 [244]. Pharmacokinetic studies also showed the rapid oral absorption and high bioavailability of BAY 12-9566 [245]. This compound has shown anti-invasive and antimetastatic activity in several experimental tumor models, including the human colon carcinoma HCT 116 [246], mammary carcinoma MDA-MB-435 [247], murine B16-F10 melanoma, and Lewis lung carcinoma [244]. In vitro, BAY 12-9566 also prevented matrix invasion by endothelial cells, a key process of angiogenesis mediated by MMP, in a concentration-dependent manner without affecting cell proliferation [248]. In vivo, oral daily administration of BAY 12-9566 (50-200 mg/kg) inhibited angiogenesis induced by basic fibroblast growth factor (bFGF) in the Matrigel plug assay, reducing the hemoglobin content of the pellets [248].

In phase I and pharmacologic study of BAY 12-9566 in patients with solid malignancies, BAY 12-9566 was well tolerated on all dose schedules and the recommended dose for further testing was concluded as 800 mg p.o. b.i.d. [249, 250]. In another phase I clinical trials, BAY 12-9566 was well tolerated with only mild and reversible adverse effects, but without the remarkable musculoskeletal effects observed with other MMP inhibitors [251]. At the recommended dose of 800 mg p.o. twice daily, steady-state plasma levels sufficient to demonstrate preclinical activity were achieved [251]. However, in a clinical trial of patients with advanced pancreatic cancer, BAY 12-9566 was significantly inferior to gemcitabine in relation to a disease-free and overall survival rate [252]. Furthermore, phase III studies of patients with in SCLC, NSCLC, ovarian and pancreatic cancer were all cancelled because, when treated with BAY12-9566, patients with SCLC unfortunately did worse than the placebo control patients in term of survival [253].

ONO-4817

ONO-4817 is a novel orally active and selective-spectrum synthetic MMP inhibitor which acts at nanomolar concentrations against the zinc ion catalytic site [254]. In a nude mouse model of experimental lung micrometastasis, either intravenous injection of ONO-4817 or a cytotoxic anticancer drug DOC inhibited the formation of lung metastasis by human NSCLC cancer cell PC14PE6 (adenocarcinoma) and H226 cells (squamous cell carcinoma), by suppressing the activity of these cell-derived MMP-2 and MMP-9 [254]. In addition, combined use of ONO-4817 with DOC significantly suppressed the tumor burden of H226 and PC14PE6 cells in the lung and prolonged the survival of PC14PE6-bearing mice compared to ONO-4817 or DOC alone [254]. These results suggest the possibility that the combined use of ONO-4817 with cytotoxic anticancer drugs can control established lung micrometastasis by inhibiting MMPs.

OJ-R11793

A series of phosphonamide-based compounds recently disclosed by Nippon Organon includes dual MMP/ADAM inhibitors, which are under development for the treatment of psoriasis [255, 256, 257]. These compounds strongly inhibit the activity of MMP-1, -3, -9, ADAM-17, and shedding of growth factors such as heparin-binding epidermal growth factor and amphiregulin. These compounds dose-dependently suppressed TPA-induced epidermal hyperplasia in mice when topically applied. In addition, they proposed a new approach to developing MMP inhibitors, by introducing an antedrug concept, to eliminate concerns about the unwanted toxicity of broad MMP inhibitors arising from nonspecific inhibition of MMPs required for homeostatic control. The use of antedrug strategy may result in locally effective MMP inhibitors with no systemic toxicity as observed in conventional MMP inhibitors. OJ-R11793 is the lead compound in these series, and showed the most rapid decomposition in plasma with a half-life <1 min. Topical application of OJ-R11793 at a dose of 100 μg/head in mice effectively suppressed TPA-induced inflammation with a 81.3 % decrease. These results suggest that OJ-R11793, although promptly metabolized in plasma, existed in its active form at the target site and could regulate EGF production to suppress phorbol-induced inflammation and epidermal hyperplasia. Further investigation of this new type of MMP inhibitor is expected in the cancer research field.

SC-77964

SC-77964 (SC-964), an MMP-1-sparing MMP inhibitor, has been developed for inhibition of angiogenesis and tumor growth [258]. SC-77964 is now in the preclinical stage. Oral SC-77964 showed an inhibitory effect on angiogenesis in mouse experimental model [259].

S-3304

S-3304 is an oral MMP inhibitor, which has been developed by Shionogi Pharmaceutical Co. Ltd [260]. It is in phase I clinical trial, and the phase II clinical trial has been prepared in the USA [260]. Detailed information on this inhibitor has not been published yet.

9.3. Others

Neovastat (AE-941)

Neovastat (AE-941) is an orally bioavailable antiangiogenic and antimetastatic drug isolated from marine cartilage extract. AE-941 markedly inhibits the gelatinolytic activity of MMP-2, and to a lesser extent those of MMP-1, MMP-7, MMP-9 and MMP-13 [261]. AE-941 also inhibited the elastinolytic activities of MMP-12 (metalloelastase), porcine pancreatic elastase, and human leukocyte elastase [261].

Oral administration of Neovastat significantly inhibited bFGF-induced angiogenesis in the Matrigel mouse model, and it also dose-dependently decreased lung metastases in the Lewis lung carcinoma model [262]. Furthermore, combined use of Neovastat with a sub-optimal dose of cisplatinum improved the therapeutic index by increasing the antimetastatic efficacy and by exerting a protective action against cisplatinum-induced body weight loss and myelosuppression [262]. Neovastat blocked the VEGF-dependent microvessel sprouting of endothelial cells from Matrigel-embedded rat aortic rings, an ex vivo model of angiogenesis, and it also strongly inhibited the VEGF-induced migration of endothelial cells [263]. Oral administration of Neovastat also inhibited VEGF-induced blood vessel hyperpermeabilization [263]. Neovastat competes against the binding of VEGF to its receptor in endothelial cells and significantly inhibits the VEGF-dependent tyrosine phosphorylation of VEGF receptor-2, whereas it has no significant effect on the VEGF receptor-1 activity [263]. Neovastat induced bovine aortic endothelial cell death with characteristics of apoptosis including chromatin condensation and DNA fragmentation, which was specifically induced by the activation of caspase-3, -8 and -9 in endothelial cell [264]. The activation of caspases by Neovastat appeared to be essential for its proapoptotic effects, which was associated with the cleavage of the nuclear substrate poly (ADP-ribose) polymerase, and by a concomitant release of cytochrome c from mitochondria to the cytoplasm [264]. Another recent study showed that Neovastat prevented the experimental metastatic bone tumor model in vitro [265].

Neovastat was confirmed to be safe to administer to humans after toxicology studies in rats and monkeys with no dose-limiting toxicity or target organ damage after 1 year of chronic exposure. An excellent safety profile with few side effects has been monitored in more than 800 patients who have been exposed to Neovastat, some of them for more than 4 years, suggesting that Neovastat is suitable for long-term use [266]. Accordingly, Neovastat is currently under evaluation in three pivotal clinical studies with two phase III clinical trials in patients with lung and renal carcinoma, and a phase II clinical trial in patients with multiple myeloma is ongoing [266]. A phase III double-blind placebo-controlled study is investgating the efficacy of Neovastat in addition to induction chemotherapy/radiotherapy combined modality treatment in patients with unresectable stage IIIA and IIIB of NSCLC [267]. Another phase III randomized, double-blind placebo-controlled study is being conducted to evaluate the efficacy of Neovastat as a monotherapy in metastatic renal cell carcinoma patients who have followed a first-line immunotherapy [267]. Detailed information on Neovastat has been reviewed by Gingras D et al [266, 268].

Metastat (Col-3, CMT-3)

Golub et al discovered that some tetracyclines could inhibit collagenase [267]. Metastat (Col-3, CMT-3), a novel oral MMP inhibitor, was synthesized by modifying some functionalities on the basic tetracycline structure [270]. Metastat shows anti-tumor activity conferred by its combined broad inhibition of several MMPs (MMP-1, -2, -8, -9 and –13). As well, the compound activates down-regulation of various inflammatory cytokines such as TNF-alpha and IL-8, which are implicated in metastasis. The proposed mechanism of action for metastat includes the inhibition of MMPs due to divalent chelation of the zinc ion at the active site of the enzyme, the downregulation of production of pro-MMPs, the inhibition of oxidative activation of pro-MMPs, an increase in degradation of pro-MMPs. Some in vitro studies also demonstrated the MMP-based mechanisms. Metastat inhibited the invasive activity of PC-3 and DU-145 (human prostate cancer cell lines) across a Matrigel-coated filter at concentrations of less than 3 μg/mL [271]. Metastat also inhibited ECM degradation mediated by the human colon carcinoma cell line COLO 205 or its conditioned medium [272]. In addition, metastat decreased the number and size of lung metastases in SCID mice inoculated with C8161 cells in vivo [273]. Another in vivo study demonstrated that daily oral lavage with metastat inhibited tumor growth and metastasis in the Dunning MAT LyLu rat prostate tumor [271]. This oral anti-angiogenesis compound is currently undergoing some clinical trials [274]. In a phase I clinical study conducted by the National Cancer Institute, metastat was well tolerated, but photosensitivity was found to be the dose-limiting toxicity [275]. With concurrent use of prophylactic sunblock, metastat was well tolerated at 70 $mg/m^2/d$ [275]. In another phase I clinical study conducted by the National Institute of Health, 3 of 35 patients with refractory metastatic cancer developed phototoxicity followed by clinical and laboratory features of drug-induced lupus [276]. Another phase I clinical trial at the National Cancer Institute reported that 8 of 35 patients with cancer developed anemia while on treatment with metastat, and 3 of them had bone marrow examinations that revealed ringed sideroblasts [277]. Metastat is now in a Phase I/II study for astrocytoma and glioblastoma muliforme, and a Phase II trial for HIV-related Kaposi's sarcoma [278].

10. Consideration

Although it is still unclear at present exactly how MMPs contribute to cancer progression, our knowledge in this field is rapidly expanding. In this chapter, much experimental and clinical evidence was provided which indicates that MMPs play a pivotal role in cancer cell invasion and metastasis via ECM degradation, but also in tumorigenesis, neoangiogenesis, and apoptosis. The pathogenic contribution of MMPs to lung cancer, in particular MMP-2 and MMP-9 to NSCLC was also shown. Considering the pathogenic participation of MMPs in the whole processes of cancer progression, inhibition of MMPs activities should be a reasonable and favorable therapeutic target. A number of synthetic MMP inhibitors have been developed and then their development terminated because of as side effects and poor anti-cancer efficacy. However, some prominent components, as shown in this chapter, are continuing to be developed under phase II or III clinical trials, and a few of them will possibly be commercialized in the near future. Although successful development of MMP inhibitors may provide us a novel insight into cancer therapy and open a new gate to overcoming cancers, there remain many clinical hurdles to establish the optimum therapeutic method in cancer therapy. When these problems are solved, MMP inhibitors will become an effective therapeutic weapon against cancers, improving the prognosis and quality of life of patients with tumors including lung cancer.

Acknowledgements

The author would like to thank Dr. Masaaki Sawa, Dr. Fuminori Sato, Dr. Hiroshi Okazaki and Dr. Jun-ichi Tsuji (Dainippon Pharmaceutical Co.Ltd.) for their useful information on new drugs.

References

[1] Herbst TJ, McCarthy JB, Tsilibary EC, Furcht LT. Differential effects of laminin, intact type IV collagen, and specific domains of type IV collagen on endothelial cell adhesion and migration. *J Cell Biol.* 1988;106(4):1365-73.

[2] Raghow R. The role of extracellular matrix in postinflammatory wound healing and fibrosis. *FASEB J.* 1994;8(11):823-31.

[3] Dogic D, Eckes B, Aumailley M. Extracellular matrix, integrins and focal adhesions. *Curr Top Pathol.* 1999;93:75–83.

[4] Streuli C. Extracellular matrix remodelling and cellular differentiation. *Curr Opin Cell Biol.* 1999;11(5):634-40.

[5] Xu J, Rodriguez D, Petitclerc E, Kim JJ, Hangai M, Moon YS, Davis GE, Brooks PC, Yuen SM. Proteolytic exposure of a cryptic site within collagen type IV is required for angiogenesis and tumor growth in vivo. *J Cell Biol.* 2001;154(5):1069-79.

[6] Brooks PC, Stromblad S, Sanders LC, von Schalscha TL, Aimes RT, Stetler-Stevenson WG, Quigley JP, Cheresh DA. Localization of matrix metalloproteinase MMP-2 to the surface of invasive cells by interaction with integrin alpha v beta 3. *Cell.* 1996;85(5):683-93.

[7] Brooks PC, Silletti S, von Schalscha TL, Friedlander M, Cheresh DA. Disruption of angiogenesis by PEX, a noncatalytic metalloproteinase fragment with integrin binding activity. *Cell.* 1998;92(3):391-400.

[8] Giannelli G, Antonaci S. Biological and clinical relevance of Laminin-5 in cancer. *Clin Exp Metastasis.* 2000;18(6):439-43.

[9] Giannelli G, Falk-Marzillier J, Schiraldi O, Stetler-Stevenson WG, Quaranta V. Induction of cell migration by matrix metalloprotease-2 cleavage of laminin-5. *Science.* 1997;277(5323):225-8.

[10] Koshikawa N, Giannelli G, Cirulli V, Miyazaki K, Quaranta V. Role of cell surface metalloprotease MT1-MMP in epithelial cell migration over laminin-5. *J Cell Biol.* 2000;148(3):615-24.

[11] Adair-Kirk TL, Atkinson JJ, Broekelmann TJ, Doi M, Tryggvason K, Miner JH, Mecham RP, Senior RM. A site on laminin alpha5, AQARSAASKVKVSMKF, induces inflammatory cell production of matrix metalloproteinase-9 and chemotaxis. *J Immunol.* 2003;171(1):398-406.

[12] Bode W, Gomis-Ruth FX, Stockler W. Astacins, serralysins, snake venom and matrix metalloproteinases exhibit identical zinc-binding environments (HEXXHXXGXXH and Met-turn) and topologies and should be grouped into a common family, the 'metzincins'. *FEBS Lett.* 1993;331(1-2):134-40.

[13] Kamiguti AS, Zuzel M, Theakston RD. Snake venom metalloproteinases and disintegrins: interactions with cells. *Braz J Med Biol Res.* 1998;31(7):853-62.

[14] Jia LG, Shimokawa K, Bjarnason JB, Fox JW. Snake venom metalloproteinases: structure, function and relationship to the ADAMs family of proteins. *Toxicon.* 1996;34(11-12):1269-76.

[15] Stone AL, Kroeger M, Sang QX. Structure-function analysis of the ADAM family of disintegrin-like and metalloproteinase-containing proteins (review). *J Protein Chem.* 1999;18(4):447-65.

[16] Nagase H, Woessner JF Jr. Matrix metalloproteinases. *J Biol Chem.* 1999;274:21491-4.

[17] Stamenkovic I. Extracellular matrix remodelling: the role of matrix metalloproteinases. *J Pathol.* 2003;200(4):448-64.

[18] Van den Steen PE, Dubois B, Nelissen I, Rudd PM, Dwek RA, Opdenakker G. *Biochemistry* and molecular biology of gelatinase B or matrix metalloproteinase-9 (MMP-9). *Crit Rev Biochem Mol Biol.* 2002;37(6):375-536.

[19] Sternlicht MD, Werb Z. How matrix metalloproteinases regulate cell behavior. *Annu Rev Cell Dev Biol.* 2001;17:463-516.

[20] Tokuraku M, Sato H, Murakami S, Okada Y, Watanabe Y, Seiki M. Activation of the precursor of gelatinase A/72 kDa type IV collagenase/MMP-2 in lung carcinomas

correlates with the expression of membrane-type matrix metalloproteinase (MT-MMP) and with lymph node metastasis. *Int J Cancer.* 1995;64(5):355-9.

[21] Knauper V, Will H, Lopez-Otin C, Smith B, Atkinson SJ, Stanton H, Hembry RM, Murphy G. Cellular mechanisms for human procollagenase-3 (MMP-13) activation. Evidence that MT1-MMP (MMP-14) and gelatinase a (MMP-2) are able to generate active enzyme. *J Biol Chem.*1996;271:17124-31.

[22] The novel information concerning the ADAM gene family is available at the following internet address: *http://www.people.virginia.edu/~jw7g/Table_of_the_ADAMs.html*

[23] The novel information concerning the ADAMTSs gene family is available at the following internet address: *http://www.gene.ucl.ac.uk/nomenclature/genefamily/adamts.html*

[24] Primakoff P, Myles DG. The ADAM gene family: surface proteins with adhesion and protease activity. *Trends Genet.* 2000;16(2):83-7.

[25] Bottomley KM, Belvisi MG. Matrix metalloproteinases and the potential therapeutic role for matrix metalloproteinase inhibitors in chronic obstructive pulmonary disease (COPD). *Ann Rep Med Chem.* 200;37:209-16.

[26] Van Eerdewegh P, Little RD, Dupuis J, Del Mastro RG, Falls K, Simon J, Torrey D, et al. Association of the ADAM33 gene with asthma and bronchial hyperresponsiveness. *Nature.* 2002; 418(6896): 426-30.

[27] Miyauchi T, Kanekura T, Yamaoka A, Ozawa M, Miyazawa S, Muramatsu T. Basigin, a new, broadly distributed member of the immunoglobulin superfamily, has strong homology with both the immunoglobulin V domain and the beta-chain of major histocompatibility complex class II antigen. *J Biochem (Tokyo).* 1990;107(2):316-23.

[28] Ellis SM, Nabeshima K, Biswas C. Monoclonal antibody preparation and purification of a tumor cell collagenase-stimulatory factor. *Cancer Res.* 1989;49(12):3385-91.

[29] Guo H, Majmudar G, Jensen TC, Biswas C, Toole BP, Gordon MK. Characterization of the gene for human EMMPRIN, a tumor cell surface inducer of matrix metalloproteinases. *Gene.* 1998;220(1-2):99-108.

[30] Li R, Huang L, Guo H, Toole BP. Basigin (murine EMMPRIN) stimulates matrix metalloproteinase production by fibroblasts. *J Cell Physiol.* 2001;186(3):371-9.

[31] Caudroy S, Polette M, Tournier JM, Burlet H, Toole B, Zucker S, Birembaut P. Expression of the extracellular matrix metalloproteinase inducer (EMMPRIN) and the matrix metalloproteinase-2 in bronchopulmonary and breast lesions. *J Histochem Cytochem.* 1999;47(12):1575-80.

[32] Guo H, Zucker S, Gordon MK, Toole BP, Biswas C. Stimulation of matrix metalloproteinase production by recombinant extracellular matrix metalloproteinase inducer from transfected Chinese hamster ovary cells. *J Biol Chem.* 1997;272(1):24-7.

[33] Zucker S, Cao J, Chen WT. Critical appraisal of the use of matrix metalloproteinase inhibitors in cancer treatment. *Oncogene.* 2000;19(56):6642-50.

[34] Kataoka H, DeCastro R, Zucker S, Biswas C. Tumor cell-derived collagenase-stimulatory factor increases expression of interstitial collagenase, stromelysin, and 72-kDa gelatinase. *Cancer Res.* 1993; 53(13):3154-8.

[35] Lim M, Martinez T, Jablons D, Cameron R, Guo H, Toole B, Li JD, Basbaum C. Tumor-derived EMMPRIN (extracellular matrix metalloproteinase inducer) stimulates collagenase transcription through MAPK p38. *FEBS Lett.* 1998; 441(1):88-92.

[36] Guo H, Li R, Zucker S, Toole BP. EMMPRIN (CD147), an inducer of matrix metalloproteinase synthesis, also binds interstitial collagenase to the tumor cell surface. *Cancer Res.* 2000; 60(4):888-91.

[37] Dalberg K, Eriksson E, Enberg U, Kjellman M, Backdahl M. Gelatinase A, membrane type 1 matrix metalloproteinase, and extracellular matrix metalloproteinase inducer mRNA expression: correlation with invasive growth of breast cancer. *World J Surg.* 2000; 24(3):334-40.

[38] Zucker S, Hymowitz M, Rollo EE, Mann R, Conner CE, Cao J, Foda HD, Tompkins DC, Toole BP. Tumorigenic potential of extracellular matrix metalloproteinase inducer. *Am J Pathol.* 2001; 158(6):1921-8.

[39] Yang JM, Xu Z, Wu H, Zhu H, Wu X, Hait WN. Overexpression of extracellular matrix metalloproteinase inducer in multidrug resistant cancer cells. *Mol Cancer Res.* 2003; 1(6):420-7.

[40] Betsuyaku T, Tanino M, Nagai K, Nasuhara Y, Nishimura M, Senior RM. Extracellular matrix metalloproteinase inducer is increased in smokers' bronchoalveolar lavage fluid. *Am J Respir Crit Care Med.* 2003; 168(2):222-7.

[41] van den Oord JJ, Paemen L, Opdenakker G, de Wolf-Peeters C. Expression of gelatinase B and the extracellular matrix metalloproteinase inducer EMMPRIN in benign and malignant pigment cell lesions of the skin. *Am J Pathol.* 1997; 151(3):665-70.

[42] Rosenthal EL, Shreenivas S, Peters GE, Grizzle WE, Desmond R, Gladson CL. Expression of extracellular matrix metalloprotease inducer in laryngeal squamous cell carcinoma. *Laryngoscope.* 2003; 113(8):1406-10

[43] Si AI, Huang L, Xu J, Kumta SM, Wood D, Zheng MH. Expression and localization of extracellular matrix metalloproteinase inducer in giant cell tumor of bone. *J Cell Biochem.* 2003; 89(6):1154-63.

[44] Gomez DE, Alonso DF, Yoshiji H, Thorgeirsson UP. Tissue inhibitors of metalloproteinases: structure, regulation and biological functions. *Eur J Cell Biol.* 1997;74(2):111-22.

[45] Brew K, Dinakarpandian D, Nagase H. Tissue inhibitors of metalloproteinases: evolution, structure and function. *Biochim Biophys Acta.* 2000;1477(1-2):267-83.

[46] Yu WH, Yu S, Meng Q, Brew K, Woessner JF Jr. TIMP-3 binds to sulfated glycosaminoglycans of the extracellular matrix. *J Biol Chem.* 2000;275(40):31226-32.

[47] Olson MW, Bernardo MM, Pietila M, Gervasi DC, Toth M, Kotra LP, Massova I, Mobashery S, Fridman R. Characterization of the monomeric and dimeric forms of latent and active matrix metalloproteinase-9. Differential rates for activation by stromelysin 1. *J Biol Chem.* 2000 ;275(4):2661-8

[48] Goldberg GI, Marmer BL, Grant GA, Eisen AZ, Wilhelm S, He CS. Human 72-kilodalton type IV collagenase forms a complex with a tissue inhibitor of metalloproteases designated TIMP-2. *Proc Natl Acad Sci U S A.* 1989;86(21):8207-11.

[49] Strongin AY, Marmer BL, Grant GA, Goldberg GI.Plasma membrane-dependent activation of the 72-kDa type IV collagenase is prevented by complex formation with TIMP-2. *J Biol Chem.* 1993;268(19):14033-9.

[50] Bigg HF, Shi YE, Liu YE, Steffensen B, Overall CM. Specific, high affinity binding of tissue inhibitor of metalloproteinases-4 (TIMP-4) to the COOH-terminal hemopexin-like domain of human gelatinase A. TIMP-4 binds progelatinase A and the COOH-terminal domain in a similar manner to TIMP-2. *J Biol Chem.* 1997;272(24):15496-500.

[51] Amour A, Slocombe PM, Webster A, Butler M, Knight CG, Smith BJ, Stephens PE, Shelley C, Hutton M, Knauper V, Docherty AJ, Murphy G. TNF-alpha converting enzyme (TACE) is inhibited by TIMP-3. *FEBS Lett.* 1998;435(1):39-44.

[52] Lee MH, Knauper V, Becherer JD, Murphy G. Full-length and N-TIMP-3 display equal inhibitory activities toward TNF-alpha convertase. *Biochem Biophys Res Commun.* 2001;280(3):945-50.

[53] Loechel F, Fox JW, Murphy G, Albrechtsen R, Wewer UM. ADAM 12-S cleaves IGFBP-3 and IGFBP-5 and is inhibited by TIMP-3. *Biochem Biophys Res Commun.* 2000;278(3):511-5.

[54] Kashiwagi M, Tortorella M, Nagase H, Brew K. TIMP-3 is a potent inhibitor of aggrecanase 1 (ADAM-TS4) and aggrecanase 2 (ADAM-TS5). *J Biol Chem.* 2001;276(16):12501-4.

[55] Murphy G, Willenbrock F. Tissue inhibitors of matrix metalloendopeptidases. *Methods Enzymol.* 1995;248:496-510.

[56] Blavier L, Henriet P, Imren S, Declerck YA. Tissue inhibitors of matrix metalloproteinases in cancer. *Ann N Y Acad Sci.* 1999;878:108-19.

[57] Jiang Y, Goldberg ID, Shi YE. Complex roles of tissue inhibitors of metalloproteinases in cancer. *Oncogene.* 2002;21(14):2245-52.

[58] Sottrup-Jensen L. Alpha-macroglobulins: structure, shape, and mechanism of proteinase complex formation. *J Biol Chem.* 1989;264(20):11539-42.

[59] Baker AH, Edwards DR, Murphy G. Metalloproteinase inhibitors: biological actions and therapeutic opportunities. *J Cell Sci.* 2002;115(Pt 19):3719-27.

[60] Bein K, Simons M. Thrombospondin type 1 repeats interact with matrix metalloproteinase 2. Regulation of metalloproteinase activity. *J Biol Chem.* 2000;275(41):32167-73.

[61] Rodriguez-Manzaneque JC, Lane TF, Ortega MA, Hynes RO, Lawler J, Iruela-Arispe ML. Thrombospondin-1 suppresses spontaneous tumor growth and inhibits activation of matrix metalloproteinase-9 and mobilization of vascular endothelial growth factor. *Proc Natl Acad Sci U S A.* 2001;98(22):12485-90.

[62] Taraboletti G, Morbidelli L, Donnini S, Parenti A, Granger HJ, Giavazzi R, Ziche M. The heparin binding 25 kDa fragment of thrombospondin-1 promotes angiogenesis and modulates gelatinase and TIMP-2 production in endothelial cells. *FASEB J.* 2000;14(12):1674-6.

[63] Lee T, Esemuede N, Sumpio BE, Gahtan V. Thrombospondin-1 induces matrix metalloproteinase-2 activation in vascular smooth muscle cells. *J Vasc Surg.* 2003;38(1):147-54.

[64] Yang Z, Strickland DK, Bornstein P. Extracellular matrix metalloproteinase 2 levels are regulated by the low density lipoprotein-related scavenger receptor and thrombospondin 2. *J Biol Chem.* 2001;276(11):8403-8.

[65] Oh J, Takahashi R, Kondo S, Mizoguchi A, Adachi E, Sasahara RM, Nishimura S, Imamura Y, Kitayama H, Alexander DB, Ide C, Horan TP, Arakawa T, Yoshida H, Nishikawa S, Itoh Y, Seiki M, Itohara S, Takahashi C, Noda M. The membrane-anchored MMP inhibitor RECK is a key regulator of extracellular matrix integrity and angiogenesis. *Cell.* 2001;107(6):789-800.

[66] Noda M, Oh J, Takahashi R, Kondo S, Kitayama H, Takahashi C. RECK: a novel suppressor of malignancy linking oncogenic signaling to extracellular matrix remodeling. *Cancer Metastasis Rev.* 2003;22(2-3):167-75.

[67] Kahari VM, Saarialho-Kere U. Matrix metalloproteinases and their inhibitors in tumour growth and invasion. *Ann Med.* 1999;31(1):34-45.

[68] Itoh Y, Nagase H. Matrix metalloproteinases in cancer. *Essays Biochem.* 2002;38:21-36.

[69] Egeblad M, Werb Z. New functions for the matrix metalloproteinases in cancer progression. *Nat Rev Cancer.* 2002;2(3):161-74.

[70] Engbring JA, Kleinman HK. The basement membrane matrix in malignancy. *J Pathol.* 2003;200(4):465-70.

[71] Liotta LA, Thorgeirsson UP, Garbisa S. Role of collagenases in tumor cell invasion. *Cancer Metastasis Rev.* 1982;1(4):277-88.

[72] Galateau-Sallе FB, Luna RE, Horiba K, Sheppard MN, Hayashi T, Fleming MV, Colby TV, Bennett W, Harris CC, Stetler-Stevenson WG, Liotta L, Ferrans VJ, Travis WD. Matrix metalloproteinases and tissue inhibitors of metalloproteinases in bronchial squamous preinvasive lesions. *Hum Pathol.* 2000;31(3):296-305.

[73] Foda HD, Zucker S. Matrix metalloproteinases in cancer invasion, metastasis and angiogenesis. *Drug Discov Today.* 2001;6(9):478-482.

[74] Kim D, Kim S, Koh H, Yoon SO, Chung AS, Cho KS, Chung J. Akt/PKB promotes cancer cell invasion via increased motility and metalloproteinase production. *FASEB J.* 2001;15(11):1953-62.

[75] Park BK, Zeng X, Glazer RI. Akt1 induces extracellular matrix invasion and matrix metalloproteinase-2 activity in mouse mammary epithelial cells. *Cancer Res.* 2001;61(20):7647-53.

[76] Zhang D, Brodt P. Type 1 insulin-like growth factor regulates MT1-MMP synthesis and tumor invasion via PI 3-kinase/Akt signaling. *Oncogene.* 2003;22(7):974-82.

[77] Chen WT. Proteases associated with invadopodia, and their role in degradation of extracellular matrix. *Enzyme Protein.* 1996;49(1-3):59-71.

[78] Chen WT, Wang JY. Specialized surface protrusions of invasive cells, invadopodia and lamellipodia, have differential MT1-MMP, MMP-2, and TIMP-2 localization. *Ann N Y Acad Sci.* 1999;878:361-71.

[79] Thompson EW, Paik S, Brunner N, Sommers CL, Zugmaier G, Clarke R, Shima TB, Torri J, Donahue S, Lippman ME, et al. Association of increased basement membrane invasiveness with absence of estrogen receptor and expression of vimentin in human breast cancer cell lines. *Cell Physiol.* 1992;150(3):534-44.

[80] Kelly T, Yan Y, Osborne RL, Athota AB, Rozypal TL, Colclasure JC, Chu WS. Proteolysis of extracellular matrix by invadopodia facilitates human breast cancer cell invasion and is mediated by matrix metalloproteinases. *Clin Exp Metastasis.* 1998;16(6):501-12.

[81] Nakahara H, Howard L, Thompson EW, Sato H, Seiki M, Yeh Y, Chen WT. Transmembrane/cytoplasmic domain-mediated membrane type 1-matrix metalloprotease docking to invadopodia is required for cell invasion. *Proc Natl Acad Sci U S A.* 1997;94(15):7959-64.

[82] Chen WT, Kelly T. Seprase complexes in cellular invasiveness. *Cancer Metastasis Rev.* 2003;22(2-3):259-69.

[83] Monsky WL, Lin CY, Aoyama A, Kelly T, Akiyama SK, Mueller SC, Chen WT. A potential marker protease of invasiveness, seprase, is localized on invadopodia of human malignant melanoma cells. *Cancer Res.* 1994;54(21):5702-10.

[84] Artym VV, Kindzelskii AL, Chen WT, Petty HR. Molecular proximity of seprase and the urokinase-type plasminogen activator receptor on malignant melanoma cell membranes: dependence on beta1 integrins and the cytoskeleton. *Carcinogenesis.* 2002;23(10):1593-601.

[85] Mueller SC, Ghersi G, Akiyama SK, Sang QX, Howard L, Pineiro-Sanchez M, Nakahara H, Yeh Y, Chen WT. A novel protease-docking function of integrin at invadopodia. *J Biol Chem.* 1999;274(35):24947-52.

[86] Bowden ET, Barth M, Thomas D, Glazer RI, Mueller SC. An invasion-related complex of cortactin, paxillin and PKCmu associates with invadopodia at sites of extracellular matrix degradation. *Oncogene.* 1999;18(31):4440-9.

[87] Keely P, Parise L, Juliano R. Integrins and GTPases in tumour cell growth, motility and invasion. *Trends Cell Biol.* 1998;8(3):101-6.

[88] Naot D, Sionov RV, Ish-Shalom D. CD44: structure, function, and association with the malignant process. *Adv Cancer Res.* 1997;71:241-319.

[89] Sneath RJ, Mangham DC. The normal structure and function of CD44 and its role in neoplasia. *Mol Pathol.*1998;51:191-200.

[90] Okamoto I, Kawano Y, Tsuiki H, Sasaki J, Nakao M, Matsumoto M, Suga M, Ando M, Nakajima M, Saya H. CD44 cleavage induced by a membrane-associated metalloprotease plays a critical role in tumor cell migration. *Oncogene.* 1999;18(7):1435-46.

[91] Guo YJ, Liu G, Wang X, Jin D, Wu M, Ma J, Sy MS. Potential use of soluble CD44 in serum as indicator of tumor burden and metastasis in patients with gastric or colon cancer. *Cancer Res.* 1994;54:422-46.

[92] Masson D, Denis MG, Denis M, Blanchard D, Loirat MJ, Cassagnau E, Lustenberger P. Soluble CD44: quantification and molecular repartition in plasma of patients with colorectal cancer. *Br J Cancer.* 1999;80(12):1995-2000.

[93] Yamane N, Tsujitani S, Makino M, Maeta M, Kaibara N. Soluble CD44 variant 6 as a prognostic indicator in patients with colorectal cancer. *Oncology.* 1999;56(3):232-8.

[94] Jalkanen S, Joensuu H, Soderstrom KO, Klemi P. Lymphocyte homing and clinical behavior of non-Hodgkin's lymphoma. *J Clin Invest.* 1991;87(5):1835-40.

[95] Seiki M. Membrane-type matrix metalloproteinases. APMIS. 1999;107(1):137-43.

[96] Kajita M, Itoh Y, Chiba T, Mori H, Okada A, Kinoh H, Seiki M. Membrane-type 1 matrix metalloproteinase cleaves CD44 and promotes cell migration. *J Cell Biol.* 2001;153(5):893-904.

[97] Yu Q, Stamenkovic I. Localization of matrix metalloproteinase 9 to the cell surface provides a mechanism for CD44-mediated tumor invasion. *Genes Dev.* 1999;13(1):35-48.

[98] Bremnes RM, Veve R, Hirsch FR, Franklin WA. The E-cadherin cell-cell adhesion complex and lung cancer invasion, metastasis, and prognosis. *Lung Cancer.* 2002;36(2):115-24.

[99] Fei Q, Zhang H, Chen X, Wang JC, Zhang R, Xu W, Zhang Z, Zou W, Zhang K, Qi Q, Wang M, Tao S, Luo Z. Defected expression of E-cadherin in non-small cell lung cancer. *Lung Cancer.* 2002;37(2):147-52.

[100] Bremnes RM, Veve R, Gabrielson E, Hirsch FR, Baron A, Bemis L, Gemmill RM, Drabkin HA, Franklin WA. High-throughput tissue microarray analysis used to evaluate biology and prognostic significance of the E-cadherin pathway in non-small-cell lung cancer. *J Clin Oncol.* 2002;20(10):2417-28

[101] Ohira T, Gemmill RM, Ferguson K, Kusy S, Roche J, Brambilla E, Zeng C, Baron A, Bemis L, Erickson P, Wilder E, Rustgi A, Kitajewski J, Gabrielson E, Bremnes R, Franklin W, Drabkin HA. WNT7a induces E-cadherin in lung cancer cells. *Proc Natl Acad Sci U S A.* 2003;100(18):10429-34.

[102] Al Moustafa AE, Yen L, Benlimame N, Alaoui-Jamali MA. Regulation of E-cadherin/catenin complex patterns by epidermal growth factor receptor modulation in human lung cancer cells. *Lung Cancer.* 2002;37(1):49-56.

[103] Soo Choi Y, Mog Shim Y, Kim SH, Soon Son D, Lee HS, Young Kim G, Han J, Kim J. Prognostic significance of E-cadherin and beta-catenin in resected stage I non-small cell lung cancer. *Eur J Cardiothorac Surg.* 2003;24(3):441-9.

[104] Nakashima T, Huang C, Liu D, Kameyama K, Masuya D, Kobayashi S, Kinoshita M, Yokomise H. Neural-cadherin expression associated with angiogenesis in non-small-cell lung cancer patients. *Br J Cancer.* 2003;88(11):1727-33.

[105] Kren L, Hermanova M, Goncharuk VN, Kaur P, Ross JS, Pavlovsky Z, Dvorak K. Downregulation of plasma membrane expression/cytoplasmic accumulation of beta-catenin predicts shortened survival in non-small cell lung cancer. A clinicopathologic study of 100 cases. *Cesk Patol.* 2003;39(1):17-20.

[106] Rodriguez-Salas N, Palacios J, de Castro J, Moreno G, Gonzalez-Baron M, Gamallo C. Beta-catenin expression pattern in small cell lung cancer: correlation with clinical and evolutive features. *Histol Histopathol.* 2001;16(2):353-8.

[107] Pirinen RT, Hirvikoski P, Johansson RT, Hollmen S, Kosma VM. Reduced expression of alpha-catenin, beta-catenin, and gamma-catenin is associated with high cell proliferative activity and poor differentiation in non-small cell lung cancer. *J Clin Pathol.* 2001;54(5):391-5.

[108] Noe V, Fingleton B, Jacobs K, Crawford HC, Vermeulen S, Steelant W, Bruyneel E, Matrisian LM, Mareel M. Release of an invasion promoter E-cadherin fragment by matrilysin and stromelysin-1. *J Cell Sci.* 2001;114(Pt 1):111-118.

[109] Nawrocki-Raby B, Gilles C, Polette M, Bruyneel E, Laronze JY, Bonnet N, Foidart JM, Mareel M, Birembaut P. Upregulation of MMPs by soluble E-cadherin in human lung tumor cells. *Int J Cancer*. 2003;105(6):790-5.

[110] Lochter A, Sternlicht MD, Werb Z, Bissell MJ. The significance of matrix metalloproteinases during early stages of tumor progression. Ann N Y Acad Sci. Kahari VM, Saarialho-Kere U. Matrix metalloproteinases and their inhibitors in tumour growth and invasion. *Ann Med.* 1999;31(1):34-45.

[111] Kahari VM, Saarialho-Kere U. Matrix metalloproteinases and their inhibitors in tumour growth and invasion. *Ann Med.* 1999;31(1):34-45.

[112] D'Armiento J, DiColandrea T, Dalal SS, Okada Y, Huang MT, Conney AH, Chada K. Collagenase expression in transgenic mouse skin causes hyperkeratosis and acanthosis and increases susceptibility to tumorigenesis. *Mol Cell Biol.* 1995;15(10):5732-9.

[113] Bergers G, Brekken R, McMahon G, Vu TH, Itoh T, Tamaki K, Tanzawa K, Thorpe P, Itohara S, Werb Z, Hanahan D. Matrix metalloproteinase-9 triggers the angiogenic switch during carcinogenesis. *Nat Cell Biol.* 2000;(10):737-44.

[114] Wilson CL, Heppner KJ, Labosky PA, Hogan BL, Matrisian LM. Intestinal tumorigenesis is suppressed in mice lacking the metalloproteinase matrilysin. *Proc Natl Acad Sci U S A*. 1997;94(4):1402-7.

[115] Masson R, Lefebvre O, Noel A, Fahime ME, Chenard MP, Wendling C, Kebers F, LeMeur M, Dierich A, Foidart JM, Basset P, Rio MC. In vivo evidence that the stromelysin-3 metalloproteinase contributes in a paracrine manner to epithelial cell malignancy. *J Cell Biol.* 1998;140(6):1535-41.

[116] Itoh T, Tanioka M, Yoshida H, Yoshioka T, Nishimoto H, Itohara S. Reduced angiogenesis and tumor progression in gelatinase A-deficient mice. *Cancer Res.* 1998;58(5):1048-51.

[117] Rudolph-Owen LA, Chan R, Muller WJ, Matrisian LM. The matrix metalloproteinase matrilysin influences early-stage mammary tumorigenesis. *Cancer Res.* 1998;58(23):5500-6.

[118] Sternlicht MD, Lochter A, Sympson CJ, Huey B, Rougier JP, Gray JW, Pinkel D, Bissell MJ, Werb Z. The stromal proteinase MMP3/stromelysin-1 promotes mammary carcinogenesis. *Cell.* 1999;98(2):137-46.

[119] Ha HY, Moon HB, Nam MS, Lee JW, Ryoo ZY, Lee TH, Lee KK, So BJ, Sato H, Seiki M, Yu DY. Overexpression of membrane-type matrix metalloproteinase-1 gene induces mammary gland abnormalities and adenocarcinoma in transgenic mice. *Cancer Res.* 2001;61(3):984-90.

[120] Sternlicht MD, Bissell MJ, Werb Z. The matrix metalloproteinase stromelysin-1 acts as a natural mammary tumor promoter. *Oncogene*. 2000;19(8):1102-13.

[121] Khokha R, Waterhouse P, Yagel S, Lala PK, Overall CM, Norton G, Denhardt DT. Antisense RNA-induced reduction in murine TIMP levels confers oncogenicity on Swiss 3T3 cells. *Science*. 1989;243(4893):947-50.

[122] Kruger A, Fata JE, Khokha R. Altered tumor growth and metastasis of a T-cell lymphoma in Timp-1 transgenic mice. *Blood.* 1997;90(5):1993-2000.

[123] Koop S, Khokha R, Schmidt EE, MacDonald IC, Morris VL, Chambers AF, Groom AC. Overexpression of metalloproteinase inhibitor in B16F10 cells does not affect extravasation but reduces tumor growth. *Cancer Res.* 1994;54(17):4791-7.

[124] Montgomery AM, Mueller BM, Reisfeld RA, Taylor SM, DeClerck YA. Effect of tissue inhibitor of the matrix metalloproteinases-2 expression on the growth and spontaneous metastasis of a human melanoma cell line. *Cancer Res.* 1994;54(20):5467-73.

[125] Werb Z, Vu TH, Rinkenberger JL, Coussens LM. Matrix-degrading proteases and angiogenesis during development and tumor formation. *APMIS.* 1999;107(1):11-8.

[126] Hiraoka N, Allen E, Apel IJ, Gyetko MR, Weiss SJ. Matrix metalloproteinases regulate neovascularization by acting as pericellular fibrinolysins. *Cell.* 1998;95(3):365-77.

[127] Stetler-Stevenson WG. Matrix metalloproteinases in angiogenesis: a moving target for therapeutic intervention. *J. Clin. Invest.* 1999;103:1237–1241.

[128] Murphy AN, Unsworth EJ, Stetler-Stevenson WG. Tissue inhibitor of metalloproteinase-2 inhibits bFGF-induced human microvascular endothelial cell proliferation. *J. Cell. Physiol.* 1993;157:351-358.

[129] Benelli R, Adatia R, Ensoli B, Stetler-Stevenson WG, Santi L, Albini A. Inhibition of AIDS-Kaposi's sarcoma cell induced endothelial cell invasion by TIMP-2 and a synthetic peptide from the metalloproteinase propeptide: implications for an anti-angiogenic therapy. *Oncol Res.* 1994;6(6):251-7.

[130] Anand-Apte B, Pepper MS, Voest E, Montesano R, Olsen B, Murphy G, Apte SS, Zetter B. Inhibition of angiogenesis by tissue inhibitor of metalloproteinase-3. Invest. Ophthalmol. *Vis. Sci.* 1997;38:817-823.

[131] Fang J, Shing Y, Wiederschain D, Yan L, Butterfield C, Jackson G, Harper J, Tamvakopoulos G, Moses MA. Matrix metalloproteinase-2 is required for the switch to the angiogenic phenotype in a tumor model. *Proc Natl Acad Sci U S A.* 2000;97(8):3884-9.

[132] Bergers G, Brekken R, McMahon G, Vu TH, Itoh T, Tamaki K, Tanzawa K, Thorpe P, Itohara S, Werb Z, Hanahan D. Matrix metalloproteinase-9 triggers the angiogenic switch during carcinogenesis. *Nat Cell Biol.* 2000;2(10):737-44.

[133] Coussens LM, Tinkle CL, Hanahan D, Werb Z. MMP-9 supplied by bone marrow-derived cells contributes to skin carcinogenesis. *Cell.* 2000;103(3):481-90.

[134] Zhou Z, Apte SS, Soininen R, Cao R, Baaklini GY, Rauser RW, Wang J, Cao Y, Tryggvason K. Impaired endochondral ossification and angiogenesis in mice deficient in membrane-type matrix metalloproteinase I. *Proc Natl Acad Sci U S A.* 2000;97(8):4052-7.

[135] Hiraoka N, Allen E, Apel IJ, Gyetko MR, Weiss SJ. Matrix metalloproteinases regulate neovascularization by acting as pericellular fibrinolysins. *Cell.* 1998;95(3):365-77.

[136] Galvez BG, Matias-Roman S, Albar JP, Sanchez-Madrid F, Arroyo AG. Membrane type 1-matrix metalloproteinase is activated during migration of human endothelial cells and modulates endothelial motility and matrix remodeling. *J Biol Chem.* 2001;276(40):37491-500.

[137] Trochon V, Mabilat C, Bertrand P, Legrand Y, Smadja-Joffe F, Soria C, Delpech B, Lu H. Evidence of involvement of CD44 in endothelial cell proliferation, migration and angiogenesis in vitro. *Int J Cancer.* 1996;66(5):664-8.

[138] Koolwijk P, Sidenius N, Peters E, Sier CF, Hanemaaijer R, Blasi F, van Hinsbergh VW. Proteolysis of the urokinase-type plasminogen activator receptor by metalloproteinase-12: implication for angiogenesis in fibrin matrices. *Blood.* 2001;97(10):3123-31.

[139] Dong Z, Kumar R, Yang X, Fidler IJ. Macrophage-derived metalloelastase is responsible for the generation of angiostatin in Lewis lung carcinoma. *Cell.* 1997;88(6):801-10.

[140] Gorrin-Rivas MJ, Arii S, Furutani M, Mizumoto M, Mori A, Hanaki K, Maeda M, Furuyama H, Kondo Y, Imamura M. Mouse macrophage metalloelastase gene transfer into a murine melanoma suppresses primary tumor growth by halting angiogenesis. *Clin Cancer Res.* 2000;6(5):1647-54.

[141] Cornelius LA, Nehring LC, Harding E, Bolanowski M, Welgus HG, Kobayashi DK, Pierce RA, Shapiro SD. Matrix metalloproteinases generate angiostatin: effects on neovascularization. *J Immunol.* 1998;161(12):6845-52.

[142] O'Reilly MS, Holmgren L, Shing Y, Chen C, Rosenthal RA, Moses M, Lane WS, Cao Y, Sage EH, Folkman J. Angiostatin: a novel angiogenesis inhibitor that mediates the suppression of metastases by a Lewis lung carcinoma. *Cell.* 1994 Oct 21;79(2):315-28.

[143] Hanford HA, Wong CA, Kassan H, Cundiff DL, Chandel N, Underwood S, Mitchell CA, Soff GA. Angiostatin(4.5)-mediated apoptosis of vascular endothelial cells. *Cancer Res.* 2003;63(14):4275-80.

[144] O'Reilly MS, Boehm T, Shing Y, Fukai N, Vasios G, Lane WS, Flynn E, Birkhead JR, Olsen BR, Folkman J. Endostatin: an endogenous inhibitor of angiogenesis and tumor growth. *Cell.* 1997;88(2):277-85.

[145] Ferreras M, Felbor U, Lenhard T, Olsen BR, Delaisse J. Generation and degradation of human endostatin proteins by various proteinases. *FEBS Lett.* 2000 Dec 15;486(3):247-51.

[146] Kim YM, Jang JW, Lee OH, Yeon J, Choi EY, Kim KW, Lee ST, Kwon YG. Endostatin inhibits endothelial and tumor cellular invasion by blocking the activation and catalytic activity of matrix metalloproteinase. *Cancer Res.* 2000;60(19):5410-3.

[147] O'Reilly M S, Boehm T, Shing Y, Fukai N, Vasios G, Lane WS, Flynn E, Birkhead JR, Olsen BR, Folkman J. Endostatin: an endogenous inhibitor of angiogenesis and tumor growth. *Cell.* 1997; 88: 277-85.

[148] Yamaguchi N, Anand-Apte B, Lee M, Sasaki T, Fukai N, Shapiro R, Que I, Lowik C, Timpl R, Olsen BR. Endostatin inhibits VEGF-induced endothelial cell migration and tumor growth independently of zinc binding. *EMBO J.* 1999; 18: 4414-23.

[149] Dhanabal M, Ramchandran R, Waterman MJ, Lu H, Knebelmann B, Segal M, Sukhatme VP. Endostatin induces endothelial cell apoptosis. *J Biol Chem.* 1999; 274:11721-6.

[150] Galligioni E, Ferro A. Angiogenesis and antiangiogenic agents in non-small cell lung cancer. *Lung Cancer.* 2001;34 Suppl 4:S3-7.

[151] Takanami I, Tanaka F, Hashizume T, Kodaira S. Vascular endothelial growth factor and its receptor correlate with angiogenesis and survival in pulmonary adenocarcinoma. *AntiCancer Res.* 1997;17(4A):2811-4.

[152] Mattern J, Koomagi R, Volm M. Coexpression of VEGF and bFGF in human epidermoid lung carcinoma is associated with increased vessel density. *AntiCancer Res.* 1997;17(3C):2249-52.

[153] Shou Y, Hirano T, Gong Y, Kato Y, Yoshida K, Ohira T, Ikeda N, Konaka C, Ebihara Y, Zhao F, Kato H. Influence of angiogenetic factors and matrix metalloproteinases upon tumour progression in non-small-cell lung cancer. *Br J Cancer.* 2001;85(11):1706-12.

[154] Koukourakis MI, Giatromanolaki A, O'Byrne KJ, Comley M, Whitehouse RM, Talbot DC, Gatter KC, Harris AL. Platelet-derived endothelial cell growth factor expression correlates with tumour angiogenesis and prognosis in non-small-cell lung cancer. *Br J Cancer.* 1997;75(4):477-81.

[155] Koukourakis MI, Giatromanolaki A, O'Byrne KJ, Whitehouse RM, Talbot DC, Gatter KC, Harris AL. Potential role of bcl-2 as a suppressor of tumour angiogenesis in non-small-cell lung cancer. *Int J Cancer.* 1997;74(6):565-70.

[156] Thompson CB. Apoptosis in the pathogenesis and treatment of disease. *Science.*1995;267: 1456-1462.

[157] Suda T, Takahashi T, Golstein P, Nagata S. Molecular cloning and expression of the Fas ligand, a novel member of the tumor necrosis factor family. *Cell.* 1993;75(6):1169-78.

[158] Schulze-Osthoff K, Ferrari D, Los M, Wesselborg S, Peter ME. Apoptosis signaling by death receptors *European Journal of Biochemistry.* 1998;254:439-459.

[159] Lee SH, Shin MS, Park WS, Kim SY, Dong SM, Lee HK, Park JY, Oh RR, Jang JJ, Lee JY, Yoo NJ. Immunohistochemical analysis of Fas ligand expression in normal human tissues. *APMIS.* 1999;107(11):1013-9.

[160] Lee SH, Shin MS, Kim HS, Lee HK, Park WS, Kim SY, Lee JH, Han SY, Park JY, Oh RR, Jang JJ, Han JY, Lee JY, Yoo NJ. Alterations of the DR5/TRAIL receptor 2 gene in non-small cell lung cancers. *Cancer Res.* 1999;59(22):5683-6.

[161] Owen-Schaub LB, van Golen KL, Hill LL, Price JE. Fas and Fas ligand interactions suppress melanoma lung metastasis. *J Exp Med.* 1998;188(9):1717-23.

[162] Lee SH, Shin MS, Park WS, Kim SY, Kim HS, Lee JH, Han SY, Lee HK, Park JY, Oh RR, Jang JJ, Lee JY, Yoo NJ. Immunohistochemical localization of FAP-1, an inhibitor of Fas-mediated apoptosis, in normal and neoplastic human tissues. *APMIS.* 1999;107(12):1101-8.

[163] Boise LH, Gottschalk AR, Quintans J, Thompson CB. Bcl-2 and Bcl-2-related proteins in apoptosis regulation. *Curr Top Microbiol Immunol.* 1995;200:107-21.

[164] Lee SH, Shin MS, Lee HS, Bae JH, Lee HK, Kim HS, Kim SY, Jang JJ, Joo M, Kang YK, Park WS, Park JY, Oh RR, Han SY, Lee JH, Kim SH, Lee JY, Yoo NJ. Expression of Fas and Fas-related molecules in human hepatocellular carcinoma. *Hum Pathol.* 2001;32(3):250-6

[165] Powell WC, Fingleton B, Wilson CL, Boothby M, Matrisian LM. The metalloproteinase matrilysin proteolytically generates active soluble Fas ligand and potentiates epithelial cell apoptosis. *Curr Biol.* 1999;9(24):1441-7.

[166] Mitsiades N, Yu WH, Poulaki V, Tsokos M, Stamenkovic I. Matrix metalloproteinase-7-mediated cleavage of Fas ligand protects tumor cells from chemotherapeutic drug cytotoxicity. *Cancer Res.* 2001;61(2):577-81.

[167] Yu WH, Woessner JF Jr, McNeish JD, Stamenkovic I. CD44 anchors the assembly of matrilysin/MMP-7 with heparin-binding epidermal growth factor precursor and ErbB4 and regulates female reproductive organ remodeling. *Genes Dev.* 2002;16(3):307-23.

[168] Witty JP, Lempka T, Coffey RJ Jr, Matrisian LM. Decreased tumor formation in 7,12-dimethylbenzanthracene-treated stromelysin-1 transgenic mice is associated with alterations in mammary epithelial cell apoptosis. *Cancer Res.* 1995;55(7):1401-6.

[169] Alexander CM, Howard EW, Bissell MJ, Werb Z. Rescue of mammary epithelial cell apoptosis and entactin degradation by a tissue inhibitor of metalloproteinases-1 transgene. *J Cell Biol.* 1996;135(6 Pt 1):1669-77.

[170] Vu TH, Shipley JM, Bergers G, Berger JE, Helms JA, Hanahan D, Shapiro SD, Senior RM, Werb Z. MMP-9/gelatinase B is a key regulator of growth plate angiogenesis and apoptosis of hypertrophic chondrocytes. *Cell.* 1998;93(3):411-22.

[171] Wu E, Mari BP, Wang F, Anderson IC, Sunday ME, Shipp MA. Stromelysin-3 suppresses tumor cell apoptosis in a murine model. *J Cell Biochem.* 2001;82(4):549-55.

[172] Boulay A, Masson R, Chenard MP, El Fahime M, Cassard L, Bellocq JP, Sautes-Fridman C, Basset P, Rio MC. High cancer cell death in syngeneic tumors developed in host mice deficient for the stromelysin-3 matrix metalloproteinase. *Cancer Res.* 2001;61(5):2189-93.

[173] LeRoith D, Roberts CT Jr. The insulin-like growth factor system and cancer. *Cancer Lett.* 2003;195(2):127-37.

[174] Manes S, Mira E, Barbacid MM, Cipres A, Fernandez-Resa P, Buesa JM, Merida I, Aracil M, Marquez G, Martinez-A C. Identification of insulin-like growth factor-binding protein-1 as a potential physiological substrate for human stromelysin-3. *J Biol Chem.* 1997;272(41):25706-12.

[175] Ishizuya-Oka A, Li Q, Amano T, Damjanovski S, Ueda S, Shi YB. Requirement for matrix metalloproteinase stromelysin-3 in cell migration and apoptosis during tissue remodeling in Xenopus laevis. *J Cell Biol.* 2000;150(5):1177-88.

[176] Ahonen M, Baker AH, Kahari VM. Adenovirus-mediated gene delivery of tissue inhibitor of metalloproteinases-3 inhibits invasion and induces apoptosis in melanoma cells. *Cancer Res.* 1998 ;58(11):2310-5.

[177] Baker AH, George SJ, Zaltsman AB, Murphy G, Newby AC. Inhibition of invasion and induction of apoptotic cell death of cancer cell lines by overexpression of TIMP-3. *Br J Cancer.* 1999;79(9-10):1347-55.

[178] Fata JE, Leco KJ, Voura EB, Yu HY, Waterhouse P, Murphy G, Moorehead RA, Khokha R. Accelerated apoptosis in the Timp-3-deficient mammary gland. *J Clin Invest.* 2001;108(6):831-41.

[179] Ahonen M, Poukkula M, Baker AH, Kashiwagi M, Nagase H, Eriksson JE, Kahari VM. Tissue inhibitor of metalloproteinases-3 induces apoptosis in melanoma cells by stabilization of death receptors. *Oncogene*. 2003;22(14):2121-34.

[180] Swinson DE, Jones JL, Richardson D, Cox G, Edwards JG, O'Byrne KJ. Tumour necrosis is an independent prognostic marker in non-small cell lung cancer: correlation with biological variables. *Lung Cancer*. 2002;37(3):235-40.

[181] Suzuki M, Iizasa T, Fujisawa T, Baba M, Yamaguchi Y, Kimura H, Suzuki H. Expression of matrix metalloproteinases and tissue inhibitor of matrix metalloproteinases in non-small-cell lung cancer. *Invasion Metastasis*. 1998;18(3):134-41.

[182] Pritchard SC, Nicolson MC, Lloret C, McKay JA, Ross VG, Kerr KM, Murray GI, McLeod HL. Expression of matrix metalloproteinases 1, 2, 9 and their tissue inhibitors in stage II non-small cell lung cancer: implications for MMP inhibition therapy. *Oncol Rep*. 2001;8(2):421-4.

[183] Brown PD, Bloxidge RE, Anderson E, Howell A. Expression of activated gelatinase in human invasive breast carcinoma. *Clin Exp Metastasis*. 1993;11(2):183-9.

[184] Brown PD, Bloxidge RE, Stuart NS, Gatter KC, Carmichael J. Association between expression of activated 72-kilodalton gelatinase and tumor spread in non-small-cell lung carcinoma. *J Natl Cancer Inst*. 1993;85(7):574-8.

[185] Reichenberger F, Eickelberg O, Wyser C, Perruchoud AP, Roth M, Tamm M. Distinct endobronchial expression of matrix-metalloproteinases (MMP) and their endogenous inhibitors in lung cancer. *Swiss Med Wkly*. 2001;131(19-20):273-9.

[186] Hrabec E, Strek M, Nowak D, Greger J, Suwalski M, Hrabec Z. Activity of type IV collagenases (MMP-2 and MMP-9) in primary pulmonary carcinomas: a quantitative analysis. *J Cancer Res Clin Oncol*. 2002;128(4):197-204.

[187] Kodate M, Kasai T, Hashimoto H, Yasumoto K, Iwata Y, Manabe H. Expression of matrix metalloproteinase (gelatinase) in T1 adenocarcinoma of the lung. *Pathol Int*. 1997;47(7):461-9.

[188] Zhang Y, Thant AA, Machida K, Ichigotani Y, Naito Y, Hiraiwa Y, Senga T, Sohara Y, Matsuda S, Hamaguchi M. Hyaluronan-CD44s signaling regulates matrix metalloproteinase-2 secretion in a human lung carcinoma cell line QG90. *Cancer Res*. 2002;62(14):3962-5.

[189] Talvensaari-Mattila A, Paakko P, Hoyhtya M, Blanco-Sequeiros G, Turpeenniemi-Hujanen T. Matrix metalloproteinase-2 immunoreactive protein: a marker of aggressiveness in breast carcinoma. *Cancer*. 1998;83(6):1153-62.

[190] Vaisanen A, Kallioinen M, Taskinen PJ, Turpeenniemi-Hujanen T. Prognostic value of MMP-2 immunoreactive protein (72 kD type IV collagenase) in primary skin melanoma. *J Pathol*. 1998;186(1):51-8.

[191] Passlick B, Sienel W, Seen-Hibler R, Wockel W, Thetter O, Mutschler W, Pantel K. Overexpression of matrix metalloproteinase 2 predicts unfavorable outcome in early-stage non-small cell lung cancer. *Clin Cancer Res*. 2000;6(10):3944-8.

[192] Cai M, Onoda K, Takao M, Kyoko IY, Shimpo H, Yoshida T, Yada I. Degradation of tenascin-C and activity of matrix metalloproteinase-2 are associated with tumor

recurrence in early stage non-small cell lung cancer. *Clin Cancer Res.* 2002;8(4):1152-6.

[193] Yamamura T, Nakanishi K, Hiroi S, Kumaki F, Sato H, Aida S, Kawai T. Expression of membrane-type-1-matrix metalloproteinase and metalloproteinase-2 in nonsmall cell lung carcinomas. *Lung Cancer.* 2002;35(3):249-55.

[194] Fujita T, Matsui M, Takaku K, Uetake H, Ichikawa W, Taketo MM, Sugihara K. Size- and invasion-dependent increase in cyclooxygenase 2 levels in human colorectal carcinomas. *Cancer Res.* 1998;58(21):4823-6.

[195] Murata H, Kawano S, Tsuji S, Tsuji M, Sawaoka H, Kimura Y, Shiozaki H, Hori M. Cyclooxygenase-2 overexpression enhances lymphatic invasion and metastasis in human gastric carcinoma. *Am J Gastroenterol.* 1999;94(2):451-5

[196] Takahashi Y, Kawahara F, Noguchi M, Miwa K, Sato H, Seiki M, Inoue H, Tanabe T, Yoshimoto T. Activation of matrix metalloproteinase-2 in human breast cancer cells overexpressing cyclooxygenase-1 or -2. *FEBS Lett.* 1999;460(1):145-8.

[197] Callejas NA, Casado M, Diaz-Guerra MJ, Bosca L, Martin-Sanz P. Expression of cyclooxygenase-2 promotes the release of matrix metalloproteinase-2 and -9 in fetal rat hepatocytes. *Hepatology.* 2001;33(4):860-7.

[198] Tsujii M, Kawano S, DuBois RN. Cyclooxygenase-2 expression in human colon cancer cells increases metastatic potential. *Proc Natl Acad Sci U S A.* 1997;94(7):3336-40.

[199] Pan MR, Chuang LY, Hung WC. Non-steroidal anti-inflammatory drugs inhibit matrix metalloproteinase-2 expression via repression of transcription in lung cancer cells. *FEBS Lett.* 2001;508(3):365-8.

[200] Dohadwala M, Batra RK, Luo J, Lin Y, Krysan K, Pold M, Sharma S, Dubinett SM. Autocrine/paracrine prostaglandin E2 production by non-small cell lung cancer cells regulates matrix metalloproteinase-2 and CD44 in cyclooxygenase-2-dependent invasion. *J Biol Chem.* 2002;277(52):50828-33.

[201] Shishodia S, Potdar P, Gairola CG, Aggarwal BB. Curcumin (diferuloylmethane) down-regulates cigarette smoke-induced NF-kappaB activation through inhibition of IkappaBalpha kinase in human lung epithelial cells: correlation with suppression of COX-2, MMP-9 and cyclin D1. *Carcinogenesis.* 2003;24(7):1269-79.

[202] Itoh T, Tanioka M, Matsuda H, Nishimoto H, Yoshioka T, Suzuki R, Uehira M. Experimental metastasis is suppressed in MMP-9-deficient mice. *Clin Exp Metastasis.* 1999;17(2):177-81.

[203] Ylisirnio S, Hoyhtya M, Turpeenniemi-Hujanen T. Serum matrix metalloproteinases -2, -9 and tissue inhibitors of metalloproteinases -1, -2 in lung cancer--TIMP-1 as a prognostic marker. *AntiCancer Res.* 2000;20(2B):1311-6.

[204] Iizasa T, Fujisawa T, Suzuki M, Motohashi S, Yasufuku K, Yasukawa T, Baba M, Shiba M. Elevated levels of circulating plasma matrix metalloproteinase 9 in non-small cell lung cancer patients. *Clin Cancer Res.* 1999;5(1):149-53.

[205] Laack E, Kohler A, Kugler C, Dierlamm T, Knuffmann C, Vohwinkel G, Niestroy A, Dahlmann N, Peters A, Berger J, Fiedler W, Hossfeld DK. Pretreatment serum levels of matrix metalloproteinase-9 and vascular endothelial growth factor in non-small-cell lung cancer. *Ann Oncol.* 2002;13(10):1550-7.

[206] Cox G, Louise Jones J, Andi A, Abrams KR, O'Byrne KJ. Bcl-2 is an independent prognostic factor and adds to a biological model for predicting outcome in operable non-small cell lung cancer. *Lung Cancer*. 2001;34(3):417-26.

[207] Hrabec E, Strek M, Nowak D, Hrabec Z. Elevated level of circulating matrix metalloproteinase-9 in patients with lung cancer. *Respir Med.* 2001;95(1):1-4.

[208] Fujise N, Nanashim A, Taniguchi Y, Matsuo S, Hatano K, Matsumoto Y, Tagawa Y, Ayabe H. Prognostic impact of cathepsin B and matrix metalloproteinase-9 in pulmonary adenocarcinomas by immunohistochemical study. *Lung Cancer.* 2000;27(1):19-26.

[209] Murray GI, Duncan ME, O'Neil P, Melvin WT, Fothergill JE. Matrix metalloproteinase-1 is associated with poor prognosis in colorectal cancer. *Nat Med.* 1996;2(4):461-2.

[210] Murray GI, Duncan ME, O'Neil P, McKay JA, Melvin WT, Fothergill JE. Matrix metalloproteinase-1 is associated with poor prognosis in oesophageal cancer. *J Pathol.* 1998;185(3):256-61.

[211] Thomas P, Khokha R, Shepherd FA, Feld R, Tsao MS. Differential expression of matrix metalloproteinases and their inhibitors in non-small cell lung cancer. *J Pathol.* 2000;190(2):150-6.

[212] Zhu Y, Spitz MR, Lei L, Mills GB, Wu X. A single nucleotide polymorphism in the matrix metalloproteinase-1 promoter enhances lung cancer susceptibility. *Cancer Res.* 2001;61(21):7825-9.

[213] Delebecq TJ, Porte H, Zerimech F, Copin MC, Gouyer V, Dacquembronne E, Balduyck M, Wurtz A, Huet G. Overexpression level of stromelysin 3 is related to the lymph node involvement in non-small cell lung cancer. *Clin Cancer Res.* 2000;6(3):1086-92.

[214] Fong KM, Kida Y, Zimmerman PV, Smith PJ. TIMP1 and adverse prognosis in non-small cell lung cancer. *Clin Cancer Res.* 1996;2(8):1369-72.

[215] Michael M, Babic B, Khokha R, Tsao M, Ho J, Pintilie M, Leco K, Chamberlain D, Shepherd FA. Expression and prognostic significance of metalloproteinases and their tissue inhibitors in patients with small-cell lung cancer. *J Clin Oncol.* 1999;17(6):1802-8.

[216] Zhang Y, Thant AA, Hiraiwa Y, Naito Y, Sein TT, Sohara Y, Matsuda S, Hamaguchi M. A role for focal adhesion kinase in hyluronan-dependent MMP-2 secretion in a human small-cell lung carcinoma cell line, QG90. *Biochem Biophys Res Commun.* 2002;290(3):1123-7.

[217] Ginsberg RJ, Rubinstein LV. Randomized trial of lobotomy versus limited resection for T_1N_0 non-small cell lung cancer. Lung Cancer Study Group. *Ann Thorac Surg.* 1995;60: 615-22.

[218] Mountain CF. Revisions in the International System for Staging Lung Cancer. *Chest.* 1997;111: 1710-17.

[219] Hidalgo M, Eckhardt SG. Development of matrix metalloproteinase inhibitors in cancer therapy. *J Natl Cancer Inst.* 2001;93(3):178-93.

[220] Beattie GJ, Smyth JF. Phase I study of intraperitoneal metalloproteinase inhibitor BB94 in patients with malignant ascites. *Clin Cancer Res.* 1998;4(8):1899-902.

[221] Macaulay VM, O'Byrne KJ, Saunders MP, Braybrooke JP, Long L, Gleeson F, Mason CS, Harris AL, Brown P, Talbot DC. Phase I study of intrapleural batimastat (BB-94), a matrix metalloproteinase inhibitor, in the treatment of malignant pleural effusions. *Clin Cancer Res.* 1999;5(3):513-20.

[222] Kruger A, Soeltl R, Sopov I, Kopitz C, Arlt M, Magdolen V, Harbeck N, Gansbacher B, Schmitt M. Hydroxamate-type matrix metalloproteinase inhibitor batimastat promotes liver metastasis. *Cancer Res.* 2001;61(4):1272-5.

[223] Wojtowicz-Praga SM, Dickson RB, Hawkins MJ. Matrix metalloproteinase inhibitors. *Invest New Drugs*. 1997;15(1):61-75.

[224] Wojtowicz-Praga S, Torri J, Johnson M, Steen V, Marshall J, Ness E, Dickson R, Sale M, Rasmussen HS, Chiodo TA, Hawkins MJ. Phase I trial of Marimastat, a novel matrix metalloproteinase inhibitor, administered orally to patients with advanced lung cancer. *J Clin Oncol.* 1998;16(6):2150-6.

[225] Tierney GM, Griffin NR, Stuart RC, Kasem H, Lynch KP, Lury JT, Brown PD, Millar AW, Steele RJ, Parsons SL. A pilot study of the safety and effects of the matrix metalloproteinase inhibitor marimastat in gastric cancer. *Eur J Cancer.* 1999;35(4):563-8.

[226] Primrose JN, Bleiberg H, Daniel F, Van Belle S, Mansi JL, Seymour M, Johnson PW, Neoptolemos JP, Baillet M, Barker K, Berrington A, Brown PD, Millar AW, Lynch KP. Marimastat in recurrent colorectal cancer: exploratory evaluation of biological activity by measurement of carcinoembryonic antigen. *Br J Cancer.* 1999;79(3-4):509-14.

[227] Rosemurgy A, Harris J, Langleben A, Casper E, Goode S, Rasmussen H. Marimastat in patients with advanced pancreatic cancer: a dose-finding study. *Am J Clin Oncol.* 1999;22(3):247-52.

[228] Miller KD, Gradishar W, Schuchter L, Sparano JA, Cobleigh M, Robert N, Rasmussen H, Sledge GW. A randomized phase II pilot trial of adjuvant marimastat in patients with early-stage breast cancer. *Ann Oncol.* 2002;13(8):1220-4.

[229] Shepherd FA, Giaccone G, Seymour L, Debruyne C, Bezjak A, Hirsh V, Smylie M, Rubin S, Martins H, Lamont A, Krzakowski M, Sadura A, Zee B. Prospective, randomized, double-blind, placebo-controlled trial of marimastat after response to first-line chemotherapy in patients with small-cell lung cancer: a trial of the National Cancer Institute of Canada-Clinical Trials Group and the European Organization for Research and Treatment of Cancer. *J Clin Oncol.* 2002;20(22):4434-9.

[230] Shepherd FA, Sridhar SS. Angiogenesis inhibitors under study for the treatment of lung cancer. *Lung Cancer.* 2003;41 Suppl 1:S63-72.

[231] Bramhall SR, Rosemurgy A, Brown PD, Bowry C, Buckels JA; Marimastat Pancreatic Cancer Study Group. Marimastat as first-line therapy for patients with unresectable pancreatic cancer: a randomized trial. *J Clin Oncol.* 2001;19(15):3447-55.

[232] British Biotech. *Results of marimastat Study 186 in patients with advanced ovarian cancer.* Press release, 2000;September 26.

[233] Phuphanich S, Levin VA, Yung WK, Forsyth P, Maestro R, Perry J, et al. A multicenter, randomized, double-blind, placebo controlled trials of marimastat in

patients with ganglioma multiforme of gliosarcama following completion of conventional, first-line treatment. *Proc ASCO*. 2001;20:52a (abstract 205).

[234] Bramhall SR, Hallissey MT, Whiting J, Scholefield J, Tierney G, Stuart RC, Hawkins RE, McCulloch P, Maughan T, Brown PD, Baillet M, Fielding JW. Marimastat as maintenance therapy for patients with advanced gastric cancer: a randomised trial. *Br J Cancer*. 2002;86(12):1864-70.

[235] British Biotech. *Marimastat update*. Press release, 2001; May 2.

[236] Naglich JG, Jure-Kunkel M, Gupta E, Fargnoli J, Henderson AJ, Lewin AC, Talbott R, Baxter A, Bird J, Savopoulos R, Wills R, Kramer RA, Trail PA. Inhibition of angiogenesis and metastasis in two murine models by the matrix metalloproteinase inhibitor, BMS-275291. *Cancer Res*. 2001;61(23):8480-5.

[237] Douillard J, Petersen V, Shepherd F, Paz-Ares L, Arnold A, Tonato M, Ottaway J, Davis M, Van Vreckem A, Humphrey J, Seymour L. Randomized phase II study of BMS-275291 versus placebo in patients with stage IIIB or IV non-small cell lung cancer receiving paclitaxel + carboplatin (PC): National Cancer Institute of Canada Clinical Trials Group (NCIC CTG) br. 18. *Eur J Cancer*. 2001;37:S19-20. (abstract 63)

[238] Poulaki V. BMS-275291 Bristol-Myers Squibb. *Curr Opin Investig Drugs*. 2002;3(3):500-4.

[239] Shinoda K, Shibuya M, Hibino S, Ono Y, Matsuda K, Takemura A, Zou D, Kokubo Y, Takechi A, Kudoh S. A novel matrix metalloproteinase inhibitor, FYK-1388 suppresses tumor growth, metastasis and angiogenesis by human fibrosarcoma cell line. *Int J Oncol*. 2003;22(2):281-8.

[240] Press release, *Arriva*, 12 Feb 2001.

[241] Trifilieff A, Walker C, Keller T, Kottirsch G, Neumann U. Pharmacological profile of PKF242-484 and PKF241-466, novel dual inhibitors of TNF-alpha converting enzyme and matrix metalloproteinases, in models of airway inflammation. *Br J Pharmacol*. 2002;135(7):1655-64.

[242] Smylie M, Mercier R, Aboulafia D, Tucker R, Bonomi P, Collier M, et al. Phase III study of the matrix metalloproteinase (MMP) inhibitor prinomastat in patients having advanced non-small cell lung carcinoma. *Proc ASCO*. 2001;20:307a. (abstract 1226)

[243] Bissett D, Bissett D, von Pawel J, Mercier R, Prince A, Nicolson M, Shephherd F, Mazabel E, Penning C, Zhang MH, Collier MA. Phase III study of the matrix metalloproteinase (MMP) inhibitor prinomastat (P) in combination with gemcitibine (G) and cisplatin (C) in non-small cell lung carcinoma (NSCLS). *Proc ASCO*.2002;21:296a. (abstract 1183)

[244] Hibner B, Bull C, Flynn C, Eberwein D, Garrison T, Casazza A, Carter C, Gibson N. Activity of the matrix metalloproteinase inhibitor BAY 12-9566 against murine subcutaneous and metastatic in vivo models. *Ann Oncol*. 1998;9 (Suppl. 2): 75.

[245] Brubaker WF, Perrino P, Wu Y, Jaworski S, Town C, Jones L, Ward D, Chien DS. Pharmacokinetics of BAY 12-9566 in animals: species comparison. *Proc Am Assoc Cancer Res*. 1999;40:391.

[246] Flynn C, Bull C, Eberwein D, Matherne C, Hibner B. Anti-metastatic activity of BAY 12-9566 in human colon carcinoma HCT116 orthotopic model. *Proc Am Assoc Cancer Res*. 1998;39: 30.

[247] Nozaki S, Sissons S, Casazza AM, Sledge GW. Inhibition of human breast cancer regrowth and pulmonary metastases by BAY 12-9566 in athymic mice. *Proc Am Assoc Cancer Res.* 1998;39:301.

[248] Gatto C, Rieppi M, Borsotti P, Innocenti S, Ceruti R, Drudis T, Scanziani E, Casazza AM, Taraboletti G, Giavazzi R. BAY 12-9566, a novel inhibitor of matrix metalloproteinases with antiangiogenic activity. *Clin Cancer Res.* 1999;5(11):3603-7.

[249] Rowinsky EK, Humphrey R, Hammond LA, Aylesworth C, Smetzer L, Hidalgo M, Morrow M, Smith L, Garner A, Sorensen JM, Von Hoff DD, Eckhardt SG. Phase I and pharmacologic study of the specific matrix metalloproteinase inhibitor BAY 12-9566 on a protracted oral daily dosing schedule in patients with solid malignancies. *J Clin Oncol.* 2000;18(1):178-86.

[250] Erlichman C, Adjei AA, Alberts SR, Sloan JA, Goldberg RM, Pitot HC, Rubin J, Atherton PJ, Klee GG, Humphrey R. Phase I study of the matrix metalloproteinase inhibitor, BAY 12-9566. *Ann Oncol.* 2001;12(3):389-95.

[251] Goel R, Hirte H, Major P, Waterfield B, Holohan S, Bennett K, Elias I, Seymour L. Clinical pharmacology of the metalloproteinase (MMP) and angiogenesis inhibitor Bayer 12-9566 in cancer patients. *Proc Am Soc Clin Oncol.* 1999;18:160a.

[252] Moore MJ, Hamm J, Eisenberg P et al. A comparison between gencitabine (GEM) and the matrix metalloproteinase (MMP) inhibitor BAY12-9566 in patients with advanced pancreatic cancer. *Proc ASCO.*2000;19: 240a. (abstract 930).

[253] Press release, *Bayer* 30. Sep. 2003.

[254] Yamamoto A, Yano S, Shiraga M, Ogawa H, Goto H, Miki T, Zhang H, Sone S. A third-generation matrix metalloproteinase (MMP) inhibitor (ONO-4817) combined with docetaxel suppresses progression of lung micrometastasis of MMP-expressing tumor cells in nude mice. *Int J Cancer.* 2003;103(6):822-8.

[255] Sawa M, Kiyoi T, Kurokawa K, Kumihara H, Yamamoto M, Miyasaka T, Ito Y, Hirayama R, Inoue T, Kirii Y, Nishiwaki E, Ohmoto H, Maeda Y, Ishibushi E, Inoue Y, Yoshino K, Kondo H. New type of metalloproteinase inhibitor: design and synthesis of new phosphonamide-based hydroxamic acids. *J Med Chem.* 2002;45(4):919-29.

[256] Sawa M, Tsukamoto T, Kiyoi T, Kurokawa K, Nakajima F, Nakada Y, Yokota K, Inoue Y, Kondo H, Yoshino K. New strategy for antedrug application: development of metalloproteinase inhibitors as antipsoriatic drugs. *J Med Chem.* 2002;45(4):930-6.

[257] Phosphonamide-based metalloproteinase inhibitors: a new approach to the development of safer metalloproteinase inhibitors. *Curr Med Chem anti-inflammatory and anti-allergy agents.* 2003;2: in print.

[258] Villamil CI, Becker DP, Barta TE, Bedell LJ, Talley JJ, Hockerman SL, Munie GE, Boyce SY, et al. Design and synthesis of MMP-13 selective alpha-sulphone hydroxamates. *224th ACS (Boston)*, 2002, MEDI 309.

[259] Villamil CI, Barta TE, Becker DP, Bedell LJ, DeCrescenzo G, Freskos JN, et al. Design and synthesis of 4,4-disubstituted piperidine alpha-sulphone hydroxamates as potent and selective MMP inhibitors: The discovery of SC-77964. *222nd ACS (Chicago),* 2001, MEDI 258.

[260] Shionogi & Co., Ltd *Annual report* 2003.

[261] Gingras D, Renaud A, Mousseau N, Beaulieu E, Kachra Z, Beliveau R. Matrix proteinase inhibition by AE-941, a multifunctional antiangiogenic compound. *AntiCancer Res.* 2001;21(1A):145-55.

[262] Dupont E, Falardeau P, Mousa SA, Dimitriadou V, Pepin MC, Wang T, Alaoui-Jamali MA. Antiangiogenic and antimetastatic properties of Neovastat (AE-941), an orally active extract derived from cartilage tissue. *Clin Exp Metastasis.* 2002;19(2):145-53.

[263] Beliveau R, Gingras D, Kruger EA, Lamy S, Sirois P, Simard B, Sirois MG, Tranqui L, Baffert F, Beaulieu E, Dimitriadou V, Pepin MC, Courjal F, Ricard I, Poyet P, Falardeau P, Figg WD, Dupont E. The antiangiogenic agent neovastat (AE-941) inhibits vascular endothelial growth factor-mediated biological effects. *Clin Cancer Res.* 2002;8(4):1242-50.

[264] Boivin D, Gendron S, Beaulieu E, Gingras D, Beliveau R. The antiangiogenic agent Neovastat (AE-941) induces endothelial cell apoptosis. *Mol Cancer Ther.* 2002;1(10):795-802.

[265] Weber MH, Lee J, Orr FW. The effect of Neovastat (AE-941) on an experimental metastatic bone tumor model. *Int J Oncol.* 2002;20(2):299-303.

[266] Gingras D, Boivin D, Deckers C, Gendron S, Barthomeuf C, Beliveau R. Neovastat-a novel antiangiogenic drug for cancer therapy. *Anticancer Drugs.* 2003;14(2):91-6.

[267] Falardeau P, Champagne P, Poyet P, Hariton C, Dupont E.. Neovastat, a naturally occurring multifunctional antiangiogenic drug, in phase III clinical trials. *Semin Oncol.* 2001;28(6):620-5.

[268] Gingras D, Batist G, Beliveau R. AE-941 (Neovastat): a novel multifunctional antiangiogenic compound. *Expert Rev Anticancer Ther.* 2001;1(3):341-7.

[269] Golub LM, Lee HM, Lehrer G, Nemiroff A, McNamara TF, Kaplan R, Ramamurthy NS. Minocycline reduces gingival collagenolytic activity during diabetes: preliminary observations and a proposed new mechanism of action. *J Periodontal Res.* 1983;18(5):516-26.

[270] Greenwald RA, Golub LM. Biologic Properties of Non-Antibiotic, Chemically Modified Tetracyclines (CMTs): A Structured, Annotated Bibliography. *Curr Med Chem.* 2001;8(3):305-16.

[271] Lokeshwar BL, Selzer MG, Zhu BQ, Block NL, Golub LM. Inhibition of cell proliferation, invasion, tumor growth and metastasis by an oral non-antimicrobial tetracycline analog (COL-3) in a metastatic prostate cancer model. *Int J Cancer.* 2002;98(2):297-309.

[272] Gu Y, Lee HM, Roemer EJ, Musacchia L, Golub LM, Simon SR. Inhibition of tumor cell invasiveness by chemically modified tetracyclines. *Curr Med Chem.* 2001;8(3):261-70.

[273] Seftor RE, Seftor EA, De Larco JE, Kleiner DE, Leferson J, Stetler-Stevenson WG, McNamara TF, Golub LM, Hendrix MJ. Chemically modified tetracyclines inhibit human melanoma cell invasion and metastasis. *Clin Exp Metastasis.* 1998;16(3):217-25.

[274] Lush RM, Rudek MA, Figg WD. Review of Three New Agents That Target Angiogenesis, Matrix Metalloproteinases, and Cyclin-Dependent Kinases. *Cancer Control.* 1999;6(5):459-465.

[275] Rudek MA, Figg WD, Dyer V, Dahut W, Turner ML, Steinberg SM, Liewehr DJ, Kohler DR, Pluda JM, Reed E. Phase I clinical trial of oral COL-3, a matrix metalloproteinase inhibitor, in patients with refractory metastatic cancer. *J Clin Oncol.* 2001;19(2):584-92.
[276] Ghate JV, Turner ML, Rudek MA, Figg WD, Dahut W, Dyer V, Pluda JM, Reed E. Drug-induced lupus associated with COL-3: report of 3 cases. *Arch Dermatol.* 2001;137(4):471-4.
[277] Rudek MA, Horne M, Figg WD, Dahut W, Dyer V, Pluda JM, Reed E. Reversible sideroblastic anemia associated with the tetracycline analogue COL-3. *Am J Hematol.* 2001;67(1):51-3.
[278] Press release, *CollaGenex Pharmaceuticals, Inc.*, 7 March 2002.

In: Focus on Lung Cancer Research
Editor: Robert L. Carafaro, pp. 121-159

ISBN 1-59454-082-9

Chapter IV

NON-SMALL CELL LUNG CANCER AND ANGIOGENESIS

P. Sardari Nia and P. Van Schil
Department of Thoracic and Vascular Surgery
University Hospital of Antwerp
Edegem, Belgium
e-mail : paul.van.schil@uza.be

ABSTRACT

In the last few decades cancer research has generated an enormous amount of information regarding the molecular biologic processes that take place in cancer tissue, one of which is the formation of new blood vessels, angiogenesis. More than 100 papers have been published so far, studying various components of angiogenesis and their relation to lung cancer. Many anti-angiogenic agents have been tested or are currently evaluated in clinical trials. However, the results are inconclusive or disappointing and clinical practice has not been altered to a great extent. The hypothesis that tumor growth is obligatory dependent on angiogenesis, which prevailed for many years, has been challenged with the description of nonangiogenic growth. An essential prerequisite for nonangogenic growth appears to be the ability of the tumor to preserve the parenchymal structures of the host tissue. This morphologic feature, growth pattern, is visible on a routine tissue section and is a surrogate marker of angiogenesis. Heterogeneity of the patient population with regards to the angiogenic dependency of the individual tumors might be responsible for the failure of some anti-angiogenic trials. Pre-treatment patient selection based on these growth patterns might therefore be useful. This chapter reviews the existing literature in the field of angiogenesis and lung cancer and provides a new model based on recent publications.

ABBREVIATIONS

aMVD	activated Microvessel Density
Ang-1 and –2	Angiopoietin-1 and –2
ARNT	Aryl Hydrocarbon Receptor Nuclear Translocator
bFGF	basic Fibroblast Growth Factor
bFGF-BP	basic Fibroblast Growth Factor Binding Protein
CA9	Carbonic Anhydrase 9
COX	Cyclooxygenase
ECM	Extracellular Matrix
ECS	single Endothelial Cell Score
EGFR	Epidermal Growth Factor Receptor
ECOG	Eastern Cooperative Oncology Group
EORTC	European Organization for the Research and Treatment of Cancer
FGF	Fibroblast Growth Factor
GLUT1 and 3	Glucose Transporter-1 and –3
HIF	Hypoxia-Inducible Factor
HB-GAM	Heparin-Binding-Growth-Associated Molecule
HGF	Hepatocyte Growth Factor
hMVD	hot spot Microvessel Density
HREs	Hypoxia Response Elements
ICAM	Intercellular Adhesion Molecule
Id1/Id3	Inhibitors of differentiation 1 and 3
IFN	Interferon
IL	Interleukin
IP-10	Interferon-gamma inducible Protein-10
MCP-1	Monocyte Chemoattractant Protein-1
Meth-1 and –2	Methamphetamine
MMP	Matrix Metalloproteinase
MT-1-MMP	Membrane Type 1 Matrix Metalloproteinase
MVD	Microvessel Density
NCIC-CTG	National Cancer Institute of Canada-Clinical Trials Group
NOS	Nitric Oxide Synthase
NSCLC	Non-Small Cell Lung Cancer
PAI-1	Plasminogen Activator Inhibitor-1
PDECGF	Platelet-Derived Endothelial Cell Growth Factor
PDGFR	Platelet-Derived Growth Factor Receptor
P1GF	Placenta Growth Factor
RCCC	Renal Clear Cell Carcinoma
SCLC	Small Cell Lung Cancer
SPARC	Secreted Protein Acidic and Rich in Cystein
TF	Tissue Factor
TIMP	Tissue Inhibitor of Metalloproteinase
TGF-α	Transfoming Growth Factor-α
TP	Thymidine Phosphorylase
TSP-1 and –2	Thrombospondin-1 and -2
uPAR	urokinase Plasminogen Activator Receptor
VEGF	Vascular Endothelial Growth Factor
VEGFR	Vascular Endothelial Growth Factor Receptor
VEGI	Vascular Endothelial Growth Inhibitor
VHL	Von Hippel-Lindau

1. Introduction

Over the last decades cancer research has generated an enormous amount of information adding further complexity to the scientific literature. Despite the enormous wealth of scientific literature, the translation of knowledge to clinical practice has been limited.

There are some conceptional problems in the current scientific methodology, which govern the final understanding of a complex phenomenon like cancer. First, it must be emphasized that science has always been reductionistic in essence, reducing and analyzing the composing elements of a specific system, forgetting that the interrelation between a set of simple determinants creates a new dimension of characteristics and functions. This is inherent to every system, from quantum physics and cosmology to cancer. In cancer biology the cancer cell, and some of its specific characteristics like its proliferative capacity, have long been the focuses of all of our attention. This view is translated to existing treatment modalities, like chemotherapy and radiotherapy, which target these specific characteristics.

The last decades have been characterized by a move in cancer research from a reductionistic approach focusing mainly on the cancer cell itself to a greater appreciation of the importance of interactions between cancer cells and stroma. This has resulted in much new information concerning molecular-biological processes that take place in stroma, one of which is the formation of new blood vessels, angiogenesis.

Although there is now a greater focus on processes that take place in cancer tissue, the principal analysis is still reductionistic. The interrelation of different processes remains unexplored. New processes are analyzed in more depth, loosing the view of the whole picture. More than three decades, the process of angiogenesis has been the subject of extensive studies, but angiogenesis-inhibitors which are being tested in different clinical trials, have failed to show a substantial improvement in survival.

The second problem that has been ignored is heterogeneity. This heterogeneity exists at different levels. Only by viewing the scientific literature one can see that, at a patient level, every possible clinical characteristic can contribute to the overall prognosis.

If we consider surgically resected human tumor sections, the existing literature reveals heterogeneity of every existing parameter besides the classical parameters like histiotype and grading. Moreover, there are also differences at the level of dynamic parameters like growth kinetics, which have not yet been the subjects of extensive studies.

This heterogeneity is important since the differences in biological properties determine the response to a specific treatment modality and the clinical outcome of our patients. The effectiveness of selective therapies, like anti-angiogenic therapy, is determined by our exact knowledge of the biological profile of the targeted tissue, for example angiogenic profile.

The existing animal models in which a new molecule is tested use a malignant, fast growing tumor with homogeneous characteristics in growth kinetics and biological behavior. The failure in clinical practice is then the result of the existing heterogeneity in the human that is not addressed in animal models.

The third problem that results from the latter, is the lack of integrating parameters. The heterogeneity among tumors, even of the same histiotype, obliges us to look for such parameters that represent a biological sample of the tumor. For example, if we search the literature for prognostic factors, we find enormous amount of data, but the anatomical TNM-staging is still the most important prognostic factor on which we base our choice of treatment. TNM-staging is in essence a holistic integrating parameter, giving information about the progression of the disease as a whole. However there is an urgent need for biological integrating parameters which give complementary information to the TNM-staging. In this chapter we will discuss a new possible biological integrating parameter, growth pattern.

Finally, although most cancer deaths are the results of metastases, cancer research has mainly focused on the primary tumor. More research on human metastases models is therefore needed for a better understanding of the biological profile of metastases.

2. Angiogenesis

2.1 Angiogenic Process

Angiogenesis is a physiological process involved in the development, growth and repair of tissues and organs. During embryogenesis blood vessels are formed de novo from endothelial-cell precursors or angioblasts -the process of vasculogenesis- that assemble into a primary capillary plexus. This primitive network then differentiates, and new blood vessels sprout and branch from pre-existing capillaries- the process of angiogenesis [1].

Adult tissues that undergo physiological angiogenesis are female reproductive organs, organs that demonstrate physiological growth or injured tissues [2]. Abnormal or excessive angiogenesis is associated with many pathological conditions. The best known are cancer, psoriasis, arthritis and blindness, but also many other common disorders such as obesity, asthma, atherosclerosis and infectious diseases [3].

2.2 Angiogenesis and Tumor Growth

Judah Folkman in 1971 [4] first emphasized the importance of angiogenesis in tumor biology. His experiments showed that a tumor without vascularization would grow only to a few thousand cells in size or around 1-2 mm^3, which is the distance that nutrients can enter tumor cells by passive diffusion. To grow beyond this passive diffusion-limited size, the growing tumor must switch to the angiogenic phenotype that provides the tumor with newly formed vessels and sets the conditions for rapid growth.

Induction of the angiogenic switch depends on the balance between angiogenic activators and inhibitors [5]. Up- and down regulation of angiogenic factors is induced by physiological stimuli, such as hypoxia, which results from increased tissue mass [6], and also by *Oncogene* activation or tumor-suppressor mutation [7].

Tumor angiogenesis is a multistep process of degradation of the extracellular matrix, proliferation, differentiation and migration of endothelial cells from postcapillary venules, and, finally tube formation [8]. More than 20 endogenous activators and inhibitors have been identified (table 1) [9]. This process is initiated by the activation of quiescent endothelial cells by the binding of growth factors, produced either by tumor or stromal cells, to endothelial cell receptors. VEGF (vascular endothelial growth factor) is the most potent and specific growth factor for endothelial cell activation. VEGF is also known as vascular permeability factor, based on its ability to induce vascular leakage [10-11]. This permeability enhancing activity is important since it allows extravasation of plasma proteins, which lay down a provisional matrix on which activated endothelial cells migrate. VEGF is secreted by almost all solid tumors [12] and even hematological malignancies have shown to express VEGF [13]. Evidence for the importance of VEGF-induced angiogenesis in tumor growth has been demonstrated by use of neutralizing antibodies or a dominant-negative soluble receptor to inhibit VEGF action and growth of primary and metastatic experimental tumors [14].

Table 1: Activators and inhibitors of angiogenesis

Activator	Function	Inhibitor	function
VEGF	Stimulation angio-/vasculo-genesis, permeability	Soluble VEGFR-1	Inhibition of VEGF, VEGF-B, PIGF.
VEGFR	Integration of angiogenic and survival signals	Ang2.	Antagonist of Ang1
Ang1 and Tie2	Stabilization of blood vessels, inhibition of permeability	TSP-1,-2	Inhibition of endothelial cell migration, growth, adhesion and survival
PDGF-BB and receptors	Recruitment of smooth muscle cells	Angiostatin	Suppression of angiogenesis
TGF-beta1, endoglin, TGF-beta receptors	Stimulation of production of extracellular matrix	Endostatin	Inhibition of survival and migration of endothelial cells
FGF, HGF, MCP-1	Stimulation of angiogenesis	Vasostatin	Inhibition of endothelial growth
Integrins	Receptors for matrix macromolecules and proteinases	Platelet factor-4	Inhibition of binding of bFGF and VEGF
VE-cadherin, PECAM	Endothelial junction molecules	TIMPs (inhibitors of MMPs)	Suppression of pathological angiogenesis
Ephrins	Regulation of arterial venous characteristics	Meth-1;meth-2	Inhibition of MMP, TSP and disintegrin domains
Plasminogen activators, MMPs	Reconstruction of matrix, release and activation of growth factors	IFN-α,-β,-gamma: IP-10,IL-4,IL-12,IL-18	Inhibition of endothelial migration; downregulation of bFGF
PAI-1	Stabilisation growing blood vessels	Prothrombin 2; antithrombine III fragment	Suppression endothelial growth
NOS, COX-2	Stimulation of angiogenesis and vasodilatation	Prolactin	Inhibition bFGF/VEGF
AC133	Regulation of angioblast differentiation	VEGI	Modulation of cell growth
Chemokines	Multiple effects on angiogenesis	Fragment of SPARC	Inhibition of endothelial binding and activation of VEGF
Id1/Id3	Regulation of endothelial plasticity	Osteopontin fragment	Interference with Integrin
		Maspin	Protease inhibitor
		Canstatin, proliferin related protein, restin	Unknown mechanism

Hypoxia is the most potent stimulus for induction of VEGF expression, but *Oncogenes*, tumor suppressor genes, cytokines, hormones and other mediators can also a play a role in control of its expression [11]. Experimental studies have shown that cells in hypoxic conditions induce the expression of certain genes, hypoxia-inducible genes, which are involved in rising the oxygen level, adaptation of the cell's metabolism or neutralizing the byproducts of hypoxic conditions (table 2)[15]. Under hypoxic conditions, cells switch from aerobic to anaerobic metabolism [16]. Hypoxic cancer cells use glycolysis as a primary mechanism of ATP production. So, in hypoxic conditions the expression of enzymes involved in glycolytic pathway, as well as the glucose transporters GLUT1 and GLUT3, which mediate cellular glucose uptake, are induced [17]. Glycolysis is considered to be the main mechanism by which tumors lower their pH, through generation of lactic acid. Carbonic anhydrases, which reversibly convert carbon dioxide and water to carbonic acid, are expressed during hypoxia [18-19]. Carbonic anhydrase 9 is expressed in perinecrotic areas in a wide range of tumor types, and high expression levels have been associated with poor prognosis [20]. Its possible role in tumor cell growth is neutralization of the acidotic intracellular pH, which has a negative effect on survival. By lowering the extracellular pH tumor cell progression and invasion are promoted. Hypoxia also induces the expression of genes involved in oxygen transport and iron metabolism, like erythropoietin [15].

The expression of these hypoxia-inducible genes are modulated by a transcription factor, hypoxia-inducible transcription factor 1 (HIF-1) [15, 21]. HIF-1 is a heterodimer that consists of the hypoxic response factor HIF-1α and the constitutively expressed aryl hydrocarbon receptor nuclear translocator (ARNT) –also known as HIF-1β [22]. Both the HIF-α and HIF-β subunits exist as a series of isoforms encoded by distinct genetic loci. HIF-β subunits are constitutive nuclear proteins, whereas HIF-α subunits are inducible by hypoxia. Among three HIF-α isoforms, HIF-1α and HIF-2α appear closely related and are each able to interact with hypoxia response elements (HREs) to induce transcriptional activity [23-24]. In contrast, HIF-3α appears to be involved in negative regulation of the response, through an alternately spliced transcript termed inhibitory PAS domain protein [25]. In the presence of oxygen, HIF-1α is hydroxylated by prolyl hydroxylase, an enzyme that requires oxygen, ferrous iron and 2-oxoglutarate for its activity. The hydroxylated form of HIF-1α then binds to the tumor suppressor Von Hippel-Lindau (VHL) protein. This interaction causes HIF-1α to become ubiquitylated and targeted to the proteasome, where it is degraded [26-28]. Under hypoxic conditions, this post-transcriptional hydroxylation no longer occurs and HIF-1α and HIF-1β form a complex that then diffuses to the nucleus and induces the expression of its targeted genes.

2.3 Tumor versus Physiological Angiogenesis

A balance between pro- and anti-angiogenic signals tightly regulates the physiological angiogenesis. The new vessels rapidly mature and become stable. In contrast, tumors - considered as "wounds that never heal"-[29] have lost the balance between positive and negative controls of angiogenesis. Blood vessels of tumor tissue fail to become quiescent, enabling constant growth and remodeling. This leads to architecturally different blood vessels: they are irregularly shaped, dilated, tortuous and can have dead ends. They are not organized into definitive venules, arterioles and capillaries, but rather share chaotic features of all of them [30-31]. Endothelial cells lining tumor blood vessels differ in many respects with regard to gene expression from those of normal vasculature [32]. The tumor blood vessels are often leaky and hemorrhagic, partly due to the overproduction of VEGF. The blood flows irregularly in tumor vessels, moving more slowly and sometimes even oscillating [33]. This leads to dysfunctional capillaries. Consequently, increased tumor angiogenesis, as indicated by increased microvessel density or by increased VEGF expression, does not necessarily correlate with increased blood flow and oxygen availability.

Table 2: hypoxia inducible genes

Genes induced by hypoxia
Angiogenesis: Adrenomedullin, angiopoietin-2, cyclooxygenase-2, endothelin-1 and 2, fibroblast growth factor-3, , hepatocyte growth factor, histone deacetylase, monocyte chemotactic protein-1, nitric oxide synthase, osteopontin, placental growth factor, Tie-2 (an angiopoietin receptor), transforming growth factor (TGF)-α, TGF-β1, TGF-β3, Vascular endothelial growth factor (VEGF)-A and VEGF receptor-1
Cell adhesion, extracellular matrix, cytoskeleton and proteases/ coagulation CD99, collagen-5α1, Ku70, Ku80, low-density lipoprotein receptor-related protein, metalloproteinases, matrix metalloproteinase-13, neural cell-adhesion molecule L1 (L1CAM), plasminogen activator inhibitor-1, proline-4 hydroxylase, tissue factor (TF), urokinase receptor, vimentin and α-integrin
Glycolysis and glucose uptake Aldolase-A, enolase-1, glucose transporter-1,-3 (GLUT1, GLUT3), glyceraldehyde-3-phosphate dehydrogenase, hexokinase-1, hexokinase-2, lactate dehydrogenase-A, phosfructokinase-C, phosfructokinase-L, phosphoglycerate kinase-1 and pyruvate kinase-M
Growth factor and cytokines IGF-2 (insuline-like growth factor-2), interleukin-6, interleukin-8, intestinal trefoil factor, macrophage inhibitory factor, platelet-derived growth factor-B and staniocalcin
Metabolism, pH and neurotransmitters Acetoacetyl CoA thiolase, adenylate kinase-3, aminopeptidase-A, carbonic anhydrase-9,-12, phosphoribosyl pyrophosphate synthetase, spermidine N1-acetyltransferase, tyrosine hydroxylase and α-adrenergic receptor
Oxygen transport and iron metabolism Ceruloplasmin, erythropoietin, ferritin light chain, heme oxygenase-1 transferrin and transferrin receptor
Stress-response pathways 150-kDa ORP (oxygen-regulated protein), glucose-related protein, growth arrest- and DNA damage-induced gene (GADD153), human apurinic apyrmidinic site endonuclease (HAP-1) and thioredoxin
Transcription factors Annexin V, BCL-interacting Killer (BIK), cyclin G2, differentiated embryo-chondrocyte expressed gene 1 (DEC1), FOS, heat-shock factor, hypoxia-inducible factor (HIF)-1α, HIF-2α, insulin-like growth factor (IGF) binding protein-1,-2,-3, JUN, KIP1, lipocortin, nuclear factor-κB (NF-κB), NIP3, NIX, transgelin, transglutiminase-2 and WAF1

2.4 Methodology of Angiogenesis Quantification in Solid Tumor Sections

Microvessel Density

Counting microvessels in microscopic fields of tumor tissues has been applied for estimation of the net result of different phases of angiogenesis. In carcinomas, and not necessarily in sarcomas, microvessels cluster in so-called 'vascular hot spots' [34]. Immunohistochemical staining of endothelial cells with pan-endothelial cell markers, factor VIII, CD31 and CD34, are used to stain blood vessels. The rationale of counting microvessels in vascular "hot spots" is that these areas originated from tumor cell clones with the highest angiogenic potential and, consequently, with easiest access to blood stream and with an increased probability of producing metastases capable of becoming angiogenic and growing tumors [35]. Microvessel density has been shown to be a predictor of poor prognosis in many solid tumors including breast, prostate, ovarian, colorectal and gastric carcinoma [36-41].

Classical Method

The proposed standard method for counting microvessels in consensus methodology of quantification of angiogenesis consists of a systematic scan of tumor tissue at low magnification (e.g. 10x), selection of at least 3 vascular hot spots, and subsequently counting blood vessels at a higher magnification (200x-400x)

Chalkley

Chalkley count is a morphometric method that gives a relative estimate of an area rather than a true vessel count. It consists of a grid of 25 points. The chalkley count is the number of grid points that hit stained microvessels. This technique has abolished one of the highly observer-dependent steps of measuring microvessel density, namely the frequent decision an observer has to make whether two immunostained and adjacent structures are the reflection of single or two separate blood vessels [42]. The use of this quantification technique has led to large studies of breast cancer patients showing a very significant and independent prognostic value of Chalkley microvessel count in vascular hot spots for survival [43].

Quantitative Image Analysis

Automated image analysis algorithms has also been used in combination with a motorized scanning stage microscope and an autofocus device to scan whole tumor sections [44]. The developers of the method mentioned a throughput of the system of an average of 3.5 hour per square centimeter, reducible by optimization of the system to 1.4 hour per square centimeter. The time-consuming nature together with the specialized equipment needed for analyses are the major drawbacks of this method.

Counting Endothelial Cell Proliferation Fraction

Using double immunostaining techniques, antibodies directed at an endothelial cell marker and a marker of proliferating cells, the endothelial cells in proliferation can be visualized. This technique allows for the simultaneous assessment of endothelial and tumor cell proliferation and has been applied for breast and colorectal adenocarcinomas and liver metastases [45-46].

Other Techniques

Pericyte recruitment, as parameter reflecting the functional status of the tumor, vascular differentiation, activation markers and different factors of hypoxia pathway have also been used for assessing the angiogenic profile of the tumor [35].

2.5 Rationale of Anti-Angiogenic Therapy

The rationale of anti-angiogenic therapy is based on two assumptions: firstly, the obligatory dependency of tumor growth on angiogenesis and secondly, the notion that inhibition of angiogenesis inhibits tumor growth [4]. Additional theoretical advantages of anti-angiogenic therapy are as follows: 1) endothelial cells are genetically stable cells compared to unstable mutating tumor cells, and therefore are least likely to induce drug resistance 2) endothelial cells are easily accessible by anti-angiogenic agents compared to drugs that act directly on tumor cells and have to penetrate large bulky masses 3) physiological angiogenesis occurs in limited quantities in adults (wound healing and ovulation), thus selectively targeting endothelial cells is theoretically safe and should avoid normal tissue toxicity 4) as each tumor capillary supplies hundreds of tumor cells, targeting of tumor vascularization should lead to a potentiation of the anti-tumorigenic effect [7,9].

Table 3: direct angiogenesis inhibitors

Drug	Target	Effect
Endostatin Tumstatin Canstatin Arresten Vitaxin	Integrin $\alpha v\beta 3$	Inhibition of endothelial cell proliferation, migration, tube formation, neovascularization and induction of apoptosis of endothelial cells
Angiostatin	APT synthase Angiomotin Annexin II	Inhibition of endothelial cell proliferation and migration
Combrestatin	Microtubules	Induces reorganization of the actin of cytoskleton and early membrane blebbing in human endothelial cells
Bevacizumab (avastin)	VEGF	Inhibits the effects of VEGF
NM-3	VEGF	Inhibits the effects of VEGF
Thrombospondin		Blocks endothelial-cell migration and neovascularization in the cornea, but might not be specific for endothelial cells
2-methoxyestradiol	microtubuline	Inhibits microtubuline function in proliferating endothelial cells, resulting in endothelial cell apoptosis

There are two classes of angiogenesis inhibitors-: direct and indirect [7]. Direct angiogenesis inhibitors prevent the endothelial cells from proliferating, migrating or cell death in response to a spectrum of pro-angiogenic proteins, including VEGF (table 3). Indirect angiogenesis inhibitors prevent the expression or block the activity of a tumor protein that activates angiogenesis, or block the expression of its receptor on endothelial cells (table 4).

Table 4: indirect angiogenesis inhibitors

Drug	Cancer-cell target	Pro-angiogenic proteins
ZD1839, ZD6474, OSI774, CI1033, PKI1666, IMC225	EGF receptor tyrosine kinase	VEGF; bFGF, TGFα
PTK787, ZD6474, SU6668, SU11248	VEGF receptor	VEGF receptor on endothelial cell
PTK787, SU11248	PDGF receptor	PDGF receptor
Herceptin	ERBB-2 (HER-2/neu receptor tyrosine kinase)	VEGF, angiopoietin-1, TGF-β, PAI1; upregulates thrombospondin-1
Interferon (IFN)-α	INF-α receptor	Inhibits expression of bFGF by cancer cells

2.6 Heterogeneity and Angiogenesis

2.6.1 Angiogenesis Independent Vascularization

2.6.1.1 Co-option

The prevailing view has been that malignancies and metastases initially grow as small avascular masses. To grow beyond this diffusion-limited size, a switch to the angiogenic phenotype is needed. In a study of gliomas in a rat model, well-vascularized tumors were formed after 1 week of implantation of tumor cells. The tumor cells had co-opted the blood vessels of the surrounding brain tissue. There was no angiogenic switch to this phase and VEGF expression in tumor cells was either absent or low. Later on, the regression of co-opted vessels, subsequent tumor cell death and hypoxia resulted in intense angiogenesis at the tumor margin. In this model, co-option was restricted to the early phase of tumor growth [47].

In a study of 500 non-small cell lung cancers (NSCLC), an alveolar growth pattern was described, in which the tumor cell nests simply filled the alveolar spaces without destruction of lung parenchyma, and were co-opting the septal blood vessels. In the tumor cell nests, no associated desmoplastic stroma or new blood vessels were present [48]. The co-option has also been described in liver metastases of colorectal adenocarcinoma [46]. In the replacement growth pattern, tumor cells replaced the hepatocytes of the liver cell plates, while conserving the supportive tissue including the sinusoidal blood vessels. The co-opted vessels did not express CD34, a marker present on nearly all blood vessels in primary tumors, but not on normal sinusoidal liver blood vessels. There was also a low fraction of proliferating endothelial cells.

The vascular co-opting non-angiogenic growth patterns have also been described in lymph node metastases [49], skin metastases [50] and lung metastases [51].

2.6.1.2 Vasculogenic Mimicry

Vasculogenic mimicry was first described in aggressive human uveal and cutaneous melanoma [52]. The tumor cells were found to line vascular channels forming a perfused network in the absence of the endothelial cells. They also expressed genes associated with vascular development, such as the endothelial receptor kinase Tie-1 and the endothelial cell adhesion molecule VE-cadherin. The gene expression profile of aggressive cutaneous and uveal melanoma cells revealed that these cells resemble undifferentiated, embryonic-like cells [53]. This indicates that aggressive melanoma cells revert to an embryonic-like phenotype, explaining their ability to mimic the activities of endothelial cells [54].

2.6.1.3 Mosaic Blood Vessels

In the mosaic blood vessels the luminal surface of the vessels is formed by both endothelial cells and tumor cells [55]. This is different in respect to vasculogenic mimicry, as the tumor cells of mosaic blood vessels do not show an endothelial phenotype. In fact, the tumor cells might be in transit, entering or exiting the vessels.

2.6.1.4 Vasculogenesis

The process of vasculogenesis, formation of blood vessels out of angioblasts, seems also to occur in tumor tissue. In a murine bone-marrow transplantation model, bone marrow derived endothelial cell progenitors or angioblasts were abundant in the highly vascularized peripheral regions of implanted colon cancer. An increase in circulating endothelial cell progenitors was observed following VEGF administration in this model [56].

2.6.1.5 Intussusceptive Vascular Growth

Intussusceptive vascular growth is formation of a vascular network by insertion of interstitial tissue columns into the vascular lumen and subsequent growth of these columns resulting in partitioning of the vessel lumen. Endothelial cell division is not required for this form of vascular remodeling [57].

2.6.2 Heterogeneity in Angiogenic Tumors

Beside the existence of angiogenesis-independent vascularization, heterogeneity even exists within the subgroup of angiogenic tumors. Compared with the physiological angiogenesis in the cyclic bovine ovarian corpus luteum, measurements of microvessel density (MVD), endothelial cell proliferation and recruitment of pericytes in human, renal cell, colon, mammary, lung and prostate carcinomas, have shown that there are significant differences in angiogenesis between the tumor types and even within each tumor group [58].

3. Angiogenesis and Non-Small Cell Lung Cancer (NSCLC)

3.1 Microvessel Density (MVD)

The prognostic value of MVD has not been clearly shown in NSCLC and remains a controversial subject. A systematic review of the literature of the role of microvessel density on the survival of patients with lung cancer with a meta-analysis has been performed [59]. In total, 32 studies were selected, 14 were found evaluating the MVD count by factor VIII, 10 by CD34 and 8 by CD31. The overall conclusion was that a high microvessel count in NSCLC was a significant poor prognostic factor for survival in NSCLC. However it is worth mentioning that only in 5 studies more than 200 patients were included. Out of these 5 studies, MVD had a prognostic value in only three. In the largest study of 515 patients with the longest follow-up time, no prognostic value of MVD was demonstrated [60].

Four studies deserve special attention. In the first, tissue sections of 116 patients were analyzed. Microvessel counting was used for angiogenesis assessment. Microvessel counting was performed in three consecutive areas; peripheral at the invading front, intermediate, and inner tumor area. Each area was estimated to cover a course of 2 mm, covering each 3 optical fields of 200x. The mean microvessel score of each area was determined. Also microvessel counting was performed in the normal lung proximal to the tumor periphery. Analysis showed that MVD decreased progressively from the tumor periphery to the intermediate and inner tumor area. The mean MVD in normal lung was significantly higher than the mean MVD in all the tumor areas. All the differences were statistically significant.

Analyzing the changing patterns of MVD from the invading front to the inner tumor areas, three patterns of vascular growth were identified: the edvin (edge vs. inner) type1, where a low MVD was observed in both peripheral and inner tumor areas; the edvin type 2, where a high MVD was noted in the invading front but a low MVD in inner areas; and edvin type 3, where both peripheral and inner tumor areas had a high MVD. The investigators also determined the mean single endothelial cell score (ECS) in different areas of the tumor. This single endothelial cell component is close to zero in all normal tissues including lungs. The ECS was high in the invading edge in edvin type 2 and 3 cases and decreased sharply in both types in inner areas, suggesting that endothelial cell migration is unlikely to contribute to the angiogenic process in areas away from the tumor front. The immunohistochemical staining of the tumor sections of VEGF and thymidine phosphorylase (TP) showed that VEGF and TP expression was associated with a high MVD at the invading edge. Patients with edvin type 2 and 3 vascular growth showed an increased incidence of node metastasis and patients with edvin type 3 vascular growth had a poorer prognosis in univariate survival analysis [61].

In the second study, the heterogeneity of MVD was examined at different levels in NSCLC. For each specimen of 60 lung tumors and 9 normal lung tissues, one representative block was selected and 47 blocks were taken from three different regions of 4 tumors: periphery, center and midway between the periphery and the center. The tissue sections were stained with antibodies against Von Willebrand Factor and MVD was quantified in vascular hot spots (h-MVD) as well as average MVD throughout the section. Statistical analysis showed that h-MVD values were similar to h-MVD values of normal bronchus, whereas average MVD was higher in the latter ($p<0.01$). This suggests that elevated MVD doesn't necessarily represent angiogenesis in NSCLC. Analyses of the 47 blocks taken from 4 lung tumors showed significant differences in MVD among multiple blocks taken from the same region ($p<0.05$). There was also a significant difference between different regions within the same tumor in 50 % of cases with a trend of a higher MVD towards the center, suggesting that the highest MVD was not necessarily found in the periphery of the tumor. Although there was a considerable variation in the MVD of blocks within each tumor and within each region, the variation between the tumors was even more pronounced. The investigators also assessed whether determining the MVD in a single block was sufficient to provide an estimate of the overall MVD in a given tumor. When only one block per tumor was examined, the chance of obtaining an accurate estimate of the vascularity of that tumor was less than 68% [62].

In another study MVD was assessed using anti-CD34 antibodies and anti-CD105 antibodies. CD105 (endoglin) is a homodimeric membrane glycoprotein expressed on endothelial cells that can bind TGF-β1 and -β3. It has been shown that anti-CD105 antibodies have a greater affinity for "activated" endothelial cells in tissues participating in angiogenesis, in contrast to pan-endothelial antibodies, such anti-CD34, anti-CD31 and anti-vWf, which react not only with newly formed vessels but also with pre-existing vessels.

Tumor tissues of a total of 236 patients with NSCLC were analyzed. MVD was determined in tumor sections stained with anti-CD34 (CD34-MVD) and with anti-CD105 (CD105-MVD) antibodies, by selecting the 10 most vascularized areas within each section and counting the blood vessels. The average counts were recorded as CD105-MVD or CD105-MVD. Both CD34-MVD as well as CD105-MVD correlated with the expression of VEGF, although CD105-MVD correlated more closely with VEGF. A high CD105-MVD was a predictor of poor prognosis in univariate as well as in multivariate survival analysis. CD-34-MVD did not reach statistical significance [63].

In the fourth study, the microvessel density was assessed using 11B5 monoclonal antibody recognizing the VEGF/KDR complex to assess the VEGF expression in cancer cells and the VEGF/KDR activated microvessel density (aMVD). KDR or VEGF receptor 2 is one of the two identified VEGF receptors- the other is Flt-1 or VEGF receptor 1- and is almost exclusively expressed on endothelial cells. The anti-CD31 was used to assess the standard MVD. The aMVD was significantly higher at the invading front of the tumor and was an independent prognostic factor in a multivariate Cox analysis. The standard MVD was higher in the normal lung and decreased from the invading front to the inner tumor area [64].

3.2 Vascular Endothelial Growth Factor (VEGF)

VEGF-A is a member of a family of dimeric glycoproteins that belongs to the platelet-derived growth factor (PDGF) superfamily of growth factors. Other members of the VEGF family include VEGF-B, VEGF-C, VEGF-D, VEGF-E, and Placenta growth factor (P1GF). The VEGF-A consists of at least 6 isoforms (VEGF121, VEGF145 VEGF165, VEGF 183, VEGF189, and VEGF 206) which are regulated by splicing at the mRNA level. VEGF165 is the most prevalent isoform. VEGF-A has two conventional transmembrane tyrosine kinase receptors, VEGFR-1 (Flt-1) and VEGFR-2 (KDR, Flk-1), that are selectively but not exclusively expressed by vascular endothelium. Other receptors that also interact with VEGF-A have been described: two neuropilins (NRPs) and heparan sulfate proteoglycans [11, 65]. The VEGF-A expression by tumor cells has been found to have a prognostic value in many types of tumors, including breast, kidney, colon, brain, ovary, cervix, thyroid, bladder, esophagus, prostate, NSCLC but also in osteogenic and soft tissue sarcomas and pediatric tumors [66-94]. In all these studies, the VEGF-A expression measured by immunohistochemistry, in situ hybridization, quantitative immunoassays, Western blotting, or reverse-transcriptase polymerase chain reaction (RT-PCR) correlated with one or more of the following prognostic factors: tumor size, metastases, and shorter disease-free and overall survival.

The VEGF-A levels can also be more conveniently measured in body fluids than in tumor homogenates, and it has been shown that increased levels of circulating VEGF-A, measured by enzyme-linked immuno-assay or other assays, is associated with a large tumor burden and widespread metastatic disease [95-97].

In NSCLC it has been documented that VEGF expression is directly correlated with MVD and inversely correlated with survival [84, 86-88]. A study of expression profiles of VEGF isoforms in 57 surgically resected NSCLC using RT-PCR has demonstrated that a high tumoral expression of VEGF189 is associated with a high MVD, shorter overall survival and early postoperative relapse. VEGF189 is a membrane-associated form, unlike VEGF121 and VEGF165 (secreted form), and represents less than 10% of the total VEGF expression [98]. This suggests that VEGF189 might be more important to angiogenesis in NSCLC than the other isoforms.

It has also been shown that the co-expression of NRP1 and NRP2 is correlated with increased vessels counts and poor prognosis in patients with NSCLC [99].

As mentioned above, beside VEGF-A there are other members of VEGF family but these have been far less studied than VEGF-A. There is currently a growing interest in the other members of VEGF family because of their possible roles in lympho-angiogenesis. VEGF-C and VEGF-D have been shown to bind VEGFR2 and VEGFR3 and to play an important role in physiological and tumoral lympho-angiogenesis. In NSCLC, VEGF-C expression is correlated with lymph node metastasis, lymphatic invasion, and poor prognosis [100-103].

3.3 Other Angiogenic Growth Factors

Platelet-derived endothelial cell growth factor (PDECGF) is an angiogenic factor secreted by platelets. PDECGF is a non-heparin-binding homodimer thymidine phosphorylase (TP) [104]. TP increases DNA synthesis, endothelial cell migration in vitro and tumor growth and angiogenesis in vivo [105]. TP is overexpressed in solid tumors and its serum level is elevated in cancer patients [106-107]. TP expression correlates with MVD in NSCLC, especially in squamous cell carcinoma [108].

Like VEGF, basic fibroblast growth factor (bFGF) consists of different isoforms. bFGF induces protease and urokinase plasminogen activator receptor (uPAR) expression and also modulates the expression of integrins [109-111]. In vitro bFGF leads to formation of capillary-like structures in collagen [112]. bFGF stimulates VEGF secretion and the effects of VEGF and bFGF appear to be synergistic in vitro and in vivo [113-116]. The angiogenic effect of bFGF can be inhibited in vivo by using bFGF antibody [117]. The secretion of bFGF binding protein (bFGF-BP) seems also to be important, because its upregulation increases tumor growth and angiogenesis [118]. The secreted bFGF adheres to the extracellular matrix (ECM) where it is bound to heparan sulphate and released by proteolytic enzymes. The increased secretion of bFGF-BP in tumor cells probably results in an increased concentration of bFGF-BP into the ECM with binding of bFGF-BP to bFGF and subsequent release of soluble active bFGF [119].

Angiopoietin (Ang-)-1 and –2 have recently been identified as potent angiogenic factors that function in concert with VEGF. Ang-1 and Ang-2 have been identified as ligands for Tie2, which is a receptor tyrosine kinase selectively, expressed on endothelial cells. The binding of Ang-1 to Tie2 stabilizes mature vessels by promoting the interaction between endothelial cells and surrounding extracellular matrix. Ang-2 competitively binds to Tie2, and antagonizes the stabilizing action of Ang-1, which results in destabilization of vessels. In absence of angiogenic factors vessel regression may occur whereas in the presence of VEGF these destabilized vessels may undergo an angiogenic switch [120-123]. It has been shown that the expression of Ang-2 is significantly correlated with poor prognosis in NSCLC that is enhanced in the presence of high VEGF expression [124].

There are several other growth factors which are thought to be involved in angiogenesis in NSCLC, like hepatocyte growth factor (HGF), tissue factor (TF), heparin-binding-growth-associated molecule (HB-GAM), interleukin-8, epithelial-neutrophil activating peptide and interferon-γ-inducible protein 10, which are not well studied until now [126-130].

3.4 Proteases

Plasminogen activators and matrix metalloproteinases (MMP) are part of a proteolytic cascade capable of degrading the ECM. This proteolytic apparatus is important since the degradation of ECM promotes the migration of endothelial cells participating in angiogenesis and facilitates tumor cell invasion. The expression of these proteases is under transcriptional control of angiogenic cytokines and growth factors, and their activity is partly controlled by their endogenous inhibitors [131].

MMPs are a family of zinc-dependent degradative enzymes that are capable of degrading basement membranes and components of ECM, and have been classified into subgroups depending on their substrates, i.e., collagenases, gelatinases, stromelysins, membrane-type, and non-classified. MMPs are known to be expressed by both cancer and stromal cells. Several studies have shown that MMPs, especially MMP-2 and MMP-9 (gelatinase A and B), membrane type 1 MMP (MT1-MMp), the activator of MMP-2, and stromelysin-3 are overexpressed in various types of tumors, and their level of expression is correlated with poor histological grade, advanced clinical stage and poor clinical outcome [132]. Tissue inhibitors of metalloproteinases (TIMPs) are endogenous inhibitors of MMP and are generally inhibitors of angiogenesis [133]. Four TIMPs have been described to date.

Stromelysin-3 is overexpressed by stromal elements (normal pulmonary fibroblasts) of NSCLC [134-135]. In a study of NSCLC patients, the plasma concentration of MMP-9 was 71.0 +/- 60.2 ng/ml, which was significantly elevated compared to that of healthy volunteers ($p<0.0001$) [136].

Both cancer cell lines and NSCLC tumor samples frequently express MMP-2, MMP-9, TIMP-1, and TIMP-2. In particular MMP-2 is highly expressed in malignant cells and surrounding fibroblasts [137]. Increased immunohistochemical expression of MMP-2 has also been shown to be associated with poor prognosis in early stage NSCLC [132].

3.5 Adhesion

There are four adhesion molecule families consisting of cadherins, selectins, integrins and the immunoglobulin super-family. E-cadherin is a transmembrane adhesion molecule involved with α-caterin, β-caterin and plakoglobin in the formation of cell-cell junctions. Dysfunction of these junctions may increase the ability of a tumor cell to invade and metastasize. In NSCLC reduced expression of E-cadherin is associated both with stage and lymph node involvement [138-139].

Integrins are a family of transmembrane proteins involved in cell-cell and cell-matrix adhesion. They are composed of linkage of two chains, α and β, in more than 20 combinations. They are important for cellular anchorage, migration and signaling. Their binding to ECM alters gene expression and cellular proliferation and differentiation. It has been shown that integrins containing the β1 chain bind to ECM elements including fibronectin, laminin and type IV collagen. Proteolysis of the ECM will release these components allowing them to bind to the β1 chain and induce signal transduction [140]. The β1 chain is involved in the expression of several MMPs [141].

The integrin αvβ3 is required for angiogenesis and is expressed by growing vessels. Antibodies to αvβ3 decrease blood vessel growth in chick chorioallantoic membrane assays [142]. The expression of integrins α5 and β1 is shown to be significantly associated with lymph node metastasis in NSCLC [143].

3.6 Growth Factor Receptors

The erb/HER type I family of tyrosine kinase receptors are involved in cell proliferation and differentiation. Two important members of this family are epidermal growth factor receptor (EGFR) and c-erbB-2 (neu or Her-2). EGFR is a transmembrane protein that binds ligands such as EGF and transforming growth factor α (TGF-α). EGFR signaling facilitates tumor-cell cycling, proliferation, invasion and decreased apoptosis [144]. As EFGR is detected in dividing endothelial cells, it is likely to be involved in the regulation of angiogenesis [145]. Its blockage leads to downregulation of pro-angiogenic cytokines, including VEGF and IL-8, in several tumor cell lines expressing EGFR [146].

EGFR is commonly overexpressed in various types of malignancies, including NSCLC [144]. EGFR overexpression has been shown to be associated with poor prognosis in NSCLC in some studies [144, 147].

Membranous and cytoplasmatic expression of HER-2 has been demonstrated in NSCLC and found to be associated with a poor prognosis in adenocarcinomas [147, 148,149].

3.7 Apoptosis

The induction of a malignant growth is initiated by activation of *Oncogene*s or the inactivation of tumor suppressor genes that lead to dysregulation of circuits that govern normal cell proliferation and homeostasis. The rate of tumor growth is determined by the balance between cell proliferation and cell loss. The latter occurs by necrosis and apoptosis or programmed cell death. An effective anti-tumor therapy relies largely on induction of endogenous apoptotic pathway [150]. Lung cancer is associated with the expression of several genes including p53, bcl-2, myc, ras and Rb [151].

The p53 gene encodes a nuclear phosphoprotein that has a prominent role in regulation of cell proliferation and apoptosis. A mutation of p53 gene is the most common event in human malignancies. p53 causes the arrest of the cell cycle at the G1-phase, increases DNA repair time, decreases replication DNA synthesis and induces apoptosis. The induced apoptosis by p53 is triggered by DNA damage, hypoxia, cytokines and growth factor-deprivation [152-153]. Wild-type p53 decreases VEGF expression whilst mutant p53 increases protein kinase C induced VEGF expression [154-155]. Mutations of the p53 gene enable a cell to survive longer under hypoxic condition [156]. Loss of p53 expression leads to increase angiogenesis by decreasing the matrix glycoprotein thrombospondin-1 [157]. The prognostic value of p53 expression has been a controversial subject in NSCLC. p53 expression has been shown to be associated with good prognosis, a poor prognosis or to have no prognostic significance [158-168]. However, a recent prospective study has shown that p53 mutations are statistically significant predictors of poor prognosis in patients with stage I NSCLC [169].

3.8 Hypoxia

Limited availability of oxygen and nutrients impairs tumor cell proliferation. The ability of tumors to adapt to hypoxic conditions is an important mechanism that promotes tumor growth [16].

It has been shown that increased tumor cell hypoxia, measured with a polarographic needle, is correlated with increased metastatic potential, resistance to radiotherapy, and a worse prognosis in solid tumors including NSCLC [170-172].

As mentioned above, during hypoxia a set of genes are upregulated providing adaptive tools to hypoxia. The expression of these genes is modulated by a transcriptional factor HIF-1 [15, 21].

One of the genes, which are upregulated during hypoxia, is carbonic anhydrase (CA) 9. Expression of CA9 has been found predominantly in perinecrotic areas [173-175]. In a prospective study a strong correlation was found between polarographic measurements of intratumoral oxygen tensions and CA9 immunostaining [19]. These findings indicate that CA9 expression can be used as a surrogate marker of cellular hypoxia.

There are two studies in which the immunohistochemical expression of CA9 is examined in NSCLC. In the first study, tissue sections of patients with NSCLC were analyzed for expression of CA9 and other angiogenic factors. CA9 expression was not only qualitatively scored (present or absent), but also quantitatively (percentage of positive tumor cells). Out of 107 cases analyzed, 39 (36.4%) had a strong membrane/cytoplasmatic expression of CA9 and were grouped as positive. CA9 expression was found in perinecrotic areas and was associated with the extent of necrosis ($p=0.004$). CA9 expression was found more frequently in squamous cell histology ($p=0.001$). Double-immunohistochemical staining for CA9 and CD31 revealed an overall higher MVD in the areas expressing CA9 than in negative areas ($p=0.0005$). There was no association between CA9 expression and MVD, VEGF, bFGF,

Hif-1α and Hif-1β. A direct association of CA9 expression was found with EGFR, c-erB-2 and MUC1 expression ($p<0.04$). Survival analysis showed that CA9 expression is related to poor prognosis. Multivariate analysis confirmed that CA9 expression is a significant prognostic factor [176].

In the second study, tissue sections of 175 patients with NSCLC were stained immunohistochemically for CA9. CA9 expression was evaluated in tumor cells (membranous, cytoplasmatic and perinuclear expression) and in stroma. The membranous, cytoplasmatic and stromal expression correlated with the extent of tumor necrosis. The distance to blood vessels from tumor cells or clusters was greater if they expressed CA9 than if they did not ($p<0.001$). Perinuclear CA9 expression was associated with a poor prognosis ($p=0.035$). In a multivariate Cox model perinuclear CA9 expression revealed to be an independent predictor of poor prognosis [177].

We can conclude that CA9 expression is probably a marker of hypoxia and its expression is associated with a poor prognosis in NSCLC.

3.9 Angiogenesis Inhibitors for Treatment of Lung Cancer

3.9.1 Endogenous Inhibitors of Angiogenesis

Endostatin

Endostatin is an endogenous angiogenesis inhibitor that blocks endothelial cell proliferation and increases apoptosis in tumor cells. In a murine Lewis Lung cancer model endostatin induced a nearly complete regression of fully developed tumors and its repeated systemic administration maintained tumor dormancy [178-179]. Recombinant human endostatin is well tolerated at doses ranging from 15 to 600 mg/m² with only minor evidence of anti-tumor activity and without any confirmed remission [180].

Interferons

Interferons belong to the cytokine family with immunomodulatory, anti-viral and anti-angiogenic properties. Interferons inhibit angiogenesis by inhibiting mitosis and migration of endothelial cells. The anti-angiogenic properties of interferons have been shown in the treatment of life-threatening hemangiomas of infancy [181]. They also have been effective against Kaposi's sarcoma [182]. There have been four randomized trials with interferons as adjuvant therapy in SCLC with no increase in overall survival in the interferon-treated patients [183-186]. In two of these trials interferon was associated with a poorer survival. Interferon was also associated with considerable toxicity that interfered with treatment delivery.

3.9.2 Inhibitors of Endothelial Cell Proliferation

RhuMAb VEGF (Avastin)

RhuMAb VEGF is a recombinant humanized monoclonal antibody to VEGF that has been shown to inhibit the growth of a variety of human cancer cell lines. In a phase I trial, VEGF serum concentration dropped to undetectable levels after administration of rhuMAb VEGF in a dose of 3 mg/kg per week or more. No pharmacological interactions were observed when RhuMAb VEGF was combined with a variety of chemotherapeutic agents [187-188].

In a randomized phase II trial of patients with stage IIIB/IV NSCLC, standard therapy with carboplatin and paclitaxel was compared to the same regimen with rhuMAb VEGF [189]. Response rates, time to progression and median survival time were longer in the rhuMAb arm. In the latter, unexpected life-threatening hemoptysis resulted in four fatalities. Less severe bleeding has also been noticed in trials of rhuMAb VEGF for other tumor types [190-192]. A phase III trial of rhuMAb VEGF in advanced NSCLC is now ongoing through the Eastern Cooperative Oncology Group (ECOG) [193].

SU5416

SU5416 is a quinolone derivate, that inhibits VEGFR-2 (Flk-1) and also c-kit mediated signaling [194]. It is administered parenterally and in a phase I trials, the most common adverse effects were nausea, vomiting, headache, diarrhea, pain and fever. Dose limiting toxicity's were headache and projectile vomiting [195]. SU5416 was further evaluated in combination with gemcitabine and cisplatin in 19 patients with advanced malignancies. In this study vascular events including pulmonary emboli, myocardial infarctions and cerebrovascular events occurred [196]. This agent will not be further investigated because of its significant toxicity.

SU6668

SU6668 is an oral tyrosine kinase inhibitor with multiple receptor targets including receptors of VEGF, PDGF (platelet-derived growth factor) and bFGF [197]. Although the preclinical testing clearly showed growth inhibition of established human tumor xenografts in mice, this agent will not be developed further because of its unacceptable toxicity profile seen in phase I studies [193].

ZD6474

ZD6474 is an inhibitor of VEGFR2, and to a lesser extent EGFR. It is administered orally and preclinical xenograft models have shown a dose-dependent inhibitory effect on tumor growth. In phase I study ZD6474 appeared to be well tolerated. With dose escalation, grade 3 thrombocytopenia, diarrhea and rash were observed [198]. A randomized phase II trial in small cell lung cancer (SCLC) patients is under development by the NCIC-CTG [193].

CP-547, 632 and Other Tyrosine Kinase Inhibitors

CP-547, 632 is an inhibitor of VEGFR-2 with additional activity against EGFR, PDGFR and other tyrosine kinases. It is administered orally and early phase I data suggest an encouraging safety profile and pharmacokinetic parameters [199-200]. Phase II trials have not yet started.

3.9.3 Matrix Metalloproteinase Inhibitors (MMPI)

Marimastat (BB2516)

Marimastat is a broad spectrum MMPI that has inhibitory activity against MMPs 1, 2, 3, 7 and 9 [201]. Marimastat is orally administered and in pre-clinical studies inhibited tumor growth and metastatic spread [202-204]. The NCIC-CTG (National Cancer Institute of Canada-Clinical Trials Group) and the EORTC (European Organization for the Research and Treatment of Cancer) conducted a Phase III randomized double blind, placebo controlled trial of marimastat in SCLC patients who had responded to first-line therapy and had achieved either complete or partial remission [205]. There was no survival benefit for patients treated with marimastat, and significant musculoskeletal toxicity required discontinuation of therapy in almost 20% of patients. The latter caused significant worsening of their quality of life.

Primomastat (AG3340)

Primomastat has a more targeted activity against MMP-2 and MMP-9, and has been evaluated in two Stage IIIB/IV NSCLC trials, where it was added to both paclitaxel and carboplatin, or gemcitabine and cisplatin, without any survival advantage [206-207]. As with marimastat, joint toxicity was seen frequently which was dose related.

BMS 275291

BMS 275291 has a broad activity against MMPs 1, 2, 8, 9, 13, 14 and to a lesser extent 3. It has minimal activity against sheddases, which are thought to be responsible for the dose-limiting joint toxicity [208]. The results of a phase III randomized trial in advanced NSCLC of paclitaxel and carboplatin with either BMS 275291 or placebo are awaited for. The phase II portion of the trial confirmed that the incidence of severe joint toxicity was similar in the active treatment and placebo arms [209].

BAY 12-9566

BAY 12-9566 is an inhibitor of MMP-2 and MMP-3 and has been compared with placebo in a randomized trial of patients with SCLC [210]. An interim analysis revealed no survival advantage and the active treatment arm was associated with an unexpected degree of thrombocytopenia.

Neovastat (AE-941)

Neovastat is natural agent isolated from shark cartilage. It has an inhibitory activity against MMPs 2, 9 and 12 in vitro. It also inhibits VEGF-dependent tyrosine phosphorylation and VEGF binding to endothelial cells [211]. In an animal model of Lewis lung carcinoma, neovastat reduced pulmonary metastases by 70% when given alone and by 83% when combined with cisplatin [211]. NCI and MD Anderson Cancer Center initiated a phase III, double-blind placebo-controlled trial of neovastat in locally advanced NSCLC in October 2000.

3.9.4 Other Agents

Thalidomide

Thalidomide inhibits angiogenesis induced by bFGF and VEGF. It also blocks tumor necrosis factor alpha and cycloxygenase 2 (COX2) changes intercellular adhesion molecule (ICAM) expression and modifies the ECM [212]. The main toxicities of thalidomide are fatigue, nausea and vomiting. The same toxicity profile has been seen in a dose escalation study of thalidomide given with paclitaxel and carboplatin in patients with stage III/IV NSCLC [213]. ECOG is conducting a phase III trial (ECOG E3598) with carboplatin, paclitaxel and thoracic radiotherapy with thalidomine or placebo in patients with stage IIIB NSCLC and results are not available yet. For SCLC a phase II trial of carboplatin, etoposide and thalidomide was well tolerated [214].

Squalamine

Squalamine is an aminosterol from the liver of the dogfish shark that inhibits angiogenesis by inhibition of mitogen stimulation of endothelial cells through modulation of cellular pH [215]. In a phase I trial, squalamine was well tolerated in doses approaching those required for anti-angiogenic effects in vitro [216-218]. A phase II trial in advanced NSCLC has been completed, but survival data are not yet available [219].

Celecoxib

Celecoxib is an inhibitor of cyclooxygenase 2 (COX2). This is an enzyme of the prostaglandin synthesis apparatus and is frequently upregulated in NSCLC. It also promotes angiogenesis, prevents apoptosis and induces resistance to radiotherapy [220]. Inhibitors of COX2 are widely used in the inflammatory setting, but their potential anticancer effects have only recently been recognized. In a preclinical setting celecoxib reduces the growth of NSCLC [221]. A phase II study suggests that celecoxib may enhance the response to preoperative paclitaxel and carboplatin in patients with stage I-III NSCLC [220].

ZD6126

ZD6126 selectively targets and induces direct damage to existing tumor endothelial cells by binding to tubuline of the cytoskeleton [222]. This binding leads to morphological changes with subsequent vessel occlusion and extensive central tumor necrosis. Main toxicities which are dose-related anorexia, constipation, dyspnea, fatigue, headache, nausea, vomiting and pain [223].

Integrin Antagonists

EM121974 and SCH221153 target endothelial αV integrins. Preclinical studies have shown their anti-angiogenic and growth inhibitory effects on tumor xenografts [224-225]. Preliminary phase I studies have shown that this agent is tolerated in doses up to 1200mg/m^2, with main toxicities being fatigue, rash, pruritus, nausea and vomiting [226].

TNP-470

TNP-470 is a synthetic fumagillin analog that inhibits endothelial cell proliferation by blocking methionine aminopeptidase [227]. In preclinical studies TNP-470 in single use is cytostatic, but in combination with paclitaxel or other cytotoxic agents induces tumor regression [228-230]. A phase I study of TNP-470 in combination with paclitaxel has shown that it is well tolerated with minimal pharmacokinetic interactions between the two drug [230].

4. Growth Pattern as a Surrogate Marker of Angiogenesis

Lung cancer remains the leading cause of cancer death in industrialized countries. Most patients with NSCLC present with advanced disease, and despite recent advances in multi-modality therapy, the overall 10-year survival rate remains a dismal 8-10%. The lungs are also a major site of metastatic disease [231].

Although large number of papers have been published evaluating prognostic factors in cancer [232], TNM-staging is still the most important tool to make estimates of prognosis for lung cancer patients, and to choose the best possible combination of treatment modalities such as surgery, radiation and chemotherapy. TNM-staging gives an accurate estimate of the progression of disease at the time of diagnosis. However, it does not always account for survival differences. Resected stage I NSCLC is a typical example: 35-50% of patients with stage I disease will relapse within 5 years and at the present time it is not currently possible to identify specific high-risk patients.

In the last 10 years more than 100 papers have been published studying various components of angiogenesis and their relation to prognosis in lung carcinoma, but results so far are inconclusive or awaiting confirmation and clinical practice has not so far been altered [193, 233-234].

Although reductionism has brought enormous amount of information on tumor biology, it has not provided any integrating parameter that is useful for clinical purposes.

In a study of 500 patients with NSCLC in stage I (T1, T2), 4 patterns of growth were described based on vascular profile [48]. The tissue sections of the tumors were stained with anti-CD34 antibodies. In basal growth pattern the basic structure of mucosa was reproduced and neoplastic cells were arranged in epithelial nests surrounded by connective tissue in which the blood vessels were laid. In papillary growth pattern the vessels were arranged in a stromal stalk, which is covered by neoplastic cells. In diffuse growth pattern vessels and stroma were admixed with neoplastic cells without any recognizable architectural structure. The first three growth patterns have the destruction of lung parenchyma with formation of a tumor-associated stroma in common, which is inherent to the process of angiogenesis. In alveolar growth pattern the tumor cell nests just simply filled the alveolar spaces without destruction of the alveolar septa; the only vessels evident in this pattern arise from the alveolar septa and highlight the alveolar network entrapped by the neoplastic cells. The arrangement of the vessels according to the normal lung architecture and the presence of anthracytic pigment in the surrounding stroma were strong arguments that these vessels are co-opted alveolar vessels entrapped by the tumor mass. The investigators classified as alveolar pattern only the ones presenting this feature through the whole tumor and not just on the edge. The alveolar growth pattern was considered to be putative non-angiogenic and its description confirmed the hypothesis that if an appropriate vascular bed is available, a tumor can exploit it.

There was no difference in average MVD measured by Chalkley between angiogenic and putative non-angiogenic growth patterns. Based upon frequency tables the investigators observed that the patients with an alveolar growth pattern had 25% more metastases than other patients [48]. In a subsequent study the vascular phenotype of normal lung, angiogenic and non-angiogenic growth patterns were investigated [235]. To distinguish between mature and immature vessels the expression of LH39 was assessed, which is an epitope within the lamina lucida of the basement membrane of human tissue [236]. It has been shown that LH39 is expressed on the basal membrane of capillaries and small venules in a variety of normal human tissues [237]. It has also been shown that in normal breast tissue where remodeling occurs physiologically, a proportion of the vessels is LH39 negative [238]. These data suggest that LH39 expression allow the discrimination between mature and recently formed vessels. The majority of the intratumoral vessels should therefore be negative for LH39. This has been confirmed in 3 studies of oral, breast and lung carcinoma [236, 238-239]. Integrin $\alpha v\beta 3$ which is expressed on newly formed vessels as discussed above, was also investigated. In putative non-angiogenic tumors, the vascular phenotype of all the vessels was the same as that of the alveolar vessels in normal lung: LH39 positive and $\alpha v\beta 3$ variable or negative. This is in contrast to 104 angiogenic tumors, in which only a minority of vessels (mean 13.1%; range 0-60%) expressed LH39, while $\alpha v\beta 3$ (in 45 cases) was strongly expressed on many of them (mean 55.5%; range 5-90%) [235]. This study confirmed the morphological evidence that the alveolar growth pattern is non-angiogenic.

The prognostic value of the alveolar growth pattern has also been suggested in another study of 143 patients with different stages of NSCLC [240]. The tumors were divided into two groups; alveolar (entirely or partially) and angiogenic (the remainder). In a multivariate analysis for overall survival advanced stage, higher age, adenocarcinoma and angiogenic vascular pattern were independent predictors of poor prognosis. Rather surprisingly, in this study a better prognosis was found for alveolar growth pattern! It is worth mentioning that in 46 patients (32%) no representative tissue was available to examine the interface of the tumors. The paraffin block from each patient containing the tumor tissue was chosen blindly, so no analysis of other sections was performed. Also the median time to death for 112 patients was 22 months (range 0-110 months), suggesting that operative mortality was also considered [240].

In our department lung metastases from renal clear cell carcinoma (RCCC), a hypervascular primary tumor with an angiogenic switch due to mutation of VHL-gene, were studied. It has been shown that due to mutation of VHL-gene and subsequently the inactive gene protein, there is activation of hypoxia-inducible genes related to overexpression of HIF-1α in RCCC [241]. Tissue sections of lung metastases from RCCC were analyzed. Three growth patterns were observed which were visible on routine haematoxylin-eosin stained tissue sections. In desmoplastic growth pattern -angiogenic- the parenchymal architecture of the lungs was not preserved. In alveolar and interstitial growth pattern (non-angiogenic), the vascular pattern and parenchymal architecture of the lungs were conserved within the metastases. The quantification of vascular density, hypoxia and endothelial cell proliferation confirmed that these different growth patterns represented different angiogenic profiles [242].

We have also observed different non-angiogenic and angiogenic growth patterns in a subset of lung metastases from colorectal adenocarcinoma [243]. The non-angiogenic growth patterns have also been observed in lung metastases from breast carcinoma [51].

Based on the previous observations we analyzed a subset of 100 patients with NSCLC [244]. The biological classification of NSCLC into growth patterns proposed by Pezzella et al. was modified. Tumors were classified according to growth patterns based on two fundamental considerations: firstly, conservation or destruction of lung parenchyma at the lung-tumor interface, and secondly, presence or absence of a tumor-associated stroma at the lung-tumor interface. Based on these considerations tumors were classified into three growth patterns as follows:

- Destructive growth pattern - angiogenic growth pattern: destruction of lung parenchyma with presence of tumor-associated stroma at the interface.
- Papillary growth pattern (intermediate growth pattern): conservation of the alveolar structure of the lung parenchyma at the interface with formation of stromal stalks containing capillary vessels originating from the alveolar septa with morphological evidence of angiogenesis.
- Alveolar growth pattern (non-angiogenic): conservation of the alveolar structure of lung parenchyma with co-option of septal blood vessels without evidence of angiogenesis at the interface.

The interface was defined as a field of x100 magnification at the edge of the tumor, containing only tumor tissue, next to normal lung tissue.

Survival analysis showed that patients with an alveolar growth pattern had a poor prognosis with a significant shorter disease-free survival time compared to patients with an angiogenic growth pattern [244].

The proposed classification is based on the properties of the interface, where the tumor is expanding and most active. As discussed above, the highest MVD, VEGF/KDR and activated microvessel density (aMVD) have been found at the invading front of the tumor in NSCLC [61, 64]. Expression of other angiogenic factors, like Angiopoietin I en Angiopoietin II was also observed at the edge of the tumor in NSCLC [124].

The conclusion that patients with an alveolar or non-angiogenic growth pattern have the worst prognosis seems to be paradoxical in view of numerous studies describing a correlation between high MVD and poor prognosis. Angiogenesis induces a chaotic and inefficient vascularization. The vascularization of non-angiogenic growth pattern is more efficient, implying a better growth and progression for non-angiogenic tumor tissue. The prognostic value of MVD has also been a controversial subject in NSCLC as discussed above. This is in our view due to the presence of different growth patterns with different biological properties and subsequently, different prognostic values [245]. The prognostic value of MVD can only be investigated in the subgroup with an angiogenic growth pattern. Such a study has not been performed yet.

Angiogenesis can also be considered as a specific differentiation state of a tumor. A tumor that can not induce angiogenesis can be considered "biologically" less differentiated.

Survival differences between the growth patterns in the proposed classification are due to differences in several biological properties.

An essential prerequisite for non-angiogenic growth appears to be the ability of the tumor tissue to respect the stromal architecture of the host tissue. This morphological feature, growth pattern, is visible on a routine haematoxylin-eosin tissue section and has been one of its neglected properties.

The clinical value of growth patterns is threefold. Firstly, growth patterns can be used as surrogate markers of angiogenesis and pre-treatment patient selection based on these growth patterns could increase the number of patients who respond to anti-angiogenic treatment. Secondly, growth patterns could have a prognostic value as well, which has been suggested in the above studies and finally, the mechanisms underlying these different features of growth patterns could reveal new therapeutic targets. The existing animal models use homogenous conditions to test new applications. Extrapolation to the human body is very difficult because of tumor heterogeneity. A typical example is the use of anti-angiogenic treatment that works perfectly in animal models but fails in clinical trails.

The problem of heterogeneity is also reflected by the fact that patients with tumors of the same histology respond differently to specific treatment modalities. Growth patterns represent this heterogeneity. Therefore the response rate of growth patterns to different treatment modalities could vary enormously. This opens a new window for modern oncology: selective targeting, i.e. treatment of a patient based on the biological properties of the tumor.

As Marcus Aurelius once said; *the first principle is simplicity.* Cancer research has always been focusing and reducing, forgetting the simple visible features of cancer tissue. These features, growth patterns, have a diagnostic and prognostic application, and can be used to select a specific therapy for the individual patient. Hopefully, the grim prognosis of patients with NSCLC and lung metastases may be improved in this way.

References

[1] Carmeliet P. Mechanisms of angiogenesis and arteriogenesis. *Nature Medicine* 2000; 6:389-395.

[2] Hanahan D et al. Patterns and emerging mechanisms of the angiogenic switch during tumorigenesis. Cell 1996; 86:353-364.

[3] Carmeliet P. Angiogenesis in health and disease. *Nature medicine* 2003; 9:653-660.

[4] Folkman J. Tumour angiogenesis: therapeutic implication. N Engl J Med 1971; 285: 1182-1186.

[5] Bergers G and Benjamin L. Tumorigenesis and the angiogenic switch. *Nature reviews* 2003; 3:401-410.

[6] Dor Y et al. Vascular enothelial growth factor and vascular adjustments to pertubations in Oxygen homeostasis. Physiol Cell Physiol 2001; 280:1367-1374.

[7] Kerbel R and Folkman J. Clinical translation of angiogenesis inhibitors. *Nature reviews* 2002; 2:727-739.

[8] Carmeliet P and Jain K. Angiogenesis in cancer and other diseases. *Nature* 2000; 407:249-257.

[9] Scappaticci FA. Mechanisms and future directions for angiogenesis-based cancer therapies. *J Clin Oncol* 2002; 20:3906-3927.

[10] Ferrara N. Role of vascular endothelial growth factor in regulation of physiological angiogenesis. *Am J Physiol Cell Physiol* 2001; 280:C1358-C1366.

[11] Dvorek FH. Vascular permeability factor/vascular endothelial growth factor: a critical cytokine in tumor angiogenesis and a potential target for diagnosis and therapy. *J Clin Oncol* 2002; 20:4368-4380.

[12] Stiver S et al. Vascular permeability factor/vascular endothelial growth factor (VPF/VEGF). *J Clin Ligand Assay* 2000; 23:193-205.

[13] Bellamy WT et al. Expression of vascular endothelial growth factor and its receptors in hematopoietic malignancies. *Cancer Res* 1999; 59:728-733.

[14] Asano M et al. Inhibition of tumor growth and metastasis by an immunoneutralizing monoclonal antibody to human vascular endothelial growth factor/vascular permeability factor. *Cancer Res* 1995; 55:5296-5301.

[15] Harris AL. Hypoxia-a key regulatory factor in tumour growth. *Nat Rev Cancer* 2002 Jan;2(1):38-47.

[16] Dang, CV and Semenza GL. Oncogenic alterations of metabolism. Trends Biochem Sci 1999; 24:68-72.

[17] Chen CH et al. Regulation of GLUT1 mRNA by hypoxia-inducible factor-1: interaction between H-ras and hypoxia. *J Biol Chem* 1999; 276:9519-9525.

[18] Wykoff CC et al. Hypoxia-inducible expression of tumor-associated carbonic anhydrases. *Cancer Res* 2000; 60:7075-7083.

[19] Loncaster JA et al. Carbonic anhydrase (CA IX) expression, a potential new intrinsic marker of hypoxia: correlations with tumor oxygen measurements and prognosis in locally advanced carcinoma of the cervix. *Cancer Res* 2001; 61:6394-6399.

[20] Chia SK et al. Prognostic significance of a novel hypoxia-regulated marker, carbonic anhydrase IX, in invasive breast carcinoma of the cervix. *J Clin Oncol* 2001; 19:3660-3668.

[21] Pugh CW and Ratcliffe PJ. Regulation of angiogenesis by hypoxia: role of the HIF system. *Nature Medicine* 2003; 9:677-684.

[22] Wang GL et al. Hypoxia-inducible factor 1 is a basis-helix-loop-helix-PAS heterodimer regulated by cellular O2 tension. *Proc Natl Acad Sci USA* 1995; 92:5510-5514.

[23] Tian H et al. Endothelial PAS domain protein 1 (EPAS1), a transcription factor selectively expressed in endothelial cells. *Genes Dev* 1997; 11:72-82.

[24] Wiesener MS et al. Induction of enothelial PAS domainprotein-1 by hypoxia: characterisation and comparison with hypoxia-inducible factor-1α. *Blood* 1998; 92:2260-2268.

[25] Makino Y et al. Inhibitory PAS domain protein is a negative regulator of hypoxia-inducible gene expression. *Nature* 2001; 414:550-554.

[26] Jaakkola P et al. Targeting of HIF-α to the von Hippel-Lindau ubiquitylation complex by O2-regulated prolyl hydroxylation. *Science* 2001; 292:468-472.

[27] Ivan M et al. HIF-α targeted for VHL-mediated destruction by proline hydroxylation: implication for O2 sensing. *Science* 2001; 292:464-468.

[28] Masson N et al. Independent function of two destruction domains in hypoxia-inducible factor-α chains activated by prolyl hydroxylation. *EMBO J* 2001; 20:5197-5206.

[29] Dvorek HF. Tumors: wounds that do not heal. Similarities between tumor stroma generation and wound healing. *N Engl J Med* 1986; 315:1650-1659.

[30] Vaupel PW. The influence of tumor blood flow and microenvironmental factors on the efficacy of radiation, drugs and localized hyperthermia. *Clin Paediatr* 1997; 209:243-249.

[31] Jain RK. Determinants of tumor blood flow: a review. *Cancer Res* 1988; 48:2641-2658.

[32] St Croix B et al. Genes expressed in human tumor endothelium. *Science* 2000; 289:1197-1202.

[33] Less JR et al. Microvascular architecture in a mammary carcinoma: branching patterns and vessel dimensions. *Cancer Res* 1991; 51:265-273.

[34] Tomlinson J et al. Different patterns of angiogenesis in sarcomas and carcinomas. *Clin Cancer Res* 1999; 5:3516-3522.

[35] Vermeulen PB et al. Second international consensus on the methodology and criteria of evaluation of angiogenesis in solid tumours. *Eur J Cancer*, in press

[36] Weidner N et al. Tumour angiogenesis and metastasis—correlation in invasive breast, carcinoma. *Engl J Med* 1991; 324:1-8.

[37] Toi M et al. Tumour angiogenesis is an independent prognostic indicator in primary breast carcinoma. *Int J Cancer* 1993; 55:371-374.

[38] Weidner N et al. Tumour angiogenesis correlates with metastasis in invasive prostate carcinoma. *Am J Pathol* 1993; 143:401-409.

[39] Hollingsworth HC et al. Tumour angiogenesis in advanced stage ovarian carcinoma. *Am J Pathol* 1995; 147:33-41.

[40] Saclarides TJ et al. Tumor angiogenesis and rectal carcinoma. *Dis Colon Rectum* 1994; 37:921-926.

[41] Tanigawa N et al. Extent of tumour vascularization correlates with prognosis and hematogenous metastasis in gastric carcinomas. *Cancer Res* 1996; 56:2671-2676.

[42] Fox SB et al. Quantification and prognostic value of breast cancer angiogenesis: comparison of microvessel density, Chalkley count, and computer image analysis. *J Pathol* 1995; 177:275-283.

[43] Hansen S et al. The prognostic value of angiogenesis by Chalkley counting in a confirmatory study design on 836 breast cancer patients. *Cancer Res* 2000; 6:139-146.

[44] Beliën JAM et al. Fully automated microvessel counting and hot spot selection by image processing of whole tumour sections in invasive breast cancer. *J Clin Pathol* 1999;52:184-192.

[45] Vermeulen PB et al. Correlation of the fractions of proliferation tumor and endothelial cells in breast and colorectal adenocarcinoma is independent of tumor histiotype and microvessel density. *Microvascular Res* 1997; 54:88-92.

[46] Vermeulen PB et al. Liver metastases from colorectal adenocarcinomas grow in three patterns with different angiogenesis and desmoplasia. *J Pathol* 2001; 195:336-342.

[47] Holash J et al. New model of tumor angiogenesis: dynamic balance between vessel regression and growth mediated by angiopoietins and VEGF. *Oncogene* 1999; 18:5356-5362.

[48] Pezzella F et al. Non-small-cell lung carcinoma tumor growth without morphological evidence of neo-angiogenesis. *Am J Pathol* 1997; 151:1417-1423.

[49] Vermeulen PB et al. Lack of angiogenesis in lymph node metastases of carcinomas is growth pattern dependent. *Histiopathology* 2002: 40:105-107.

[50] Colpaert C et al. Cutaneous breast cancer deposits show distinct growth patterns with different degrees of angiogenesis, hypoxia and fibrin deposition. *Histopathology* 2003;42:530-40.

[51] Pezzella F. Evidence for novel non-angiogenic pathway in breast-cancer metastasis. *Lancet* 2000; 355:1787-1788.

[52] Maniotis AJ et al. Vascular channel formation by human melanoma cells in vivo and in vitro: vasculogenic mimicry. *Am J Pathol* 1999; 155:739-752.

[53] Bittner M et al. Molecular classification of cutaneous malignant melanoma by gene expression profiling. *Nature* 2000; 406:536-540.

[54] Hendrix JC et al. Vasculogenic mimicry and tumour-cell plasticity: lessons from melanoma. *Nature reviews* 2003; 3:411-421.

[55] Chang YS et al. Mosaic blood vessels in tumors: frequency of cancer cells in contact with flowing blood. *Proc Natl Acad Sci* 2000; 97:14608-14613.

[56] Asahara T et al. Bone marrow origin of endothelial progenitor cells responsible for postnatal vasculogenesis in physiological and pathological neovascularization. *Circulation Res* 1999; 85:221-228.

[57] Patan S. Intussusceptive microvascular growth in a human colon adenocarcinoma xenograft: a novel mechanism of tumor angiogenesis. *Microvascular Res* 1996; 51:260-272.

[58] Eberhard A et al. Heterogeneity of angiogenesis and blood vessel maturation in human tumor: implication for antiangiogenic tumor therapies. *Cancer Res* 2000; 60:1388-1393.

[59] Meert AP et al. The role of mirovessel density on the survival of patients with lung cancer: a systematic review of the literature with meta-analysis. *Br J Cancer* 2002; 87:694-701.

[60] Pastorino U et al. Immunocytochemical markers in stage I lung cancer: relevance to prognosis. *J Clin Onco*logy 1997; 15:2858-2865.

[61] Giatromanolaki A et al. 'Invading edge vs. Inner' (edvin) patterns of vascularization: an interplay between angiogenic and vascular survival factors defines the clinical behaviour of non-small cell lung cancer. *J Pathol* 2000; 192: 140-149.

[62] Schor AM et al. Heterogeneity in microvascular density in lung tumours: comparison with normal bronchus. *Br J Cancer* 1998; 77:946-951.

[63] Tanaka F et al. Evaluation of angiogenesis in non-small cell lung cancer: comparison between anti-CD105 antibody and anti-CD34 antibody. *Clin Cancer Res.* 2001; 7:3410-3415.

[64] Koukourakis ML et al. Vascular endothelial growth factor/KDR activated microvessel density versus CD31 standard microvessel density in non-small cell lung cancer. *Cancer Res* 2000; 60:3088-3095.

[65] Ferrara N et al. The biology of VEGF and its receptors. *Nature Medicine* 2003; 9:669-676.

[66] Brownet LF et al. Expression of vascular permeability factor (vascular endothelial growth factor) and its receptors in breast cancer. *Hum Pathol* 1995; 26:86-91.
[67] Relf M et al. Expression of the angiogenic factors vascular endothelial growth factor, acidic and basic fibroblast growth factor, tumour growth factor -1, platelet-derived endothelial cell growth factor, placenta growth factor, and pleiotrophin in human primary breast cancer and its relation to angiogenesis. *Cancer Res* 1997; 57:963-969.
[68] Toi M et al. Vascular endothelial growth factor and platelet-derived endothelial cell growth factor are frequently coexpressed in highly vascularized human breast cancer. *Clin Cancer Res* 1995; 36:193-204.
[69] Brown LF et al. Increased expression of vascular permeability factor (vascular endothelial factor) and its receptors in kidney and bladder carcinomas. *Am J Pathol* 1993; 143:1255-1262.
[70] Takahashi Y et al. Expression of vascular endothelial growth factor and its receptor, KDR, correlates with vascularity, metastases and proliferation of human colon cancer. *Cancer Res* 1995; 55:3964-3968.
[71] Brown LF et al. Expression of vascular permeability factor (vascular endothelial factor) and its receptors in adenocarcinomas of the gastrointestinal tract. *Cancer Res* 1993; 53:4727-4735.
[72] Maeda K et al. Prognostic value of vascular endothelial growth factor expression in gastric carcinoma. *Cancer* 1996;77:858-863.
[73] Abdulrauf SI et al. Vascular endothelial growth factor expression and vascular density as prognostic markers of survival in patients with low-grade astrocytoma. *J Neurosurg* 1998; 88:513-520.
[74] Olson TA et al. Vascular permeability factor gene expression in normal and neoplastic ovaries. *Cancer Res* 1994; 54:276-280.
[75] Guidi AJ et al. Vascular permeability factor (vascular endothelial growth factor) expression and angiogenesis in cervical neoplasia. *J Natl Cancer Inst* 1995; 87:506-516.
[76] Guidi, AJ et al. Vascular permeability factor (vascular endothelial growth factor) expression and angiogenesis in cervical neoplasia. *J Natl Cancer Inst* 1995; 87:1237-1245.
[77] Shih CH et al. Vascular endothelial growth factor expression predicts outcome and lymph node metastasis in squamous cell carcinoma of the esophagus. *Clin Cancer Res* 2000; 6:1161-1168.
[78] Borre M et al. Association between immunohistochemical expression of vascular endothelial growth factor (VEGF), VEGF-expressed neuroendocrine-differentiated tumor cells, and outcome in prostate cancer patients subjected to watchful waiting. *Clin Cancer Res* 2000; 6:1882-1890.
[79] Kuniyasu H et al. Relative expression of type IV collagenase, E-cadherin, and vascular endothelial growth factor/vascular permeability factor in prostatectomy specimens distinguishes organ-confined from pathologically advanced prostate cancers. *Clin Cancer Res* 2000; 6:2295-2308.
[80] Mattern J et al. Vascular endothelial growth factor expression and angiogenesis in non-small cell lung carcinomas. *Int J Oncol* 1995; 6:1059-1062.

[81] Holm C et al. Expression of PDGF, VEGF and their receptors in non-small cell lung tumor lines. *Int J Oncol* 1996; 9:1077-1086.
[82] Ohta Y et al. Significance of vascular endothelial growth factor messenger RNA expression in primary lung cancer. *Clin Cancer Res* 1996; 2:1411–1416.
[83] Takanami I et al. Pulmonary adenocarcinoma angiogenesis: a study of factors that may influence tumor angiogenesis and survival. *Int J Oncol* 1997;10:101-106.
[84] Fontanini G et al. Vascular endothelial cell growth factor is associated with neovascularization and influences progression of non-small cell lung carcinoma. *Clin Cancer Res* 1997;3:861-865.
[85] Ohta Y et al. Vascular endothelial growth factor and lymph node metastasis in primary lung cancer. *Br J Cancer* 1997; 76:1041-1045.
[86] Mattern J et al. Association of vascular endothelial growth factor expression with intratumoral microvessel density and tumour cell proliferation in human epidermoid lung carcinoma. *Br J Cancer* 1996; 73:931-934.
[87] Imoto H et al. Vascular endothelial growth factor expression in non-small cell lung cancer: prognostic significance in squamous cell carcinoma. *J Thorac Cardiovasc Surg* 1998; 115:1007-1014.
[88] Tsao MS et al. Angiogenesis correlates with vascular endothelial growth factor expression but not with Ki-ras Oncogene activation in non-small cell lung carcinoma. *Clin Cancer Res* 1997; 3:1807-1814.
[89] Oshika Y et al. Expression of cell-associated isoform of vascular endothelial growth factor 189 and its prognostic relevance in non-small cell lung cancer. *Int J Oncol* 1998; 12:541-544.
[90] Fontanini G et al. Expression of vascular endothelial growth factor mRNA in non-small cell lung carcinomas. *Br J Cancer* 1999; 79:363-369.
[91] Mineta H et al. Prognostic value of vascular endothelial growth factor (VEGF) in head and neck squamous cell carcinomas. *Br J Cancer* 2000; 83:775-781.
[92] Kaya M et al. Vascular endothelial growth factor expression in untreated osteosarcoma is predictive of pulmonary metastasis and poor prognosis. *Clin Cancer Res* 2000; 6:572-577.
[93] Yudoh K et al. Concentration of vascular endothelial growth factor in tumour tissue as a prognostic factor of soft tissue sarcomas. *Br J Cancer* 2001; 84:1610-1615.
[94] Tabone MD et al. Are basic fibroblast growth factor and vascular endothelial growth factor prognostic indicators in pediatric patients with malignant solid tumors? *Clin Cancer Res* 2001; 7:538-543.
[95] Fuhrmann-Benzakein E et al. Elevated levels of angiogenic cytokines in plasma of cancer patients. *Int J Cancer* 2000; 80:40-45.
[96] Kraft A et al. Vascular endothelial growth factor in the sera and effusions of patients with malignant and nonmalignant disease. *Cancer* 1999; 85:178-187.
[97] Salven P et al. Serum vascular endothelial growth factor is often elevated in disseminated cancer. *Clin Cancer Res* 1997; 3:647-651.
[98] Yuan A et al. Vascular endothelial growth factor 189 mRNA isoform expression specifically correlates with tumor angiogenesis, patient survival, and postoperative relapse in non-small cell lung cancer. *J Clin Oncol* 2001; 19:432-441.

[99] Kawakami T et al. Neuropilin 1 and Neuropilin 2 co-expression is significantly correlated with increased vascularity and poor prognosis in non-small cell lung carcinoma. *Cancer* 2002; 95:2196-2201.

[100] Plate KH et al. From angiogenesis to lymphangiogenesis. *Nature Med* 2001; 7:151-152

[101] Li Q et al.Clinical significance of co-expression of VEGF-C and VEGFR-3 in non-small cell lung cancer. *Chin Med J* 2003;116:727-730.

[102] Kajita T et al. The expression of vascular endothelial growth factor C and its receptors in non-small cell lung cancer. *Br J Cancer* 2001; 85:255-260.

[103] Arinaga A et al. Clinical significance of vascular endothelial growth factor C and vascular endothelial growth factor receptor 3 in patients with non-small cell lung carcinoma. Cancer 2003; 97:457-464.

[104] Moghaddam A and Bicknell R. Expression of platelet-derived endothelial cell growth factor in Escherichia coli and confirmation of its thymidine phosphorylase activity. *Biochemistry* 1992;31:12141-12146.

[105] Moghaddam A et al. Thymidine phosphorylase is angiogenic and promotes tumour growth. *Proc Natl Acad Sci* 1995; 92:998-1002.

[106] Pauly J L et al. Identification and comparative analysis of thymidine phosphorylase in the plasma of healthy subjects and cancer patients. *J Natl Cancer Inst* 1977; 58:1587-1590.

[107] Yoshimura A et al. Purification and tissue distribution of human thymidine phosphorylase; high expression in lymphocytes, reticulocytes and tumors. *Biochim Biophys Acta* 1990; 1034:107-113.

[108] Koukourakis MI et al. Platelet-derived endothelial cell growth factor expression correlates with tumour angiogenesis and prognosis in non-small cell lung cancer. *Br J Cancer* 1997;75:477-481.

[109] Gualandris A et al. Interaction of high molecular weight basic fibroblast growth factor (bFGF) with endothelium: biological activity and intracellular fate of human recombinant Mr 24000 bFGF. *J Cell Physiol* 1994; 161:149-159.

[110] Mignatti P et al. Expression of the urokinase receptor in vascular endothelial cells is stimulated by the basic fibroblast growth factor. *J Cell Biol* 1991; 113:1193-1201.

[111] Klein S et al. Basic fibroblast growth factor modulates integrin expression in microvascular endothelial cells. *Mol Biol Cell* 1993; 4:973-982.

[112] Montesano R et al. Basic fibroblast growth factor induces angiogenesis in vitro. *Proc Natl Acad Sci* 1986; 83:7297-7300.

[113] Pepper MS et al. Potent synergism between vascular endothelial growth factor and basic fibroblast growth factor in the induction of angiogenesis in vitro. *Biochem Biophys Res Commun* 1992;189:824-831.

[114] Goto F et al. Synergistic effects of vascular endothelial growth factor and basic fibroblast growth factor on the proliferation and cord formation of bovine capillary endothelial cells within collagen gels. *Lab Invest* 1993; 69:508-517.

[115] Stavri GT et al. Basic fibroblast growth factor upregulates the expression of vascular endothelial growth factor in vascular smooth muscle cells. Synergistic interaction with hypoxia. *Circulation* 1995; 92:11-14.

[116] Ashara T et al. Synergistic effect of vascular endothelial growth factor and basic fibroblast growth factor on angiogenesis in vivo. *Circulation* 1995; 92:365-371.

[117] Hori A et al. Suppression of solid tumour growth by immunoneutralizing monoclonal antibody against human basic fibroblast growth factor. *Cancer Res* 1991;51:6180-6184.

[118] Czubayko F et al. Tumour growth and angiogenesis induced by a secreted binding protein for fibroblast growth factors. *J Biol Chem* 1994; 269:28243-28248.

[119] Czubayko F et al. A secreted FGF-binding protein can serve as the angiogenic switch in human cancer. *Nat Med* 1997; 3:1137-1140.

[120] Yancopoulos GD et al. Vascular-specific growth factors and blood vessel formation. *Nature* 2000; 407:242-248.

[121] Davis S et al. Isolation of angiopoietin-1, a ligand for the TIE2 receptor, by secretion-trap expression cloning. *Cell* 1996; 87:1161-1169.

[122] Suri C et al. Requisite role of angiopoietin-1, a ligand for the TIE2 receptor, during embryonic angiogenesis. *Cell* 1996; 87:1171-1180.

[123] Maisonpierre PC et al. Angiopoietin-2, a natural anatgonist for TIE2 that disrupts in vivo angiogenesis. *Science*; 277:55-60.

[124] Tanaka F et al. Expression of angiopoietins and its clinical significance in non-small cell lung cancer. *Cancer Res* 2002; 62:7124-7129.

[125] Siegfried JM et al. The clinical significance of hepatocyte growth factor for non-small cell lung cancer. *Ann Thor Surg* 1998;66:1915-1918.

[126] Zhang Y et al. Tissue factor controls the balance of angiogenic and anti-angiogenic properties of tumor cells in mice. *J Clin Invest* 1994; 9:1320-1327.

[127] Koomagi R and Volm M. Tissue-factor expression in human non-small cell lung carcinoma measured by immunohistochemistry: correlation between tissue factor and angiogenesis. *Int J Cancer* 1998;79:19-22.

[128] Jager R et al. Differential expression and biological activity of the heparin-binding growth-associated molecule (HB-GAM) in lung cancer cell lines. *Int J Cancer* 1997; 73:537-543.

[129] Arenberg DA et al. The role of CXC chemokines in the regulation of angiogenesis in non-small cell lung cancer. *J Leukocyte Biol* 1997; 62:554-562.

[130] Arenberg DA et al. Epithelial-neutrophil activating peptide (ENA-78) is an important angiogenic factor in non-small cell lung cancer. *J Clin Invest* 1998;102:465-472.

[131] Cox G et al. The plasmin cascade and matrix metalloproteinases in non-small cell lung cancer. *Thorax* 1999; 54:169-179.

[132] Passlick B et al. Overexpression of matrix metalloproteinase 2 predicts unfavorable outcome in early-stage non-small cell lung cancer. *Clin Cancer Res* 2000; 6:3944-3948.

[133] Hidalgo M et al. Development of matrix metalloproteinase inhibitors in cancer therapy. *J Natl Cancer Inst* 2001; 93:178-193.

[134] Mari BP et al. Stromelysin-3 is induced in tumor/stroma cocultures and inactivated via a tumor-specific and basic fibroblast growth factor-dependent mechanism. *J Biol Chem* 1998;273:618-626.

[135] Anderson IC et al. Stromelysin-3 is overexpressed by stromal elements in primary non-small cell lung cancers and regulated by retinoic acid in pulmonary fibroblasts. *Cancer Res* 1995; 55:4120-4126.

[136] Iizasa T et al. Elevated levels of circulating plasma matrix metalloproteinase 9 in non-small cell lung cancer patients. *Clin Cancer Res* 1999; 5:149-153.

[137] Suzuki M et al. Expression of matrix metalloproteinases and tissue inhibitor of matrix metalloproteinases in non-small-cell lung cancer. *Invasion Metastasis* 1998-99;18:134-141.

[138] Sulzer MA et al. Reduced E-cadherin expression is associated with increased lymph-node metastasis and unfavorable prognosis in non-small cell lung cancer. *Am J Respir Crit Care Med* 1998; 157:1319-1323.

[139] Shibanuma H et al. Influence of E-cadherin dysfunction upon local invasion and metastasis in non-small cell lung cancer. *Lung Cancer* 1998; 22:85-95.

[140] Luscinskas FW and Lawler J. Integrins as dynamic regulators of vascular function. *Fed Am Soc Exp Biol J* 1994;8:929-938.

[141] Huhtala P et al. Cooperative signalling by 51 and 41 integrins regulates metalloproteinase gene expression in fibroblasts adhering to fibronectin. *J Cell Biol* 1995;129:867-879.

[142] Brooks PC et al. Requirement of vascular integrin -v/-3 for angiogenesis. *Science* 1994; 264:569-571.

[143] Smythe WR et al. Loss of -v integrin expression and recurrence in node-negative lung carcinoma. *Ann Thorac Surg* 1997; 64:949-953.

[144] Klapper LN et al. Biochemical and clinical implications of the ErbB/HER signaling network of growth factor receptors. *Adv Cancer Res* 2000; 77:25-79.

[145] Kim SJ et al. Blockade of epidermal growth factor receptor signaling in tumor cells and tumor-associated endothelial cells for therapy of androgen-independent human prostate cancer growing in the bone of nude mice. *Clin Cancer Res* 2003; 9:1200-1209.

[146] Hirata A et al. ZD1839 (Iressa) induces antiangiogenic effects through inhibition of epidermal growth factor receptor tyrosine kinase. *Cancer Res* 2002; 62:2554-2560.

[147] Fontanini G et al. Evaluation of epidermal growth factor-related growth factors and receptors and of neoangiogenesis in completely resected stage I-IIIA non-small-cell lung cancer: imphiregulin and microvessel density count are independent prognostic indicators of survival. *Clin Cancer Res* 1998; 4:241-249.

[148] Giatromanolaki A et al. Non-small cell lung cancer: c-erbB-2 correlates with angiogenesis and poor prognosis. *AntiCancer Res* 1996; 16:3819-3825.

[149] Tateishi M et al. Prognostic value of c-erbB-2 protein expression in human lung adenocarcinoma and squamous cell carcinoma. *Eur J Cancer* 1991; 27:1372-1375.

[150] Hickman JA et al. Apoptosis and cancer chemotherapy. *Philos Trans R Soc Lond Ser B* 1995; 345:83-89.

[151] Sekido Y et al. Progress in understanding the molecular pathogenesis of human lung cancer. *Biochim Biophys Acta* 1998;F21-F59.

[152] Canman CE et al. Growth factor modulation of p53-mediated growth arrest versus apoptosis. *Genes Dev* 1995; 9:600-611.

[153] Graeber TG et al. Hypoxia induces accumulation of p53 protein, but activation of a G1-phase checkpoint by low-oxygen conditions is independent of p53 status. *Mol Cell Biol* 1994;14:6264-6277.

[154] Mukhopadhyay D et al. Wild-type p53 and v-Src exert opposing influences on human vascular endothelial growth factor gene expression. *Cancer Res* 1995; 55:6161-6165.

[155] Keiser A et al. Mutant p53 potentiates protein kinase C induction of vascular endothelial growth factor expression. *Oncogene* 1994; 9:964-969.

[156] Graeber TG et al. Hypoxia-mediated selection of cells with diminished apoptotic potential in solid tumors. *Nature* 1996; 379:88-91.

[157] Dameron KM et al. Control of angiogenesis in fibroblasts by p53 regulation of thrombospondin-1. *Science* 1994; 265:1582-1584.

[158] Lee JS et al. Expression of p53 oncoprotein in non-small cell lung cancer: a favourable prognostic indicator. *J Clin Oncol* 1995;13:1893-1903.

[159] Passlick B et al. Immunohistochemical detection of p53 is not associated with a poor prognosis in non-small cell lung cancer. *J Thor Cardiovasc Surg* 1995; 109:1205-1211.

[160] Top B et al. Comparative analysis of p53 gene mutations and protein accumulation in human non-small cell lung cancer. *Int J Cancer* 1995; 64:83-91.

[161] Quinlan DC et al. Accumulation of p53 correlates with poor prognosis in human lung cancer. *Cancer Res* 1992; 52:4828-4831.

[162] Horio Y et al. Prognostic significance of p53 mutations in primary resected non-small cell lung cancer. *Cancer Res* 1993; 53:1-4.

[163] Harpole DH et al. A prognostic model of recurrence and death in stage I non-small cell lung cancer utilizing presentation, and Oncogene expression. *Cancer Res* 1995; 55:51-56.

[164] Dalquen P et al. Nuclear p53 overexpression is an independent prognostic parameter in node-negative non-small cell lung carcinoma. *J Pathol* 1996; 178:53-58.

[165] Fukuyama Y et al. K-ras and p53 are an independent unfavourable prognostic indicator in patients with non-small cell lung cancer. *Br J Cancer* 1997; 75:1125-1130.

[166] Fontanini G et al. Neoangiogenesis and p53 protein in lung cancer: their prognostic role and their relation with vascular endothelial growth factor (VEGF) expression. *Br J Cancer* 1997; 75:1295-1301.

[167] McLaren R et al. The relationship of p53 immunostaining to survival in carcinoma of the lung. *Br J Cancer* 1992; 66:735-738.

[168] Nishio et al. Prognostic significance of abnormal p53 accumulation in primary, resected non-small cell lung cancers. *J Clin Oncol* 1996; 14:497-502.

[169] Ahrendt SA et al. p53 mutations and survival in stage I non-small-cell lung cancer: results of a prospective study. *J Natl Cancer Inst* 2003;95:961-70.

[170] Choi N et al. Predictive factors in radiotherapy for non-small-cell lung cancer: present status. *Lung Cancer* 2001; 31:43-46.

[171] Hockel M et al. Association between tumor hypoxia and malignant progression in advanced cancer of the uterine cervix. *Cancer Res* 1996; 56:4509-4515.

[172] Stadler P et al. Influence of the hypoxic subvolume on the survival of patients with head and neck cancer. *Int J Radiot Oncol Biol Phys* 1999; 44:749-754.

[173] Wykoff CC et al. Expression of the hypoxia-inducible and tumor-associated carbonic anhydrases in ductal carcinoma in situ of the breast. *Am J Pathol* 2001; 158:1011-1019.

[174] Beasley NJ et al. Carbonic anhydrase IX, an endogenous hypoxia marker, expression in head and neck squamous cell carcinoma and its relationship to hypoxia, necrosis, and microvessel density. *Cancer Res* 2001; 61:5262-5267.

[175] Chia SK et al. Prognostic significance of a novel hypoxia-regulated marker, carbonic anhydrase IX, in invasive breast carcinoma. *J Clin Oncol* 2001; 19:3660-3668.

[176] Giatromanolaki A et al. Expression of hypoxia-inducible carbonic anhydrase-9 relates to angiogenic pathways and independently to poor outcome in non-small cell lung cancer. *Cancer Res.* 2001;61:7992-7998.

[177] Swinson DE et al. Carbonic anhydrase IX expression, a novel surrogate marker of tumor hypoxia, is associated with a poor prognosis in non-small-cell lung cancer. *J Clin Oncol* 2003;21:473-482.

[178] Li S et al. The influence of tumour resection on angiostatin levels and tumour growth– an experimental study in tumour-bearing mice. *Eur J Cancer* 2001; 37:2283-2288.

[179] O'Reilly MS et al. Endostatin: an endogenous inhibitor of angiogenesis and tumor growth. *Cell* 1997; 88:277-285.

[180] Herbst RS et al. Phase I study of recombinant human endostatin in patients with advanced solid tumors. *J Clin Oncol* 2002; 20:3792-3803.

[181] Ezekowitz RA et al. Interferon alfa-2a therapy for life-threatening hemangiomas of infancy. *New Engl J Med* 1992; 326:1456-1463.

[182] Shepherd FA et al. A prospective randomized trial of tow dose levels of interferon-alpha and zidovudine for the treatment of Kaposi's sarcoma associated with human immunodeficiency virus infection. *J Clin Oncol* 1998; 16:1736-1742.

[183] Kelly K et al. Role of recombinant interferon alfa-2a maintenance in patients with limited-stage small-cell lung cancer responding to concurrent chemoradiation: a Southwest Oncology Group study. *J Clin Oncol* 1995; 13:2924-2930.

[184] Jett JR et al. Phase III trial of recombinant interferon gamma in complete responders with small-cell lung cancer. *J Clin Oncol* 1994; 12:2321-2326.

[185] Mattson K et al. Natural interferon alfa as maintenance therapy for small cell lung cancer. *Eur J Cancer* 1992;28:1387-1391.

[186] Lebeau B et al. Alpha Interferon as maintenance therapy for small cell lung cancer (SCLC). *Proc ASCO* 1999;18:475a abst. 1832.

[187] Gordon MS et al. Phase I trial of recombinant human monoclonal anti-vascular endothelial growth factor (anti-VEGF MAB) in patients with metastatic cancer. *Proc ASCO* 1998; 18:435a abstr. 1678.

[188] Margolin K et al. Phase 1b trial of intravenous recombinant humanized monoclonal antibody (Mab) to vascular endothelial growth factor (rhuMAB VEGF) in combination with chemotherapy (CHrX) in patients with advanced cancer (CA): pharmacologic and long-term safety data. *Proc ASCO* 1999;18:435a abstr. 1678.

[189] DeVore R et al. A randomized Phase II trial comparing rhuMAb VEGF (recombinant humanized monoclonal antibody to vascular endothelial cell growth factor) plus carboplatin/paclitaxel (CP) to CP alone in patients with Stage III/IV NSCLC. *Proc ASCO* 2000;19:485a abstr. 1896.

[190] Reese D et al. A phase II trial of humanized monoclonal anti-vascular endothelial growth factor antibody (rhuMAb VEGF) in hormone refractory prostate cancer (HRPC). *Proc ASCO* 1999;18:351a abstr. 1355 .
[191] Sledge G et al. A Phase II trial of single-agent rhuMAb VEGF (recombinant humanized monoclonal antibody to vascular endothelial growth factor) in patients with relapsed metastatic breast cancer. *Proc ASCO* 2000; 19:3a abstr. 5c.
[192] Bergsland E et al. A randomized Phase II trial comparing rhuMAb VEGF (recombinant humanized monoclonal antibody to vascular endothelial growth factor) plus 5-fluorouracil/leucovorin (FU/LV) to FU/LV alone in patients with metastatic colorectal cancer. *Proc ASCO* 2000;19:242a abstr. 939.
[193] Shepherd F and Sridhar SS. Angiogenesis inhibitors under study for the treatment of lung cancer. *Lung Cancer* 2003; 41:63-72.
[194] Fong TA et al. SU5416 is a potent and selective inhibitor of the vascular endothelial growth factor receptor (Flk-1/KDR) that inhibits tyrosine kinase catalysis, tumor vascularization, and growth of multiple tumor types. *Cancer Res* 1999; 59:99-106.
[195] Rosen L et al. Phase I dose-escalating trial of SU5416, a novel angiogenesis inhibitor in patients with advanced malignancies. *Proc ASCO* 1999; 18:161a abstr. 618.
[196] Kuenen BC et al. Dose-finding and pharmacokinetic study of cisplatin, gemcitibine, and SU5416 in patients with solid tumors. *J Clin Oncol* 2002; 20:1657-1667.
[197] Herbst RS et al. Angiogenesis inhibitors in clinical development for lung cancer. *Semin Oncol* 2002; 29:Suppl. 66-77.
[198] Hurwitz H et al. Clinical evaluation of ZD6474, an orally active inhibitor of VEGF signaling in patients with solid tumors. *Proc ASCO* 2002; 21:82a abstr. 325.
[199] Tolcher AW et al. A phase I and biologic correlative study of an oral endothelial vascular growth factor receptor-2 (VEGFR-2) tyrosine kinase inhibitor, CP-547,632 in patients with advanced solid tumors. *Proc ASCO* 2002; 21:84a abstr. 334.
[200] Roberts WG et al. Preclinical development of CP-547,632, a novel VEGFR-2 inhibitor for cancer therapy. *Proc ASCO* 2002; 21:119a abstr. 473.
[201] Wojtowicz-Praga SM et al. Matrix metalloproteinase inhibitors. *Invest New Drugs* 1997;15:61-75.
[202] Brown PD and Giavazzi R. Matrix metalloproteinase inhibition: a review of anti-tumour activity. *Ann Oncol* 1995; 6:967-974.
[203] Bramhall SR et al. Marimastat as maintenance therapy for patients with advanced gastric cancer: a randomised trial. *Br J Cancer* 2002; 86:1864-1870.
[204] Steward WP et al. Marimastat (BB2516): current status of development. *Cancer Chemother Pharmacol* 1999; 43:Suppl S56-S60.
[205] Shepherd FA et al. Prospective, randomized, double-blind, placebo-controlled trial of marimastat after response to first-line chemotherapy in patients with small-cell lung cancer: a trial of the national cancer institute of Canada-clinical trials group and the European organization for research and treatment of cancer. *J Clin Oncol* 2002; 20:4434-4439.
[206] Smylie M et al. Phase III study of the matrix metalloprotease (MMP) inhibitor prinomastat in patients having advanced non-small cell lung cancer. *Proc ASCO* 2001; 20:307a abstr. 1226.

[207] Bissett D et al. Phase III study of the matrix metalloproteinase inhibitor prinomastat in combination with gemcitibine and cisplatin in non-small cell lung cancer. *Proc ASCO* 2002; 21:296a abstr. 1183.
[208] Naglich JG et al. Inhibition of angiogenesis and metastasis in two murine models by the matrix metalloproteinase inhibitor, BMS-275291. *Cancer Res.* 2001; 61:8480-8485.
[209] Douillard J et al. Randomized phase II study of BMS-275291 versus placebo in patients with stage IIIB or IV non-small cell lung cancer receiving paclitaxel and carboplatin: National Cancer Institute of Canada clinical Trials Group BR18. *Eur J Cancer* 2001; 37:Suppl S19-S20 Abstract 63.
[210] Erlichman C et al. Phase I study of the matrix metalloproteinase inhibitor, BAY 12-9566. *Ann Oncol* 2001;12:389-395.
[211] Falardeau P et al. Neovastat, a naturally occurring multifunctional antiangiogenic drug, in phase III clinical trials. *Semin Oncol* 2001; 28:620-625.
[212] D'Amato RJ et al. Thalidomide is an inhibitor of angiogenesis. *Proc Natl Acad Sci* 1994; 91:4082-4085.
[213] Merchant J et al. Pilot and safety trial of carboplatin, paclitaxel and thalidomide in advanced non-small cell lung cancer. *Proc ASCO* 2000; 18:541a abst. 2130.
[214] Lee SM et al. A phase II study of carboplatin/etoposide with thalidomide in small cell lung cancer (SCLC). *Proc ASCO* 2002; 21:313a abst. 1251.
[215] Sills AK et al. Squalamine inhibits angiogenesis and solid tumor growth in vivo and perturbs embryonic vasculature. *Cancer Res* 1998; 58:2784-2792.
[216] Patnaik A et al. A phase I and pharmacokinetic (pk) study of the unique angiogenesis inhibitor Squalamine lactate (MSI1256F). *Proc ASCO* 1999; 18:162a abstr. 622.
[217] Bhargava P et al. A phase I safety, tolerance and pharmacokinetic study of rising dose, rising duration continuous infusion MSI-1256F (Squalamine Lactate) in patients with advanced malignancies. *Proc ASCO* 1999; 18:163a abstr. 623.
[218] Kalidas M et al. A phase I and pharmacokinetic study of the angiogenesis inhibitor, Squalamine Lactate (MSI1256-F). *Proc ASCO* 2000; 19:180a abstr. 698.
[219] Schiller JH et al. Phase 2A trial of Squalamine for the treatment of advanced non-small cell lung cancer. *Proc ASCO* 2001; 20:339a abstr. 1353.
[220] Altorki NK et al. Celecoxib (Celebrex), a selective COX-2 inhibitor, enhances the response to preoperative paclitaxel/carboplatin in early stage non-small cell lung cancer. *Proc ASCO* 2002; 21:26a abstr. 101.
[221] Gridelli C et al. Selective cyclooxygenase-2 inhibitors and non-small cell lung cancer. *Curr Med Chem* 2002; 9:1851-1858.
[222] Goto H et al. Activity of a new vascular targeting agent, ZD6126, in pulmonary metastases by human lung adenocarcinoma in nude mice. *Cancer Res* 2002; 62:3711-3715.
[223] Gadgeel SM et al. A dose-escalation study of the novel vascular-targeting agent, ZD6126, in patients with solid tumors. *Proc ASCO* 2002; 21:110a abstr. 438.
[224] Kumar CC et al. Inhibition of angiogenesis and tumor growth by SCH221153, a dual alpha(v)beta3 and alpha(v)beta5 integrin receptor antagonist. *Cancer Res* 2001; 61:2232-2238.

[225] Eskens F et al. Phase I and pharmacologic study of EMD 121974, an alphaV3 and alphaVB5 integrin inhibitor that perturbs tumor angiogenesis, in patients with solid tumors. *Proc ASCO* 2000; 19:206a abstr. 801.

[226] Holden SN et al. Correlative biological assays used to guide dose escalation in a phase I study of the antiangiogenic aVB3 and a VB5 integrin antagonist EMD 121974 (EMD). *Proc ASCO* 2002; 21:28a abstr. 110.

[227] Ingber D et al. Synthetic analogues of fumagillin that inhibit angiogenesis and suppress tumour growth. *Nature* 1990; 348:555-557.

[228] Teicher BA et al. Comparison of several antiangiogenic regimens alone and with cytotoxic therapies in the Lewis lung carcinoma. *Cancer Chemother Pharmacol* 1996; 38:169-177.

[229] Teicher BA et al. Antiangiogenic treatment (TNP-470/minocycline) increases tissue levels of anticancer drugs in mice bearing Lewis lung carcinoma. *Oncol Res* 1995; 7:237-243.

[230] Herbst RS et al. Paclitaxel/carboplatin administration along with antiangiogenic therapy in non-small-cell lung and breast carcinoma models. *Cancer Chemother Pharmacol* 1998; 41:497-504.

[231] Fry WA et al. Ten-year survey of lung cancer treatments and survival in hospital in the United States. *Cancer* 1999; 86:1867-1876.

[232] Cannistra SA. When is a "Prognostic factor" really prognostic? *J Clin Oncol* 2000; 18:3745-3747.

[233] Cox G et al. Angiogenesis and non-small cell lung cancer. *Lung Cancer* 2000; 27:81-100.

[234] Yano S et al. Molecular mechanisms of angiogenesis in non-small cell lung cancer, and therapeutics targeting related molecules. *Cancer Sci* 2003; 94:479-485.

[235] Passalidou E et al. Vascular phenotype in angiogenic and non-angiogenic lung non-small cell carcinomas. *Br J Cancer* 2002; 86:244-249.

[236] Almeida BM et al. A novel lamina lucida component of epithelial and endothelial basement membranes detected by LH39 monoclonal antibody. *J Pathol* 1992;166:243-253.

[237] Almeida BM et al. The distribution of LH39 basement membrane epitope in tumour stroma of oral squamous cell carcinomas. *J Pathol* 1992; 166:369-374.

[238] Kakolyris S et al. Relationship of vascular maturation in breast cancer blood vessels to vascular density and metastasis, assessed by expression of a novel basement membrane component, LH39. *Br J Cancer* 2000; 82:844-851.

[239] Kakolyris S et al. Assessment of vascular maturation in non small cell lung cancer using a novel basement membrane component, LH39: correlation with p53 and angiogenic factor expression.*Cancer Res* 1999; 59:5602-5607.

[240] Offerson B et al. Patterns of angiogenesis in non-small cell lung carcinoma. *Cancer* 2001; 91:1500-1509.

[241] Wiesener MS et al. Constitutive activation of hypoxia-inducible genes related to overexpression of hypoxia-inducible factor-1α in clear cell renal carcinomas. *Cancer Res* 2001; 61:5215-5222.

[242] Sardari Nia P et al. Distinct angiogenic and non-angiogenic growth patterns of lung metastases from renal cell carcinoma. *Eur Surg Res* 2003; 35:216-217 (Abstract).

[243] Sardari Nia P et al. Growth patterns of pulmonary metastases of renal cell carcinoma and colorectal adenocarcinoma are distinct in angiogenesis. *Eur J Cancer*: Abstract Book; ECCO 11, 2001 Abstract number 132.

[244] P Sardari Nia et al. Growth patterns (GP) of non-small-cell lung carcinoma (NSCLC) can be used as markers of angiogenesis and have a prognostic value. *Eur Surg Res* 2003; 35:216, Abstract.

[245] P Sardari Nia et al. Growth index is dependent of microvessel density in non-small-cell lung carcinomas. *Human Pathology* 2003; 34: 959-960.

In: Focus on Lung Cancer Research
Editor: Robert L. Carafaro, pp. 161-191

ISBN 1-59454-082-9

Chapter V

LABORATORY VARIABLES AND STRATIFICATION OF LUNG CANCER PATIENTS: RECOMMENDATIONS FOR THE FUTURE (THERAPEUTIC TRIALS AND CLINICAL PRACTICE GUIDELINES)

Joseph Watine[1,*], Bruno Friedberg[2] and Jean-Christophe Charet[3]
Laboratoires de Biologie Polyvalente des Centres Hospitaliers Généraux de [1]Rodez, et de [2]Wissembourg, France, [3]Service de Pneumologie, Centre Hospitalier Général de Rodez.

ABSTRACT

Objective

To identify, through a systematic review of the literature, the laboratory variables that, in addition to performance status and to stage or extent of the disease, would allow a more accurate stratification of lung cancer patients who participate in chemotherapy trials, with or without radiotherapy. Secondary aim: to compare the results of our systematic review with the recommendations made in current clinical practice guidelines.

* Corresponding author: Joseph WATINE, Laboratoire de Biologie Polyvalente, Hôpital Général, F-12027 Rodez Cédex 9, France. Tel: +33.(0)5.65.75.15.60 - Fax: +33.(0)5.65.75.19.73 - j.watine@ch-rodez.fr - watine61@hotmail.Member of the C-EBLM, EMD, IFCC-LM., *IFCC-LM, Committee on Evidence-Based Laboratory Medicine of the Education and Management Division of the International Federation of Clinical Chemistry and Laboratory Medicine.*

Method

Update of two recently published systematic reviews, without meta-analysis, following the recommendations of the *International Federation of Clinical Chemistry and Laboratory Medicine*, and taking into account the *Consolidated Standards of Reporting Trials* statement.

Results

Of 1143 publications retrieved, our exclusion and inclusion criteria allowed us to include 26 studies in our review, of which 12 evaluated small-cell lung (SCLC) cancer patients, and 14 evaluated non-small-cell lung (NSCLC) cancer patients. The three variables which were the most often found significant in multivariate statistical analysis, were: pre-therapeutic levels of laboratory variables (12/12 in SCLC, and 14/14 in NSCLC), performance status (11/12 in SCLC, and 13/13 in NSCLC), and degree of tumour invasion (9/9 in SCLC, and 14/14 in NSCLC). The recommendations made in the eight clinical practice guidelines that we retrieved, are often vague regarding laboratory variables, and sometimes they contradict each others.

Conclusion

Available evidence supports the recommendation that the following pre-treatment laboratory variables should be systematically measured in order to stratify patients in therapeutic trials: in SCLC: serum LDH, and perhaps alkaline phosphatase, sodium, and white blood cell counts; in NSCLC: blood hemoglobin, white blood cell counts with differencial, serum LDH, albumin, calcium, and NSE. Further studies would be necessary to support the addition to this list, of other tumour markers (Cyfra 21-1 for example), and/or measurements during or after treatment. Outside the particular context of therapeutic trials, blood hemoglobin would be the only laboratory variable which could be recommended on a routine basis, but only in case of NSCLC treated with radiotherapy (three studies out of three). The possible consequences in terms of therapeutic choices of systematic hemoglobin measurements remain however to be clarified (blood transfusion or not? erythropoïetin infusion or not? at which level of hemoglobin?). Our recommendations are more in agreement with the recommendations made in the clinical practice guidelines that use evidence-based methods than with the guidelines that do not.

Key words: lung cancer, clinical practice guidelines, therapeutic trials, laboratory variables, survival, prognosis, stratification, staging, laboratory variables, LDH, ALP, blood cell counts, hemoglobin, albumin, calcium, NSE, Cyfra 21-1.

Introduction

Lung cancer is the first cause of death by cancer, at least in men. There are two main types of lung cancer: small-cell lung cancer (SCLC), and non small-cell lung cancer (NSCLC). In NSCLC, surgery can offer the patients a reasonable chance of long term survival, but unfortunately it can only offer this to the most limited stages of the disease, which are but the minority. In more advanced stages of NSCLC, as well as in SCLC, chemotherapy, alone, or associated with radiotherapy, remain the only therapeutic option. These therapies mostly aim to prolong patients survival, but the majority of the patients relapse. Both in SCLC and in NSCLC, no standard therapeutic schemes exist in many settings [1-3].

This is why controlled trials are required to assess the potential contribution of new drugs and new therapeutic schemes, and there should be as many patients as possible included in these trials [4]. In these trials, it is most difficult to demonstrate the superiority of a given protocol over another if you cannot compare the prognostic features of different patient groups. Consequently, independent prognostic factors must be identified before valid therapeutic trials can be designed, conducted and interpreted [5]. Also, the medical and scientific communities have focussed on developing quality methods for therapeutic trials, in particular those methods that are used to stratify patients [6].

Two prognostic co-variables are universally used in lung cancer patients in this context: disease stage in NSCLC, or extent of the disease in SCLC, and performance status [1-3]. Among other prognostic co-variables that can be used for the stratification of lung cancer patients, some authors use patients' age and gender, and, to a lesser extent, laboratory variables. The problem is: a) there is no general agreement regarding the independent prognostic significance of laboratory variables, and, b) not all authors propose the same laboratory tests [7-13]. Thus, in two systematic reviews that we published several years ago [12, 13], we tried to answer the question of whether or not laboratory variables should be used as additional staging variables in lung cancer patients. Our conclusion was that it remained to be demonstrated whether the "new" tests (Cyfra 21-1, NSE or other tumor markers) would be superior to the "old" tests (hemoglobin, blood cell counts, LDH, albumin, calcium, sodium...) for such a purpose. The studies included in these reviews, however, were extremely heterogeneous; in particular, the prognostic significance of laboratory variables had been evaluated for very diverse reasons and often in limited subgroups of patients. This, together with the fact that new primary studies, as well as new clinical practice guidelines, have been published on this topic over the last few years, led us to update our previous systematic review, using more selective inclusion criteria in order to try to answer a more precise question, *i.e.*: which laboratory variables could or should be used to stratify lung cancer patients who participate in therapeutic trials? The secondary aim of our study is to compare the conclusions of the present updated systematic review with current clinical practice guidelines on the subject.

MATERIALS AND METHODS

General Methodology

The guidelines proposed by the Committee on Evidence-Based Laboratory Medicine of the International Federation of Clinical Chemistry and Laboratory Medicine were used for the literature review [14, 15]; we also had in mind the Consolidated Standards of Reporting Trials group [6]. The manual and electronic search strategies used were published in our previous reviews on the topic [12, 13]. Because of the very heterogeneous nature of the studies reviewed (to be explained below in the "Results" and in the "Discussion" sections), a meta-analysis would not have provided valid information.

Inclusion and Exclusion Criteria

Criteria used for study inclusion were the following: articles considering either NSCLC or SCLC patients treated with chemotherapy and/or radiotherapy, full-length original articles written in English, French, Italian, or German (the only languages understood, each by two co-authors at least), studies which evaluated the prognostic significance, in terms of overall survival, of pre-therapeutic laboratory variables which can be measured in biological fluids, studies using multivariate analysis (*i.e.* at least one Cox model [16], the most frequently used statistical model, and by far) taking into account at least performance status and stage of the disease (or disease extent), and in which at least one laboratory variable was measured in more than 50% of the patients.

The following exclusion criteria were used: abstracts, duplicate articles, and studies reporting less than 100 patients in the case of NSCLC, or less than 400 patients in the case of SCLC. Finally, in light of our objective, the only studies included in the final analysis were those which evaluated at least one laboratory variable with a demonstrated independent prognostic value in at least one study meeting our other inclusion criteria.

The first and corresponding author for this review read and classed by categories all the included or excluded studies and wrote the present paper. During this process, he regularly asked for advice to his co-authors. The first and second co-authors, read and extracted the data from all the included articles. Disagreements between co-authors were settled in discussions involving the three co-authors.

Laboratory Methods Used

We identified studies in which the pre-analytical and/or analytical methods used to measure laboratory variables were described, either in part or totally. Pre-analytical methodology included patient preparation (duration of fasting state, with or without infusions, etc.), time of blood sampling, sampling material and methods, mode and duration of sample transportation, any storage in the laboratory before assay, any methods used for separation or preservation of the plasma and/or serum samples before assay. Analytical methods corresponded to assay methods used by the laboratory. These methods were termed as "totally described" when the pre-analytical and analytical methods were detailed sufficiently in the article to allow an independent team to reproduce the methodology with precision.

RESULTS

Results of the Twenty Six Studies Included

Among the 1143 publications analysed, only 12 SCLC studies [17-28], and 14 NSCLC studies [29-42] were finally included in the present updated systematic review, 17 of which had been included in our previous systematic reviews. The full list of the 1143 publications is available upon request to the corresponding author.

None of the numerous excluded or included studies examined the independent prognostic value of a laboratory variable assayed in a biological fluid other than blood. The pre-analytical methods used for the laboratory analyses were never totally detailed. The methodologies of the laboratory techniques were never described in detail, except perhaps in one NSCLC study, and only in the case of a tumour marker [40]. A similar situation was observed in the case of pathology variables. In the same way, there are often many more "missing data" with laboratory variables, than with performance status, disease stage, or similar more clinical variables.

The characteristic features of the patients included in the 12 SCLC studies, or in the 14 NSCLC studies, are summarised in Tables 1, and 2, respectively, together with the thresholds that were used for some of the evaluated variables. These thresholds were very heterogeneous, varying from one article to another, not only for the laboratory variables, but also for the non-laboratory variables. Let us note that, in Tables 1 and 2, diverse mistakes in the original articles have been corrected. For example, the threshold for hemoglobin was 12g/mL in Fukuoka et *al.*'s [29], 11mg/dL in Shinkai et *al.*'s and in Sugiura et *al.*'s [36, 38]. The correct unit for such figures could hardly be anything else than g/dL.

Only one of the 26 included studies analysed a laboratory variable as a continuous variable [22]. None of the studies evaluated the kinetics of a laboratory variable. Only two of these 26 studies (one SCLC study and one NSCLC study) analysed the prognostic significance of laboratory variables that were measured during and after therapy [23, 29]. Only two studies [23, 29] used different statistical models to evaluate separately variables which are available before treatment and those available after, *e.g.* therapeutic responses.

The variables found to be significant in at least one of the 12 SCLC studies, or one of the 14 NSCLC studies, are indicated in tables 3, and 4, respectively. No factor was found to have an independent prognostic significance in all the studies.

1) In the Case of SCLC (Table 3)

Among the factors that were evaluated in more than half of the 12 included studies, the three ones that were found to be the most often significant, with the most significant p values or hazard ratios, were: tumour invasion (9/9, *i.e.* 100%), whether this invasion was evaluated *via* disease extent (7/8, *i.e.* 88%), nodal status, presence of pleural effusion, number of metastatic sites, and/or presence of liver, or bone, or brain, or mediastinal metastases; performance status (11/12, *i.e.* 92%), and pre-therapeutic LDH levels (8/9, *i.e.* 89%) (table 3). Five other factors were found to be often significant, but less so, and with less significant p values or hazard ratios: chemotherapy regimen (3/6, *i.e.* 50%), patient gender (5/10, *i.e.* 50%), pre-therapeutic white blood cell count (3/7, *i.e.* 43%), patient age (3/9, *i.e.* 34%), and pre-therapeutic ALP levels (3/9, i.e. 34%) (table 3). Considering all laboratory variables together, all of the studies (100%) concluded that this type of variable had independent prognostic significance. Apart from the three tests mentioned above (*i.e.* LDH, ALP, and white blood cell count), sodium (2/5, *i.e.* 40%) was the only other laboratory variable whose prognostic value was evaluated and demonstrated in more than one study. One study found that NSE performs better than LDH and ALP for prediction of patient survival [22]. Therapeutic responses were found to be significant in the only study that evaluated their independent prognostic value [23].

2) In the Case of NSCLC (Table 4)

Among the variables which were frequently evaluated in the 14 included studies, three were always "significant" in multivariate statistical analysis: performance status (13/13), tumour invasion (14/14) (this invasion being evaluated *via* TNM classification, disease extent, number of metastatic sites, hepatic, bone, or skin metastases, or pleural effusion), and pre-therapeutic levels of laboratory variables (14/14). However, no individual laboratory variable was unanimously found "significant" in the 14 studies included, except perhaps if we distinguish the studies according to the therapies given to the patients. Indeed, blood hemoglobin and NSE were respectively found "significant" in three studies evaluating patients treated with radiotherapy [33, 41, 42], and in two studies evaluating patients treated with chemotherapy [31, 35]. Therapeutic responses were found "significant" in the two studies [29, 32] that evaluated their independent prognostic value.

Recommendations Made in Clinical Practice Guidelines

During our manual and electronic searches, we retrieved eight clinical practice guidelines that addressed the topic [43-50]. In Tables 5, and 6, we summarise the recommendations which are made in these eight guidelines, regarding laboratory variables, and the results of our own systematic review, in SCLC, and in NSCLC respectively. In these tables, the term "unclear recommendation" refers to the fact that either the clinical decisions that would have to be made based on the results of the recommended laboratory investigations were not precisely specified, or that the names of the recommended laboratory variables themselves were not specified (*e.g.* "*Biochemistry* tests" is not clear to us), or that the level of evidence does not allow to recommend, or not to recommend the measurement. The recommendations from the eight guidelines are explained a little bit more in detail below.

1) In the Case of SCLC (Table 5)

The Scottish Intercollegiate Guidelines Network (SIGN), or the American College of Chest Physicians (ACCP) recommend the pre-treatment measurements of various laboratory variables for SCLC staging (table 5). Among the tests mentioned in table 5, SIGN stresses the pre-treatment prognostic significance of LDH, sodium, and liver function tests.

Table 1: description of study populations and quantitative thresholds used for statistical analysis in the 12 SCLC studies included

References	**17**	**18**	**19**	**20**	**21**	**22**	**23**	**24**	**25**	**26**	**27**	**28**
Study type[a]	CT(10)	Retros	RCT(1)	RCT(4)	CT(?)	Retros	CT(4)	CT(1)	RCT(6)	CT(4)	Retros	CRT(2)
Number of patients[b]	2580/636	411/320	458/458	407/?	411/411	787/770	1280/1280	484/475	874/746	763/714	614/614	608/487
Extent of disease[c]	ED/LD	ELD	ELD	ELD	ELD	ELD	ELD	ELD	ED/LD	ELD	ED/LD	LD
Previous therapy	R	no	no	no	no	?	no?	no	no or S	no?	no?	no?
Gender (% Male)	71		66	64	71.5	59-95	90	63	72	90	71	63
Mean or median age (years)			≤75			62	60	61-63			60	
Patients with pre-treatment LDH	?	?		?	351	560		475	799	577	288	
Patients with pre-treatment ALP	?	?		?	404	?	?		819	728	591	
Patients with pre-treatment NSE						770						
Years of inclusion	76-88	82-88	85-89	79-85	73-87		83-92	85-91	73-81	82-93	74-86	81-88
Year of publication	1990	1990	1993	1987	1990	1996	1995	1996	1986	2000	1991	1996
Countries/Study centers(n)	USA/>1	UK/1	UK/21	UK/1	USA/>1	6/9	F/≥37	2/5	DK/2	2/>10	2/4	Can/>1
Survivors after 2 years (%)			7-9					9-16			9.8	
Survivors after 5 years (%)	3-26							3-6			2.3	
Mean or median survival (months)	6.9-17.7		7.4-8.8			8.8	9.4			10.3	10	
Quantitative thresholds												
Age (years)	70	60-66							60	60	70	70
Performance status	0-1[d]	0-3[d]	0-4[d]	60[f]	0-4	80		0-1[d]	0-4	80[f]	0-1[e]	0-1[d]
Number of metastases	1				0-3					1	1	

Table 1: description of study populations and quantitative thresholds used for statistical analysis in the 12 SCLC studies included (Continued)

References	**17**	**18**	**19**	**20**	**21**	**22**	**23**	**24**	**25**	**26**	**27**	**28**
LDH (U/L)	N	362-512		450	200	N		Nx2	N	200	175-275	N
ALP (U/L)	N	90-130		165	103	N	N		N	110	N	
GGT (U/L)		30-70										
Sodium (mmol/L)		135-139		132			135		136		135	
Chlore (mmol/L)		97-101										
Bicarbonates (mmol/L)				24								
Uric acid (mmol/L) (or mg/dL)									.20			
Albumin (g/L)		37.6-41.5										
Hemoglobin (g/dL)	10						N		12	12-18	12	
WBC (G/mL)		7.75-9.75	10				12.5		10	10	10	
Neutrophils (G/mL) (or %)		5.5-8.5								(75)		
Platelets (G/mL)											150	
NSE (ng/mL)						12.5						

Legend: Study type[a]: CT=Chemotherapy Trial, RCT=Chemo-Radiotherapy Trial (n= number of different trials in the study), S= Surgery; Retros= Retrospective study (in Allan et al.'s, most patients had been included in CTs); Number of patients[b] = Total number of patients in the series/Number of patients taken into account in the multivariate statistical analysis that took into account laboratory variables; Extent of disease[c]: ED/LD= extensive disease and limited disease evaluated separately; ELD= extensive disease and limited disease evaluated together; Pre-treatment LDH, ALP, NSE: ?= numbers not provided whereas the prognostic significance of the variable was evaluated; Performance status = SWOG/WHO[d], ECOG[e], Karnofsky[f]; N= normal versus abnormal values.

Table 2: description of study populations and quantitative thresholds used for statistical analysis in the 14 NSCLC studies included

references	29	30	31	32	33	34	35	36	37	38	39	40	41	42
number of patients	203	411	261	378	456	1052	274	192	259	197	185	203	502	210
years of inclusion	86-88	84-90	75-92	78-84	87-90	80-91	90-98	82-89 (?)	81-85	89-93	85-94	?	74-81	89-93
stages	III-IV	IIIB, IV	III-IV	III	I-IV		IV	III-IV	III-IV	IIIB-IV	III-IV	III-IV	I-III	I-III
previous therapy	no	no	no	yes	no		no	no	yes or no	no (?)	no	yes or no	yes or no	yes or no
study type[a]	random	prosp.	non random	non random	retro.	random	prosp.	non random	random.	retro.	retro.	retro.	retro.	retro.
P.S.[b]	<3 (ECOG)	0-4 (Zubrod)	0-3 (ECOG)	60-100% (Karnofsky)	0-4 (ECOG)	Karnofsky		<3 (ECOG)	50-100% (Karnofsky)	0-4 (ECOG)	<4	0-4 (ECOG)	Karnofsky	Karnofsky
therapy[c]	chemo	diverse	chemo	chemo	radio	chemo	diverse	chemo	chemo	?	chemo and/or radio	diverse	radio	radio
quantitative threshhold														
tumour size													4 and 7 cm	7 cm
number of metastatic sites			3											
age (years)		45												
hemoglobin (g/dL)	12	12	12		12,7	12 and 18		11	12	11	11		12,5	12,5
leucocytes (1000/mm3)		10	9		16,5	10	10		9		10			
neutrophiles		8000/mm3			4950/mm3	75%								
lymphocytes (1000/mm3)	2	1,5			2			1,5						
platelets (1000/mm3)			150		422	440			400					
protides (g/L)		66		74,2										
albumin (g/L)	35	35	35		35		32	37		40	35			

Table 2: description of study populations and quantitative thresholds used for statistical analysis in the 14 NSCLC studies included (Continued)

references	29	30	31	32	33	34	35	36	37	38	39	40	41	42
calcium			10 mg/dL		2,6 mmol/L	10,3 mg/dL					10,5 mg/dL			
LDH[d] (U/L)	?	320	?	230	200	200	600	350	450	380	?	300		
ALP[e] (U/L)		90	?		120	110	125	230				100		
creatinin	1,5 mg/mL				6,9	10								
CEA[f] (ng/mL)	5		5		20			5 and 20			?			
NSE[g] (ng/mL)			10				12,5							

Legends: study type[a]: random.= randomised trial; prosp./retro.= prospective/ retrospective; P.S.[b]: performance status; ECOG=Eastern Cooperative Oncology Group Scale; therapy[c]: chemo= chemotherapy, radio= radiotherapy, diverse= chemo and/or radio, or palliative; LDH[d]: *lactate dehydrogenase*; ALP[e]: alkaline phosphatase; CEA[f]: Carcino-Embryonic Antigen; NSE[g]: *Neuron-Specific Enolase.*

Table 3: prognostic significance of various factors in the 12 SCLC studies included

References	17	18	19	20	21	22	23		24	25	26	27	28
							Pre-*	Post-*					
Patient gender	.004[a]			NS	.03	NS	NS		NS	<.001[a]	.02	NS	.0001[a]
Patient age		.002		NS	NS	NS	.0007		NS	<.001[b]		NS	NS
Weight loss				NS								NS	
Performance status	.002[a]	.004	1-4.55	.0121	<.0001	1.63	<.0001	.0004	<.001	<.001	<.001	.0002 .0099[b]	NS
Extent of disease	S*	<.0001	1-1.92	.0001	NS	1.26	.04	.001			<.001		
Nodal status												NS	
Metastatic sites (n)												.0004	
Liver metastasis					.0065		.03					NS	
Mediastinal metastasis												<.0001	
Brain metastasis					NS		.004	.03				.0412	
Bone metastasis												.0222	
Effusion	.051[a]			NS								NS	
Dysphagia			0.92-1.35	NS									
Study 8269	.005[a]												
Study 8606	.0008[b]												
Chemotherapy regimen		NS	NS	NS	.0047				.03	<.001[b]			
Therapeutic response								<.0001					

Table 3: prognostic significance of various factors in the 12 SCLC studies included (Continued)

References	17	18	19	20	21	22	23		24	25	26	27	28
LDH	<.00005[a] .0006[b]	.0001		<.0001	.0003	NS			<.001	<.001		.0472 .0078[a]	.0033[a]
ALP	NS	NS		.0186	.0015	NS	.0002	.0002		NS	NS	NS	
GGT		NS		NS									
Sodium		NS		.0009			NS	NS		.05[a]		NS	
Chlore		NS		NS									
Bicarbonates				.0321									
Uric acid										.05[a]			
Albumin		NS											
Hemoglobin	NS	NS		NS			NS	NS		<.01	NS	NS	
WBC		.01	1-1.93	NS			.0005	NS		NS	NS	NS	
Neutrophil count		NS									.05		
Platelet count												.0286	
NSE						1.24							

Legend: See Table 1; Pre-*, Post-*= pre- and post-treatment analysis (2nd chemotherapy session); [a,b]p values (or hazard ratios [22] or relative ratios [19]) for significant variables in the Cox multivariate statistical analysis that took into account laboratory variables, P.S., and disease extent, [a]significant in limited disease only, [b]significant in extensive disease only, S= significant in the multivariate analysis but p values or ratios not provided; NS = not significant in either univariate or multivariate analysis; Extent of disease: S*= S but limited and extensive diseases evaluated separately.

Table 4: prognostic significance of various factors in the 14 NSCLC studies included

references	29		30	31	32	33	34	35	36	37	38	39	40	41	42
	pre-	post-													
response		0,0000[a]			<0,001										
previous therapy					NS					0,0003					NS
stage	0,0000	0,0001	0,000	US		<0.001			US[b]	0,015	<0,0001	0,000209	<0,001	1,38 (1,13-1,67)	1,97 (1,36-2,84)
T status								US			NS				
tumour size														1,44 (1,14-1,82)	1,60 (1,11-2,30)
N status								0,024			0,0102				
disease extent							<0,0001		US	NS					
pleural effusion											0,0481				US
number of metastatic sites				US	<0,001				0,0002						
liver metastases				0,0014	NS[c]				US	0,025		US			
bone metastases				0,0008	US				US	US		US			
bone marrow metastases															
skin metastases							0,008								
histology	NS[c]	NS	NS	US	NS	NS		NS	NS		NS	NS	0,02		NS
P.S.	0,0009	0,0003	0,000	0,0001	<0,001		0,0003	0,0001	0,0026	<0,0001	<0,0001	<0,000001	<0,001	1,38 (1,13-1,69)	1,88 (1,35-2,63)
weight loss	0,0144	0,0057	0,000		NS	NS		US	US	US	US	NS	NS		US
sex	0,0076	0,0101	0,023	US	0,001	NS	0,03	NS	0,0009	NS	NS	NS	NS		NS
age	NS	NS	NS	US	NS	NS	0,02	NS	NS	NS	NS	NS	NS		NS
hemoglobin	0,0165	0,0445	US[b]	NS		0.006	US		NS	US	US	0,000001		1,36 (1,07-1,73)	1,35 (0,99-1,83)
leucocytes			US	NS		NS	0,0003	US		0,01		US			
neutrophiles			US			NS	0,02								
lymphocytes	US	US	0.012			0.008			NS						
albumin	US	US	(0.000)[d]	0,0037					0,0018		0,0149	US			

Table 4: prognostic significance of various factors in the 14 NSCLC studies included (Continued)

references	29		30	31	32	33	34	35	36	37	38	39	40	41	42
calcium				US		US	0,007					0,000799			
LDH	US	US	(0.040) [d]	US	<0,001	0.035			0,0026	<0,0001	US	US	US		
ALP				US		NS		NS	US	NS		US	US		
GGT[e]						0.032							NS		
GOT[f]				NS		US				0,025					
ACE	NS[c]	NS		NS		US			NS			NS			
TPS[g]													<0,001		
Cyfra 21-1								0,016							
NSE				<0,0001				0,0001							
symptoms			US							US				1,35 (1,09-1,68)	1,87 (1,34-2,60)
hoarseness			0.007												

Legend: see Table 2; [a]p values (or hazard ratios, with confidence intervals) for significant variables in the Cox multivariate statistical analysis that took into account laboratory variables, P.S. and disease extent, [a]significant in limited disease only, [b]significant in extensive disease only, S= significant in the multivariate analysis but p values or ratios not provided; NS = not significant in either univariate or multivariate analysis;; US[b]: uncertain significance, found to be significant ($p<0,05$) in univariate statistical analysis only; NS[c]: not significant; [d]: only the results of variables measured in more than 95% of the patients are mentioned in this table, except for the variables found significant in multivariate analysis; GGT[e]: *gamma glutamyl transpeptidase*; GOT[f]: *glutamic oxaloacetic transaminase*; TPS[g]: *Tissue Polypeptide Specific Antigen*.

Table 5: recommended laboratory variables in four different medical guidelines for the pre-treatment prognostic evaluation (and/or for the staging) of SCLC patients, compared with our own recommendations regarding therapeutic trials

Experts	Recommended	Unclear recommendation	Not recommended
SIGN [46]	LDH, liver function tests, sodium	other *Biochemistry* and haematology tests (not specified)	None
ACCP [47]	Complete blood counts, electrolytes, bun, creatinine, liver function tests, LDH	other *Biochemistry* tests (not specified)	None
EGTM [44]	NSE, Cyfra 21-1	None	None
SPLF [49]	None	None	NSE
Us	LDH	ALP, sodium, white blood cell counts	None

Legend: SCLC= small cell lung cancer; SIGN= Scottish Intercollegiate Guidelines Network; ACCP= American College of Chest Physicians; EGTM= European Group on Tumour Markers; SPLF= Société de Pneumologie de Langue Française; LDH= lactate dehydrogenase; ALP= Alkaline Phosphatase; NSE= Neuron-Specific Enolase; Cyfra 21-1= Fragments of Cytokeratin 19.

Table 6: recommended laboratory variables in seven different medical guidelines for the pre-treatment prognostic evaluation (and/or for the staging) of NSCLC patients, compared with our own recommendations regarding therapeutic trials

Experts	Recommended	Unclear recommendation	Not recommended
SIGN [46]	ALP	other *Biochemistry* and haematology tests (not specified)	None
ATS-ERS [43]	blood counts, electrolytes, albumin, calcium, ALP, transaminases, bilirubin, creatinine	None	Tumor markers
ACCP [48]	Hematocrit, ALP, calcium, GGT, SGOT	other routine laboratory tests (not specified)	None
ASCO [50]	ALP, calcium	hemoglobin, white blood cell counts, LDH	None
FNCLCC [45]	hemoglobin, white blood cell counts with differencial, LDH, albumin, and calcium	None	Tumor markers
EGTM [44]	Cyfra 21-1, CEA*	CA 125, TPA	None
SPLF [49]	None	Cyfra 21-1	CEA
Us	hemoglobin, white blood cell counts with differencial, LDH, albumin, calcium, NSE	None	None

Legend: NSCLC= non-small cell lung cancer; SIGN= Scottish Intercollegiate Guidelines Network; ATS-ERS= American Thoracic Society and European Respiratory Society; ACCP= American College of Chest Physicians; ASCO= American Society of Clinical Oncology; FNCLCC= Fédération Nationale des Centres de Lutte Contre le Cancer; ACCP= American College of Chest Physicians; EGTM= European Group on Tumour Markers; SPLF= Société de Pneumologie de Langue Française; LDH= lactate dehydrogenase; ALP= Alkaline Phosphatase; GGT= Gamma-Glutamyl Transferase; SGOT= Glutamic-Oxaloacetic Transpeptidase; Cyfra 21-1= Fragments of Cytokeratin 19; CEA= Carcino-Embryonic Antigen; *only in case of adeno or large cell carcinoma; CA 125= Cancer Antigen 125; TPA= Tissue-Polypeptide Antigen; NSE= Neuron-Specific Antigen.

The "Société de Pneumologie de Langue Française" (SPLF), and the European Group on Tumour Markers (EGTM) focussed on tumour markers only. SPLF considers the level of scientific evidence of Neuron-Specific Enolase (NSE), as being "not sufficient" for staging, prognosis, or surveillance of SCLC. EGTM recommends the measurements of NSE and of Cyfra 21-1 before therapy and during the post-therapy follow-up in SCLC patients. EGTM also stresses the independent prognostic value of NSE in SCLC.

2) In the Case of NSCLC (Table 6)

ACCP, or SIGN, or the American Society of Clinical Oncology (ASCO), or the American Thoracic Society and the European Respiratory Society (ATS-ERS), or the "Fédération Nationale des Centres de Lutte Contre le Cancer" (FNCLCC) recommend the pre-treatment measurement of various laboratory variables for the staging of NSCLC patients (table 6). Among these variables, ATS-ERS stresses the pre-treatment prognostic significance of serum albumin and, to a lesser extent, that of serum calcium, particularly in case of advanced disease, whereas SIGN, or ASCO stress the pre-treatment prognostic significance of LDH, sodium, liver function tests (SIGN), or LDH, hemoglobin, white blood cell counts (ASCO).

ATS-ERS and FNCLCC do not recommend the routine measurements of any other laboratory variable than those mentioned in table 6, including serum tumour markers, in NSCLC patients. Except for NSE, the list of laboratory variables whose pre-treatment prognostic value is stressed by FNCLCC, is the same as ours (Table 6).

SPLF and EGTM focussed on tumour markers only. SPLF classifies two tumour markers in NSCLC, *i.e.* Carcino-Embryonic Antigen (CEA) and Cyfra 21-1, according to their levels of scientific evidence. SPLF considers the CEA level as "not sufficient", neither for prognosis, nor for staging, nor for surveillance, whereas the Cyfra 21-1 level of evidence is considered "sufficient", but for prognosis only. EGTM recommends the measurements of Cyfra 21-1 before therapy and during the post-therapy follow-up in NSCLC patients, and also of CEA in case of adeno or large cell carcinoma. EGTM also stresses the independent prognostic value of not only Cyfra 21-1 and CEA, but also of CA 125, and stresses the value, as a tool for monitoring therapy efficacy in NSCLC, not only of Cyfra 21-1 and CEA, but also of Tissue-Polypeptide Antigen (TPA).

DISCUSSION

Rationale for Our Exclusion and Inclusion Criteria

We included only those publications analysing the patients survival (and not those which only evaluated recurrence-free survival or therapeutic responses) because some variables may help to predict or reflect therapeutic response without being able to independently predict outcome, and because survival is the most (and perhaps only) objective outcome (and also probably the most important one for most of the patients). What is more, a laboratory variable which is not correlated to survival is likely to be of limited value in order to stratify patients in therapeutic trials.

In the present updated systematic review, we chose to exclude studies with a population of less than 100 NSCLC patients since small series must be interpreted with caution even if they reach statistical significance. In the case of SCLC, we chose to exclude studies with less than 400 patients because the inclusion of smaller series of SCLC patients, as we did in our previous systematic reviews [12, 13], would not have significantly changed our conclusions, but would have resulted in at least two additional large tables in the present paper.

We only considered variables that can be measured in biological fluids, and not those variables which are measured in tissues, the so-called pathology variables, not only because pathology variables imply more aggressive procedures to the patients, but also because pathology variables are less easily measured again during and after treatment than classical laboratory variables.

In systematic reviews, the choice of inclusion criteria is crucial. Indeed, it is equally necessary to include as many studies as possible, and to exclude biased studies. In the current state of the literature, it would be almost impossible for an independent team to precisely reproduce the analytical and pre-analytical methodologies used in the 26 studies that we reviewed - a basic principle of good science. We could therefore be criticised because all studies included in our review did not respect this basic principle. However, if we had excluded such studies from our review, no study at all would have remained. What is more, even if most clinicians do not realise the importance of this, scientifically speaking, all their studies cannot be considered completely worthless just for this particular reason. This nevertheless suggests that laboratory specialists are not really involved in these studies. This impression is reinforced by the two other following facts: (i) big mistakes are made in some of these studies regarding units of laboratory variables (some examples are given in the "Results" section); (ii) among the included patients, there were often (many) more missing data with laboratory variables than with some other, more clinical, variables; (iii) except in the case of studies evaluating tumour markers, laboratory specialists were not frequently associated with co-authorship (even if the definitions of the various specialities vary from country to country). This issue will be further discussed below.

Despite the fact that our inclusion criteria were not extremely rigorous, many studies could not be included, even if some of them might be seen by some "experts" as very "prestigious". Among such "prestigious" excluded studies, one could cite, for example, the RTOG study [51] which was excluded because it did not fulfil the two following inclusion criteria: no Cox model was used in the statistical analysis, and the number of patients in whom laboratory variables were or were not measured was not indicated. This latter reason for exclusion was one of the most frequent one. Also, despite the fact that Dische *et al.*, or Wilhelm *et al.*'s studies [52, 53] demonstrated the prognostic value of hemoglobin in irradiated NSCLC patients (and thus supported our final conclusions), both these studies were excluded because they did not use multivariate statistical analysis. This reason for exclusion was also a frequent one. Among the many studies which were excluded because they evaluated less than 400 SCLC patients, we shall discuss a little bit more in detail Johnson *al.*'s, Maetsu *et al.*'s, and Quoix *et al.*'s [11, 54, 55] in the sections below. We also excluded the study of Rawson *et al.* [56] because it evaluated some patients who had also been included in Cerny *et al.*'s study [20], and because, as far as laboratory variables are concerned, data of this latter study were clearer, and therefore easier to be extracted, than those of Rawson *et al.* [56].

In fact, relatively few studies could be included despite our quite permissive inclusion criteria. This is another one of the arguments which stress the insufficient methodological quality of most of the publications available, at least as far as laboratory variables evaluation is concerned [57, 58]. Among the other arguments which would argue in the same way, and which were not mentioned in our previous systematic reviews, we must stress that only two included studies [23, 29] used distinct statistical models to evaluate laboratory variables that are available before therapy, separately from those available after therapy. This distinction is nevertheless fundamental in therapeutic trials. All these arguments, as well as others mentioned below, will lead us to be quite prudent in our conclusions.

How Could We Explain Controversial Results Observed Across the Studies?

As explained above, since we could not use too rigorous inclusion criteria, the 26 studies included do not form a homogeneous group. It would therefore not have been reasonable for us, scientifically speaking, to perform a meta-analysis of these 26 studies. In these conditions, in agreement with the recommendations of the IFCC [14, 15], we had to try to explain the reasons for heterogeneity within the 26 included studies.

The heterogeneous nature of these studies mostly results from their different patients' inclusion or exclusion criteria, the diverse group of prognostic factors or variables evaluated, the proportion of patients in whom the laboratory variables were measured compared with the inclusion population, the treatments used, the year and country of publication, the inclusion period, and the specialities of the co-authors in the different studies. In addition, as already stressed, the methodologies used to measure the laboratory variables are not really indicated in any of the studies. Taking into account the aim of our study, we shall focus here on the heterogeneous results regarding laboratory variables.

Most if not all laboratories are subject to strict quality control measures. Based on this fact, there is a common belief, particularly among non laboratory specialists, that different laboratory methods are unlikely to play a major role in the discrepancies observed across studies [59]. We can indeed understand that physicians do not wish to precisely explore the precise consequences of changing analytical procedures of laboratory tests on their diagnostic, or prognostic accuracies and utilities. However, even if this kind of question is not often explored in the biomedical literature, it has been demonstrated that not only the changing of analytical procedures, but also that of pre-analytical ones, can increase or decrease diagnostic errors [60]. It has even been demonstrated, in another type of cancer, that the level of prognostic significance of a laboratory variable can change depending on the procedures used for its measurements [61].

The simple reading of current results of national quality control surveys (this kind of document is available in all laboratories that participate in such surveys) shows that the results of the measurement of most molecules in the very same sample can vary significantly depending on the different analytical techniques that are used in various laboratories. Not to mention pre-analytical ones, which are known to be an even more important source of variation. Overall, analytical, pre-analytical, or biological events might account for the fact that random variability of more than 50% cannot be ruled out for the laboratory variables used in the 26 studies examined, particularly the multicentric ones. Several examples of such events have been explained and discussed elsewhere [62-64].

Use of threshold levels determined on the basis of unknown criteria could also explain some of the divergences. For an analysis of prognosis, laboratory variables (and also some non-laboratory variables) should probably be best used as continuous variables, but only one of the 26 studies [22] examined this approach. Likewise, even if no study appeared to provide kinetic data on laboratory variables, this other approach should also be used more often [62]. The use of arbitrary thresholds in the multivariate statistical analysis might also account for some of the discrepancies. In the case of LDH for example, these thresholds vary from 175 to 600 U/L (or UI/L) (Tables 1, and 2), whereas the way these thresholds were obtained is often unclear. Taking into account uncertainties already mentioned, as well as inter-assay, circadian or biological variations, it seems clear that arbitrary thresholds should be avoided [65-67].

Which Laboratory Tests Can be Recommended for Future Trials?

In therapeutic trials, prognostic co-variables, that are independent from each other, are indispensable, because, as already stressed in the introduction, the superiority of any given regimen over another can hardly be demonstrated if the prognostic profiles of the subgroups of patients participating in therapeutic trials cannot be compared with each others [5, 6]. In this context, if one wishes to demonstrate that laboratory variables should be used to stratify patients participating in therapeutic trials, in association with other prognostic variables that are currently being routinely used (*e.g.* stage or extent of the disease, and performance status), it is “only” necessary to demonstrate that they have a prognostic value that is independent from these variables. Taking into account the criticisms above, and looking at the overall results whatever the treatment used, is can be noted that 100% of the studies included in this review concluded that laboratory variables had significant independent prognostic value (Tables 3 and 4).

Therefore, the current state of the biomedical literature supports the recommendation that laboratory variables should be systematically measured in order to be used as prognostic co-variables in lung cancer trials. The question is: which particular tests should be recommended?

1) In Case of SCLC (Table 3):

The factors which appeared most frequently and most significantly of prognostic value were factors related to tumour extent (or disease stage), to performance status, and to laboratory variables (table 3). But the results concerning each individual laboratory variables were often quite contradictory, except perhaps for LDH (table 3). It would therefore be in the case of LDH that there are the strongest arguments that support the recommendation that this laboratory variable should be systematically assayed in order to stratify the patients who participate in therapeutic trials:

- overall p values or hazard ratios of LDH in the studies that evaluated this variable, were generally close to those of disease extent, or of performance status, which are the two co-variables whose prognostic value is the most often acknowledged by the medical community [1-3] (table 3)

- the only included study that did not conclude to the independent prognostic value of LDH [22] clearly has several sources of bias. First, in this multicenter study, it was found that NSE, but neither LDH nor ALP, were of independent prognostic significance (table 3), but NSE was measured in all the 770 patients who were taken into account in the statistical analysis, whereas LDH was measured in 560 patients only and the figure for ALP, which was probably even lower, was not provided. Second, the only laboratory method that was indicated in this study was the method used to measure NSE, which was the same (RIA) in all six centres; the authors specify that "there was more variation from centre to centre in the methods used for analysis of LDH and ALP". We can therefore reasonably conclude that the methods used to measure LDH and ALP in this retrospective and multicenter study were less rigorous, scientifically speaking, than the methods used to measure NSE. Therefore, in this study, the superiority of NSE over LDH or ALP cannot be considered as being really established. The study of Quoix *et al.* [11], which also compared the independent prognostic values of ALP, LDH, and NSE, demonstrated that both ALP, and LDH were suitable variables, whereas NSE was not. Quoix *et al.*'s study was not included in our review, because it "only" evaluated 263 patients. Another excluded study also demonstrated that LDH has independent prognostic value in SCLC whereas NSE has not, but NSE was only measured in 48 of the 341 patients evaluated in this study [55]. In fact, among the excluded studies, there is only one full article in which the superiority of NSE over LDH was demonstrated, but this study was excluded because it evaluated 101 patients "only" in its Cox model [54].

Apart from LDH, it seems that ALP, and to a lesser extent, sodium and white blood cell count, might perhaps be the best suited laboratory variables, to be measured together with LDH for the purpose of stratifying the patients in therapeutic trials, because these variables are those that were found significant in more than one study and also because the p values or hazard ratios obtained with these variables were generally quite close to those obtained with patients' age and gender. Nevertheless, taking into account the afore-mentioned criticisms, further studies, and of better methodological quality, would be necessary to clearly support this, particularly for sodium and white blood cell counts. Likewise, available evidence would not support the addition of any other laboratory variables, including NSE, to this list. This does not mean that it would not be worthwhile to evaluate the prognostic significance of other pre-treatment laboratory variables, including NSE, or other tumour markers, e.g. chromogranin A or Cyfra 21 [10], in further studies. In the same way, the potential usefulness of laboratory measurements during and/or after treatment might also be worth being further evaluated. Our list of laboratory variables must therefore be considered as a provisory one.

Although our systematic review was not restricted to English studies, let us note that we had to exclude all studies written in Italian or in German, as well as all but one study written in French [23]. The question is: would our results have been different if our systematic review had been restricted to the English language? Our threshold for recommending any laboratory variable being at least two studies finding this variable "significant", it appears that the exclusion of the only study not written in English [23] would not have changed our conclusions very much, except for the weak strength of recommendation behind ALP and WBC which would have become even weaker. However, this French study [23] is the only SCLC study included which evaluated the prognostic significance of laboratory variables that were measured during and after therapy, and it is also the only SCLC study which used different statistical models to evaluate separately variables which are available before treatment and those available after. Thus we would not fully agree with Moher *et al.* [68] that systematic reviews restricted to studies written in English are not biased.

2) In Case of NSCLC (Table 4):

Here too, it would be difficult to recommend variables which were found "significant" in less than two studies. Thus, in NSCLC, the variables whose pre-treatment measurements we recommend are: serum LDH, albumin, calcium, NSE, and blood cell counts with differencial, and hemoglobin. Some other variables, *e.g.* cyfra 21-1, were "significant" in one of the 14 included studies (Table 4). Let us note however that these latter sorts of variables were evaluated in studies which neglected to include in their multivariate statistical models, either performance status, or two (or more) of the laboratory variables that we recommend above.

The potential usefulness of measurements during and/or after therapy should also perhaps be better evaluated. Our list of recommended laboratory variables in NSCLC must therefore be considered as a provisory, and very general one. For example, we would not have many arguments against the measurements of (activation) markers of coagulation in case of chemotherapy trial with *versus* without anti-coagulant therapy [69].

Comparison of Published Recommendations with Our Own Recommendations

None of the eight guidelines mentioned in Tables 5 and 6 really specified the particular needs of (inoperable) lung cancer patients who participate in therapeutic trials, as compared with the needs of patients treated in routine general practice. It might therefore seem difficult to compare the recommendations made in these guidelines with the results of our own systematic review. Nevertheless, it seems clear that the areas where prognostic laboratory variables can potentially be useful in routine clinical practice, are either the staging of lung cancer patients, or their post-therapy follow-up, also called surveillance, or monitoring. It can also be said that staging is very akin to a pre-treatment prognostic evaluation, whereas post-therapy follow-up is very akin to a post-treatment prognostic evaluation. Thence, the possibility for us to compare the results of our systematic review with the recommendations made in these eight guidelines, but with some limitations, particularly with NSCLC, as indicated below.

Before we make such comparisons, it must also be kept in mind another difference between the patients in routine general practice, and those patients included in therapeutic trials. Indeed, if one wishes to demonstrate that laboratory variables should be used in routine general practice for the pre-treatment staging of the patients, it is necessary not only to demonstrate their independent pre-treatment prognostic value, but also that their results may influence clinical decisions about individual patients. For example, some other authors advise the routine measurements of blood hemoglobin in order for the anaemic NSCLC patients to receive erythrocyte-transfusion, or erythropoietin, before they are given radiation therapy [41, 42]. In order to make such proposals acceptable by all heath-care providers, it must be demonstrated that these particular procedures enable the patients' outcome to improve [70].

In the same way, the demonstration of the independent post-treatment prognostic significance of laboratory variables in lung cancer patients would only be one of the prerequisites to their possible use as a routine tool during the post-therapy follow up or surveillance. The current state of the biomedical literature does not even fulfil this prerequisite, as far as patients' survival is concerned. Therefore, it seems to us, that no laboratory variable can currently be recommended on a routine general basis neither for staging, nor for post-therapy follow-up, nor for surveillance of lung cancer patients, except of course when the question is to evaluate toxicity of, or tolerance to drugs, or radiations, using *e.g.* white blood cell counts, and except also, as will be argued below, for hemoglobin in patients who have to receive radiation therapy.

Finally, let us stress that the guidelines by the SPLF and by EGTM focussed on tumour markers only, and did not try to identify other laboratory variables which would be of value in lung cancer patients.

For all the reasons mentioned above, one must therefore be quite cautious in comparing, as we do below, these guidelines with the results of our systematic review.

1) In the Case of SCLC (Table 5)

The laboratory variables that we propose are quite close to those in the list proposed by SIGN, or by ACCP, which seems logical because SIGN and ACCP used a more or less evidence-based approach, as we did. In addition to the variables recommended by us, SIGN and ACCP also recommend other liver function tests, *Biochemistry* or haematology tests. Such additional tests may be useful in routine general practice, *e.g.* in order to assess patient's tolerance to drugs, or in order to diagnose paraneoplastic syndromes [71], but according to the current state of the literature, we could not say that these additional tests would be useful to better stratify patients in therapeutic trials. But, of course, the main criticism that we would have against the SIGN (and, to a lesser extent, ACCP) guidelines, is that they do not precisely indicate all the names of the laboratory variables that they recommend to measure, and which decisions should be made depending on the results of the laboratory investigations. In our view, this cannot really be called evidence-based laboratory medicine [14].

Regarding tumour markers, our recommendations are in good agreement with those of the SPLF, but we cannot agree with EGTM recommendations. This is not very surprising because the methodology used by SPLF was more evidence-based than the methodology used by EGTM. This adds weight to the recommendation that clinical practice guidelines should be evidence-based rather than be based on experts' opinions [72], particularly since it is well established that guidelines with flawed, or contradictory recommendations, not only can reinforce non compliance, and distrust with guidelines, but also can potentially be harmful [73-76].

2) In the Case of NSCLC (Table 6)

Guidelines from ATS-ERS, ACCP, ASCO, FNCLCC, and SIGN recommend the use of diverse biochemistry, and/or haematology tests for the staging of NSCLC patients. In case of abnormal result(s) in an otherwise resectable (stage IIIA) NSCLC patient, then, according to these guidelines, it is necessary to carefully investigate all putative metastatic sites, because if metastasis are found, the patient would have to be considered unresectable. Moreover, all guidelines do not agree with each others on the necessary laboratory variables in order to achieve this purpose. Other experts (*e.g.* those of EGTM, or of SPLF to a lesser extent) extrapolate this recommendation to Cyfra 21-1 [35, 44, 49]. But, according to our own systematic review, there is more evidence to support this recommendation about routine *Biochemistry* and haematology tests, or even, to a lesser extent about NSE, than about Cyfra 21-1.

According to the SPLF, or EGTM, the independent prognostic value of Cyfra 21-1 is clearly demonstrated in NSCLC, whereas that of NSE is not [44, 49]. However, there is only one study available in which the prognostic value of Cyfra 21-1 was specifically evaluated in non operated NSCLC patients [35]. NSE is the only tumour marker which was found "significant" in this context in more than one study, and its level of significance is higher than that of Cyfra 21-1 in the only study that compared these two markers (table 4) [35]. Since there are many more studies which evaluated usual laboratory tests than tumour markers, SPLF, or EGTM recommendations confirm that some "new" laboratory tests (*i.e.* tumour markers), may be introduced in routine practice before their real value, as compared with that of "old", and less expensive tests, is clearly demonstrated [14, 15, 77].

Both FNCLCC, and us insist on the fact that LDH is a more accurate prognostic variable than ALP in NSCLC, whereas ATS-ERS, ACCP, and SIGN do insist on the opposite; ASCO stands in an intermediate position (table 6). The results of our systematic review might answer this point (table 4).

As already suggested above another point can be made about the case of blood hemoglobin in irradiated NSCLC patients. All available studies suggest that this particular variable does have an independent prognostic value in this particular subgroup of patients (Table 4), supporting its systematic use in therapeutic trials. But, could we propose its systematic use for the staging of the patients in clinical routine practice? Before we can clearly answer this question, we would need to precisely know which decisions could be made depending on which levels of hemoglobin. And then we should decide if we should transfuse the patients with low levels of hemoglobin before they are irradiated, or if the patients should rather be given erythropoietin [70]. ATS-ERS, ACCP, FNCLCC and SIGN recommend the use of blood hemoglobin (or hematocrit) as a staging variable in NSCLC, but the therapeutic choices that would have to be made based on the precise results of blood hemoglobin are not precisely specified in these guidelines; therefore we do not precisely know on which rationale this particular recommendation is based.

Finally, since the list of laboratory variables whose pre-treatment prognostic value is stressed by FNCLCC, is the same as ours, except for NSE, we can hope that, when these experts published their recommendations, they had in their minds the results of our preliminary results which have been widely advertised in French [78, 79]. It seems logical that the FNCLCC experts did not mention NSE in their guidelines because the two studies which support NSE measurements [31, 35] were published after their guidelines. In our opinion, this supports our quite optimistic view regarding the future of evidence-based laboratory medicine in general, and of evidence-based guidelines in particular [14, 72].

CONCLUSION

To conclude our systematic review, and to help improve the performance of future therapeutic trials in lung cancer patients, we propose that the following points should be taken into consideration:

- Pre- and post-therapeutic prognostic factors should be evaluated separately using several multivariate statistical models;
- Precise indications concerning analytical, and pre-analytical methodologies used should be provided; if several different analytical methods are used, these methods should be perfectly correlated;
- Laboratory variables should be considered as continuous variables for statistical analysis and arbitrary threshold levels should be avoided. This latter proposition could also be applied to non-laboratory variables that can be expressed as continuous variables (patient age, or weight loss, for example);
- Whenever possible, the kinetics of the laboratory variables should also be considered;
- Due to the wide variability of potential prognostic markers, each a source of technical bias, it would be desirable to conduct therapeutic trials within the framework of a concerted multidisiplinary approach involving surgeons, clinicians, biostatisticians, biologists, pathologists, and fundamental scientists [80]. The same applies of course to systematic reviews as well as to evidence-based guidelines [72].

REFERENCES

[1] Bruderman I. Bronchogenic Carcinoma. In: Baum GL, Wolinsky E, eds. *Textbook of pulmonary diseases.* Fifth edition. Little, Brown and Company, New-York 1994:1345-92.

[2] Ginsberg RJ. Continuing controversies in staging NSCLC: an analysis of the revised 1997 staging system. *Oncology* 1998; 12(Suppl.2): 51-4.

[3] Ihde DC, Pass HI, Glatstein EJ. Small cell lung cancer. In: De Vita VT, Hellman S, Rosenberg SA, eds. *Cancer. Principles and Practice of Oncology.* Fourth Edition. Philadelphia: JB Lippincott Company, 1993:723-58.

[4] Lebeau B. Analyse bibliographique quantitative de la recherche clinique française en thérapeutique des cancers broncho-pulmonaires. *Rev Mal Respir* 1998; 15:185-9.

[5] Fielding LP, Fenoglio-Preiser CM, Freedman LS. The future of prognostic factors in outcome prediction for patients with cancer. *Cancer* 1992; 70:2367-7.

[6] Moher D, Schulz KF, Altman DG; CONSORT GROUP (Consolidated Standards of Reporting Trials). The CONSORT statement: revised recommendations for improving

the quality of reports of parallel-group randomized trials. *Ann Intern Med* 2001;134:657-62.

[7] Feld R, Abratt R, Graziano S, Jassem J, Lacquet L, Ninane V, Paesmans M, Rocmans P, Schiepers C, Stahel R, Stephens R. Pretreatment minimal staging and prognostic factors for non-small cell lung cancer. *Lung Cancer* 1997;17 Suppl 1:S3-10.

[8] Østerlind K. LDH or NSE or LDH and NSE as pretreatment prognostic factors in small cell lung cancer? A commentary. *Lung Cancer* 2000; 30:51-3.

[9] Pujol JL. Serum Cyfra 21-1 as a co-variable in future NSCLC chemotherapy trials. *Lung Cancer* 2001; 33:89-94.

[10] Pujol JL, Quantin X, Jacot W, Boher JM, Grenier J, Lamy PJ. Neuroendocrine and cytokeratin serum markers as prognostic determinants of small cell lung cancer. *Lung Cancer* 2003; 39:131-8.

[11] Quoix E, Purohit A, Faller-Beau M, Moreau L, Oster JP, Pauli G. Comparative prognostic value of lactate dehydrogenase and neuron-specific enolase in small-cell lung cancer patients treated with platinum-based chemotherapy. *Lung Cancer* 2000; 30:127-34.

[12] Watine J. Laboratory Variables as Additional Staging Parameters in Patients with Small-Cell Lung Carcinoma. A Systematic Review. *Clin Chem Lab Med* 1999; 37:931-8.

[13] Watine J. Prognostic evaluation of primary non-small cell lung carcinoma patients using biological fluid variables. A systematic review. *Scand J Clin Lab Invest* 2000; 60:259-74.

[14] Horvath AR, Watine J, Jorgensen PE, Oosterhuis WP, Sandberg S, Sanders GT. *Position statement from the Committee of Evidence-based Laboratory Medicine of the Education and Management Division of the IFCC* (in preparation).

[15] Sandberg S, Oosterhuis W, Freedman D, Kawai T. Systematic reviewing in laboratory medicine. Position paper from the IFCC committee on systematic reviewing in laboratory medicine. *J Int Fed Clin Chem* 1997; 9:154-5.

[16] Cox DR. Regression models and life-tables (with discussion). *J R Stat Soc* 1972; B34:187-202.

[17] Albain KS, Crowley JJ, Leblanc M, Livingston RB. Determinants of improved outcome in small cell lung cancer: An analysis of the 2580 patients Southwest Oncology Group data base. *J Clin Oncol* 1990; 8:1563-74.

[18] Allan SG, Stewart ME, Love S, Cornbleet MA, Smyth JF, Leonard RCF. Prognosis at presentation of small cell carcinoma of the lung. *Eur J Cancer* 1990; 26:703-5.

[19] Bleehen NM, Girling DJ, Machin D, Stephens RJ, on behalf of the Medical Research Council Lung Cancer Working Party. A randomised trial of three or six courses of etoposide cyclophosphamide methotrexate and vincristine or six courses of etoposide and ifosfamide in small cell lung cancer (SCLC). I: Survival and prognostic factors. *Br J Cancer* 1993; 68:1150-6.

[20] Cerny T, Blair V, Anderson H, Bramwell V, Thatcher N. Pretreatment prognosis factors and scoring system in 407 small-cell lung cancer patients. *Int J Cancer* 1987; 39:146-149.

[21] Dearing MP, Steinberg SM, Phelps R, Anderson MJ, Mulshine JL, Ihde DC, et al. Outcome of patients with small cell lung cancer: effects of changes in staging procedures and imaging technology on prognostic factors over 14 years. *J Clin Oncol* 1990; 8:1042-9.

[22] Jorgensen LGM, Østerlind K, Genolla J, Gom SA, Hernandez JR, Johnson PWM, et al. Serum neuron specific enolase (S-NSE) and the prognosis in small-cell lung cancer: a combined multivariable analysis on data from nine centres. *Br J Cancer* 1996; 74:463-7 (erratum: page 2043).

[23] Lebeau B, Chastang C, Schuller MP, Thiberville L, Vaylet F, Derenne JP, Caillaud D, Muir JF, Coetmeur D, Lemarie E. Chimiothérapie des cancers bronchiques à petites cellules. Importance pronostique d'une réponse complète (1280 patients). *Presse Med* 1995; 24:217-21.

[24] Lassen U, Kristjansen PE, Osterlind K, Bergman B, Sigsgaard TC, Hirsch FR, Hansen M, Dombernowsky P, Hansen HH. Superiority of cisplatin or carboplatin in combination with teniposide and vincristine in the induction chemotherapy of small-cell lung cancer. A randomized trial with 5 years follow up. *Ann Oncol* 1996; 7:365-371.

[25] Østerlind K, Andersen PK. Prognostic factors in small cell lung cancer: multivariate model based on 778 patients treated with chemotherapy with or without irradiation. *Cancer Res* 1986; 46:4189-94.

[26] Paesmans M, Sculier JP, Lecomte J, Thiriaux J, Libert P, Sergysels R, Bureau G, Dabouis G, Van Cutsem O, Mommen P, Ninane V, Klastersky J. Prognostic factors for patients with small cell lung carcinoma: analysis of a series of 763 patients included in 4 consecutive prospective trials with a minimum follow-up of 5 years. *Cancer* 2000; 89:523-33.

[27] Sagman U, Maki E, Evans WK, Warr D, Shepherd FA, Sculier JP, Haddad R, Payne D, Pringle JF, Yeoh JL, Ciampi A, DeBoer G, McKinney S, Ginsberg R, Feld R. Small-Cell Carcinoma of the Lung: Derivation of a Pronostic Staging System. *J Clin Oncol* 1991; 9: 1639-49.

[28] Siu LL, Shepherd FA, Murray N, Feld R, Pater J, Zee B. Influence of age on the treatment of limited-stage small-cell lung cancer. *J Clin Oncol* 1996; 14:821-8.

[29] Fukuoka M, Masuda N, Furuse K, Negoro S, Takada M, Matsui K, Takifuji N, Kudoh S, Kawahara M, Ogawara M, Kodama N, Kubota K, Yamamoto M, Kusunoki Y. A randomized trial in inoperable non-small cell lung cancer; Vindesine and cisplatin versus mitomycin, vindesine and cisplatin versus etoposide and cisplatin alternating with vindesine and mitomycin. *J Clin Oncol* 1991; 9:606-13.

[30] Hespanhol V, Queiroga H, Magalhaes A, Santos AR, Coelho M, Marques A. Survival predictors in advanced non-small cell lung cancer. *Lung Cancer* 1995; 13:253-67.

[31] Maeda T, Ueoka H, Tabata M, Kiura K, Shibayama T, Gemba K, Takigawa N, Hiraki A, Katayama H, Harada M. Prognostic factors in advanced non-small cell lung cancer: elevated serum levels of neuron specific enolase indicate poor prognosis. *Jpn J Clin Oncol* 2000; 30:534-41.

[32] O'Connell JP, Kris MG, Gralla RJ, Groshen S, Trust A, Fiore JJ, Kelsen DP, Heelan RT, Golbey RB. Frequency and prognostic importance of pretreatment clinical

characteristics in patients with advanced non-small cell lung cancer treated with combination chemotherapy. *J Clin Oncol* 1986; 4:1604-14.

[33] Ohlhauser C, Bülzebruck H, Ebert W, Drings P, Wannenmacher M. Prognostic factors for survival in inoperable non-small cell lung cancer: a multivariate regression analysis of 456 patients with radiation therapy. *Onkologie* 1997; 20:126-31.

[34] Paesmans M, Sculier JP, Libert P, Bureau G, Dabouis G, Thiriaux J, VanCutsem O, Sergysels R, Mommen P and Klastersky J for the European Lung Cancer Working Party. Prognostic factors for survival in advanced non-small-cell lung cancer: univariate and multivariate analyses including recursive partitioning and amalgamation algorithms in 1052 patients. *J Clin Oncol* 1995; 13:1221-30.

[35] Pujol J, Boher J, Grenier J, Quantin X. Cyfra 21-1, neuron specific enolase and prognosis of non-small cell lung cancer: prospective study in 621 patients. *Lung Cancer* 2001; 31:221-31.

[36] Shinkai T, Eguchi K, Sasaki Y, Tamura T, Ohe Y, Kojima A, Oshita F, Miya T, Okamoto H, Iemura K, Saijo N. A prognostic-factor risk index in advanced non-small cell lung cancer treated with cisplatin-containing combination chemotherapy. *Cancer Chemother Pharmacol* 1992; 30:1-6.

[37] Sorensen JB, Badsberg JH, Olsen J. Prognostic factors in inoperable adenocarcinoma of the lung: A multivariate regression analysis of 259 patients. *Cancer Res* 1989; 49:5748-54.

[38] Sugiura S, Ando Y, Minami H, Ando M, Sakai S, Shimokata K. Prognostic value of pleural effusion in patients with non-small cell lung cancer. *Clin Cancer Res* 1997; 3:47-50.

[39] Takigawa N, Segawa Y, Okahara M, Maeda Y, Takata I, Kataoka M, Fujii M. Prognostic factors for patients with advanced non-small cell lung cancer: univariate and multivariate analyses including recursive partitioning and amalgamation. *Lung Cancer* 1996; 15:67-77.

[40] Van der Gaast A, Schoenmakers CHH, Kok TC, Blijenberg BG, Hop WCJ, Splinter TAW. Prognostic significance of tissue polypeptide-specific antigen (TPS) in patients with advanced non-small cell lung cancer. *Eur J Cancer* 1994; 30A:1783-6.

[41] Wigren T, Oksanen H, Kellokumpu-Lehtinen P. A practical prognostic index for inoperable non-small cell lung cancer. J *Cancer Res Clin Oncol* 1997; 123:259-66.

[42] Wigren T. Confirmation of a prognostic index for patients with inoperable non-small cell lung cancer. *Radiotherapy and Oncology* 1997; 44:9-15.

[43] American Thoracic Society and European Respiratory Society. Pre-treatment Evaluation of Non-Small-cell Lung Cancer. *Am J Respir Crit Care Med* 1997; 156:320-32.

[44] European Group on Tumour Markers. Tumour markers in lung cancer: EGTM recommendations. *AntiCancer Res* 1999; 19:2817-9.

[45] Fédération Nationale des Centres de Lutte Contre le Cancer. Standards, Options et Recommandations 2000 pour la prise en charge des patients atteints d'un cancer bronchopulmonaire non à petites cellules. Downloadable at: *http://www.fnclcc.fr/*

[46] Scottish Intercollegiate Guidelines Network. Management of Lung Cancer, Pilot Edition, February 1998, downloadable at: *http://www.sign.ac.uk/*

[47] Simon GR, Wagner H; American College of Chest Physicians. Small cell lung cancer. *Chest.* 2003 Jan;123(1 Suppl):259S-271S.

[48] Silvestri GA, Tanoue LT, Margolis ML, Barker J, Detterbeck F; American College of Chest Physicians. The noninvasive staging of non-small cell lung cancer: the guidelines. *Chest.* 2003 Jan;123(1 Suppl):147S-156S.

[49] Société de Pneumologie de Langue Française. Recommandations concernant l'utilisation des marqueurs tumoraux sériques dans la prise en charge des cancers bronchiques primitifs. *Rev Mal Resp* 1997; 14(Suppl 3): 5-39 (Comments in: *Rev Mal Respir* 1999; 16:139-49, and in: *Rev Mal Respir* 1999; 16:1165-6).

[50] ASCO. Clinical practice guidelines for the treatment of unresectable non-small-cell lung cancer. Adopted on May 16, 1997 by the *American Society of Clinical Oncology. Journal of Clinical Oncology* 1997; 15: 2996-3018.

[51] Werner-Wasik M, Scott C, Cox JD, Sause WT, Byhardt RW, Asbell S, Russell A, Komaki R, Lee JS. Recursive partitioning analysis of 1999 radiation therapy oncology group (RTOG) patients with locally-advanced non-small-cell lung cancer (LA-NSCLC): identification of five groups with different survival. *Int J Radiat Oncol Biol Phys* 2000; 48:1475-82.

[52] Dische S, Warburton MF, Saunders MI. Radiation myelitis and survival in the radiotherapy of lung cancer. *Int J Radiat Oncol Biol Phys* 1988; 15:75-81.

[53] Wilhelm R, Kovacs G, Heinrichsohn D, Galalae R, Kimmig B. Überlebenszeiten ausschlieβlich bestrahlter Patienten. Die Bedeutung des prätherapeutischen Hämoglobinwerts. *Strahlenther Onkol* 1998; 174:128-32 (Comment in Strahlenther Onkol 1999; 175:42-43).

[54] Johnson PWM, Joel SP, Love S, Butcher M, Pandian MR, Squires L, Wrigley PFM, Slevin ML. Tumour markers for prediction of survival and monitoring of remission in small cell lung cancer. *Br J Cancer* 1993; 67:760-766.

[55] Maetsu I, Pastor M, Gomez-Codina J, Aparicio J, Oltra A, Herranz C, et al. Pretreatment prognostic factors for survival in small cell lung cancer: a new prognostic index and validation of three known prognostic indices on 341 patients. *Ann Oncol* 1997; 8:547-53.

[56] Rawson NSB, Peto J. An overview of prognostic factors in small cell lung cancer. A report from the Subcommittee for the Management of Lung Cancer of the United Kingdom Coordinating Committee on Cancer Research. *Br J Cancer* 1990; 61:597-604.

[57] Bossuyt PM, Reitsma JB, Bruns DE, Gatsonis CA, Glasziou PP, Irwig LM, Lijmer JG, Moher D, Rennie D, de Vet HC; STARD group. Towards complete and accurate reporting of studies of diagnostic accuracy: the STARD initiative. *Clin Chem Lab Med* 2003; 41:68-73.

[58] Hacini J, Watine J. Yet another example of lack of biological expertise in certain biomedical publications. *Clin Chem Lab Med* 2002; 40:426-7.

[59] Köhne CH, Hecker H. Reply to Letter to the Editor "Laboratory variables to stratify metastatic colorectal cancer patients", by J. Watine (*Ann Oncol* 2003; 14: 1450–1451). *Ann Oncol* 2003; 14:1451.

[60] Haeckel R, Wosniok W, Puentmann I. Discordance rate, a new concept for combining diagnostic decisions with analytical performance characteristics. 1. Application in method or sample system comparisons and in defining decision limits. *Clin Chem Lab Med* 2003; 41:347-55.

[61] Von Eyben FE, Petersen PH, Blaabjerg O, Madsen EL. Analytical quality specifications for serum lactate dehydrogenase isoenzyme 1 based on clinical goals. *Clin Chem Lab Med* 1999; 37:553-61.

[62] Basuyau JP, Leroy M, Brunelle P. Determination of Tumour Markers in Serum. Pitfalls and Good Practice. *Clin Chem Lab Med* 2001; 39:1227-33.

[63] Guder WG. Preanalytical factors and their influence on analytical quality specifications. *Scand J Clin Lab Invest* 1999; 59:545-9.

[64] Watine J, Miédougé M, Friedberg B. Carcinoembryonic Antigen as an Independent Prognostic Factor of Recurrence and Survival in Patients Resected for Colorectal Liver Metastases: A Systematic Review. *Dis Colon Rectum* 2001; 44:1791-9 (downloadable at: *http://www.discolrect.com).*

[65] Filella X, Cases A, Molina R, Jo J, Bedini JL, Revert L, Ballesta AM. Tumor markers in patients with chronic renal failure. *Int J Biol Markers* 1990; 5:85-8.

[66] Touitou Y, Haus E (eds.). *Biologic rhythms in clinical and laboratory medicine.* Springer-Verlag, 2nd printing, Heidelberg, Germany, 1994.

[67] Watine J, Miédougé M. Pre-analytical Variation of Laboratory Variables. *Clin Chem Lab Med* 2000; 38:263.

[68] Moher D, Pham B, Klassen TP, Schulz KF, Berlin JA, Jadad AR, Liberati A. What contributions do languages other than English make on the results of meta-analyses? *J Clin Epidemiol* 2000; 53:964-72.

[69] Watine J. Prognostic value of hypercoagulability in cancer patients. *Ann Biol Clin* 2001; 59:511 [Article in French].

[70] Watine J, Bouarioua N. Anemia as an independent prognostic factor for survival in patients with cancer (Comment on: *Cancer* 2001;91:2214-21). *Cancer* 2002; 94:2793-6; discussion 2796-7.

[71] Beckles MA, Spiro SG, Colice GL, Rudd RM. Initial Evaluation of the Patient with Lung Cancer Symptoms, Signs, Laboratory Tests, and Paraneoplastic Syndromes. *Chest.* 2003; 123:97S-104S.

[72] Oosterhuis WP, Bruns DE, Watine J, Sandberg S, Horvath AR. E*vidence-Based Guidelines in Laboratory Medicine Principles and Methods.*Clin Chem 2004;50:806-18.

[73] Lewis SJ. Further disquiet on the guidelies front. *CMAJ* 2001; 165: 180-1.

[74] Hurwitz B. Legal and political considerations of clinical practice guidelines. *BMJ* 1999;318:661-664.

[75] Watine J. Are laboratory investigations recommended in current medical practice guidelines supported by available evidence? *Clin Chem Lab Med* 2002; 40:252-5.

[76] Woolf SH, Grol R, Hutchinson A, Eccles M, Grimshaw J. Potential benefits, limitations, and harms of clinical guidelines. *BMJ* 1999; 318:527-530.

[77] Durand-Zalesky I, Rymer JC, Roudot-Thoraval F, Revuz J, Rosa J. Reducing unnecessary laboratory use with new test request form: example of tumour markers. *Lancet* 1993; 342:150-3.

[78] Watine J, Charet JC. Faut-il suivre les sociétés savantes de pneumologie dans leurs recommandations concernant l'utilisation des marqueurs tumoraux sériques dans l'évaluation pronostique des cancers bronchiques primitifs non à petites cellules? *Rev Mal Respir* 1999;16:139-149 [Comments in: *Rev Mal Respir* 1999; 16:1165-1166].

[79] Watine J, Pujol JL. Controverse sur les recommandations de la SPLF concernant les marqueurs tumoraux. *Réunion du GOLF*, Marseille, France, the 6th of October 2000 (oral communication).

[80] Gershon D. Laying a firm foundation for interdisciplinary research endeavours. *Nature* 2000; 406:107-8.

In: Focus on Lung Cancer Research
Editor: Robert L. Carafaro, pp. 193-207

ISBN 1-59454-082-9

Chapter VI

Medicinal use of Cannabis: Implications for Lung Cancer

Paul F. Smith*

Dept. of Pharmacology and Toxicology,
School of Medical Sciences,
University of Otago, Dunedin, New Zealand

Abstract

Despite limited clinical evidence to support its efficacy, cannabis is widely used for the relief of pain and spasticity by people suffering from multiple sclerosis or spinal cord injury. Unfortunately, the most common mode of ingesting cannabis is smoking, either in a cigarette or using a pipe, in order to achieve high blood levels of delta-9-tetrahydrocannabinol (Δ-9-THC) rapidly. Although cannabis is not associated with an increased cancer risk when it is used orally, when cannabis burns in a cigarette or pipe it generates a number of pro-carcinogenic substances, including vinyl chloride, dimethylnitrosamine, methylethylnitrosamine, benz(α)anthracene and benzo(α)pyrene. The levels of benz(α)anthracene and benzo(α)pyrene are significantly higher than in tobacco smoke and recent evidence indicates that Δ-9-THC facilitates the conversion of aromatic hydrocarbons to carcinogens in a dose-dependent manner. Compared to smoking tobacco, smoking cannabis also results in a larger increase in carboxyhaemoglobin, which limits the capacity of the blood to carry oxygen to the body tissues, and a larger increase in the amount of tar inhaled and retained in the respiratory tract. Cannabis smokers who do not use tobacco have been reported to show a number of pathological abnormalities in the lungs that are indicative of the early stages of the development of cancer. These include the exaggerated growth of basal cells, goblet cells and squamous cells, and abnormal cellular components, including variations in the size of the cell nuclei. Increased expression of the cellular proliferation marker, Ki-67, and the integral membrane protein, epidermal growth factor receptor, have also been reported. While the evidence to date does not prove conclusively that cannabis smoking

* Correspondence: Above address, ph and fax: 64 3 479 5747. Email: paul.smith@stonebow.otago.ac.nz

can cause lung cancer, it does suggest that the risk of cancer is high. If cannabis is to be used for therapeutic purposes, it would therefore be best if its active ingredients were delivered orally or by aerosol spray.

INTRODUCTION

The last several decades have seen increasing claims that cannabis use can offer therapeutic benefits in the treatment of vomiting and nausea, wasting, pain, glaucoma, and spasticity in multiple sclerosis and spinal trauma. Indeed, the major psychoactive constituent of cannabis, delta-9-tetrahydrocannabinol (Δ-9-THC), has been demonstrated to be effective as an anti-emetic and as an appetite stimulant, and synthetic cannabinoids such as dronabinol and nabilone are already available for clinical use in the USA and the UK (Tramer et al., 2001). The therapeutic claims for the management of pain, glaucoma and spasticity are more controversial. For example, most clinical studies to date suggest that Δ-9-THC is little more effective for acute pain than about 60 mg of codeine (Campbell et al., 2001). The use of cannabinoids for the treatment of glaucoma has been associated with adverse effects such as corneal ulceration (British Medical Association, 1997). In relation to spasticity in multiple sclerosis, the few well- controlled clinical trials suggest that Δ-9-THC has no more beneficial effect than placebo and is associated with more adverse side effects (Killestein et al., 2002; Smith, 2002; Smith, 2003). Nonetheless, many people still believe that natural and synthetic cannabinoids will prove to be effective treatments for these various medical problems. One real concern is that while research continues into natural and synthetic cannabinoids that might be therapeutically useful when delivered orally or by aerosol spray sublingually, many sufferers of chronic pain and multiple sclerosis continue to smoke cannabis in the belief that the chemicals therein will do them more good than harm. While the issue of whether there is any therapeutic benefit that cannot be achieved with other routes of administration remains to be resolved, there is considerable evidence to suggest that regular cannabis smoking presents a substantial risk for the development of lung cancer. The aim of this chapter is to summarise and critically evaluate what is currently known of this risk and to consider the alternatives for exploiting the therapeutic potential of cannabis and cannabinoids.

SMOKING CANNABIS AND LUNG FUNCTION

As recently reviewed by Tashkin (2001, 2002), there is direct evidence for a causal link between cannabis smoking and respiratory dysfunction (British Medical Association, 1997). In many case and epidemiological studies, the specific effects of cannabis smoking have been confounded by the use of tobacco. In such circumstances it is unclear whether any associated respiratory dysfunction is a result of smoking cannabis or the tobacco. However, other studies have controlled for this potential confound. Tashkin et al. (1987) evaluated respiratory function in 144 people who smoked marijuana only on a daily basis, and compared them with 135 smokers of both marijuana and tobacco, 70 smokers of tobacco only, and 97 non-smokers. Compared to non-smokers, they found that smokers of marijuana only had a significantly higher frequency of chronic cough, chronic sputum production, wheeze and acute bronchitis. On the other hand, the prevalence of acute and chronic bronchitis were comparable between the marijuana only smokers and the tobacco only smokers. Although the adverse effects of smoking marijuana and tobacco were not found to be additive in this study, another study did report more severe respiratory effects in those who smoked both (Bloom et al., 1987).

Roth et al. (1998) studied a group of 40 subjects, aged 20-49, who were either non-smokers, marijuana smokers, tobacco smokers or marijuana *and* tobacco smokers (n = 10 subjects in each group). None of the marijuana smokers routinely smoked tobacco, except for one who stopped smoking in 1980. The average marijuana use in this group was 5 cigarettes per week. Bronchial biopsies showed that inflammation was at least 2-3 times greater in the marijuana smoking group compared to the non-smokers. These rates were similar to the tobacco smokers who smoked 20 to 30 cigarettes a day (Roth et al., 1998). Roth et al. suggest that the manner in which marijuana is often smoked is partly responsible for the greater lung damage. Whereas tobacco cigarettes are rolled tightly and usually filtered, marijuana cigarettes are usually loosely packed and unfiltered, and as a result deliver hotter smoke with a high concentration of small particles from the cigarette. Also, marijuana smoke is often inhaled with a larger puff volume and a greater retention time. Bronchoalveolar lavage has been used to assay the number of inflammatory cells (i.e., alveolar macrophages) in marijuana only smokers and has shown a significant increase in their production relative to non-smokers (Barbers et al., 1987; Fligiel et al., 1988; Fligiel et al., 1997). Similar results have been reported by Sherman et al. (1995), who also reported that alveolar macrophages showed a trend toward genetic damage. Functional studies of alveolar macrophages from marijuana smokers also suggest that they have an impaired ability to produce cytokines and to destroy bacterial and tumour cells (Baldwin et al., 1997).

In a more recent study by Taylor et al. (2000), the respiratory function of 943 adults, aged 21, was studied. Again, an important aspect of this study was that tobacco use could be distinguished from cannabis use, so that the researchers could assess lung function in subjects who smoked cannabis only. Ninety-one subjects were classified as cannabis-dependent (according to the DSM-IIIR criteria) and of these 28 did not smoke tobacco. The average consumption of cannabis amongst the cannabis-dependent group was 230 times during the previous 12 months (approximately 4.8 times a week). The respiratory symptoms associated with smoking cannabis only were wheezing (in the absence of colds), shortness of breath when exercising, waking during the night with chest tightness, and the production of sputum in the early morning. Relative to subjects who did not smoke tobacco, these effects were all increased by more than 60% and were similar in frequency to tobacco smokers smoking between 1 and 10 cigarettes per day (see Figure 1). While it could be argued that this extent of respiratory dysfunction might apply only to cannabis smokers who are dependent and not to those who smoke cannabis on a more occasional basis, this kind of evidence clearly links smoking cannabis with the development of respiratory problems (Hall, 1998). Zimmer and Morgan (1997) argue that these kinds of data must be balanced against the fact that cannabis smokers often smoke less frequently than tobacco smokers. However, if cannabis is to be used for therapeutic purposes, for example to reduce spasticity in multiple sclerosis, its frequency of use is likely to be higher and the associated adverse health risks greater (Smith, 2002; Smith, 2003).

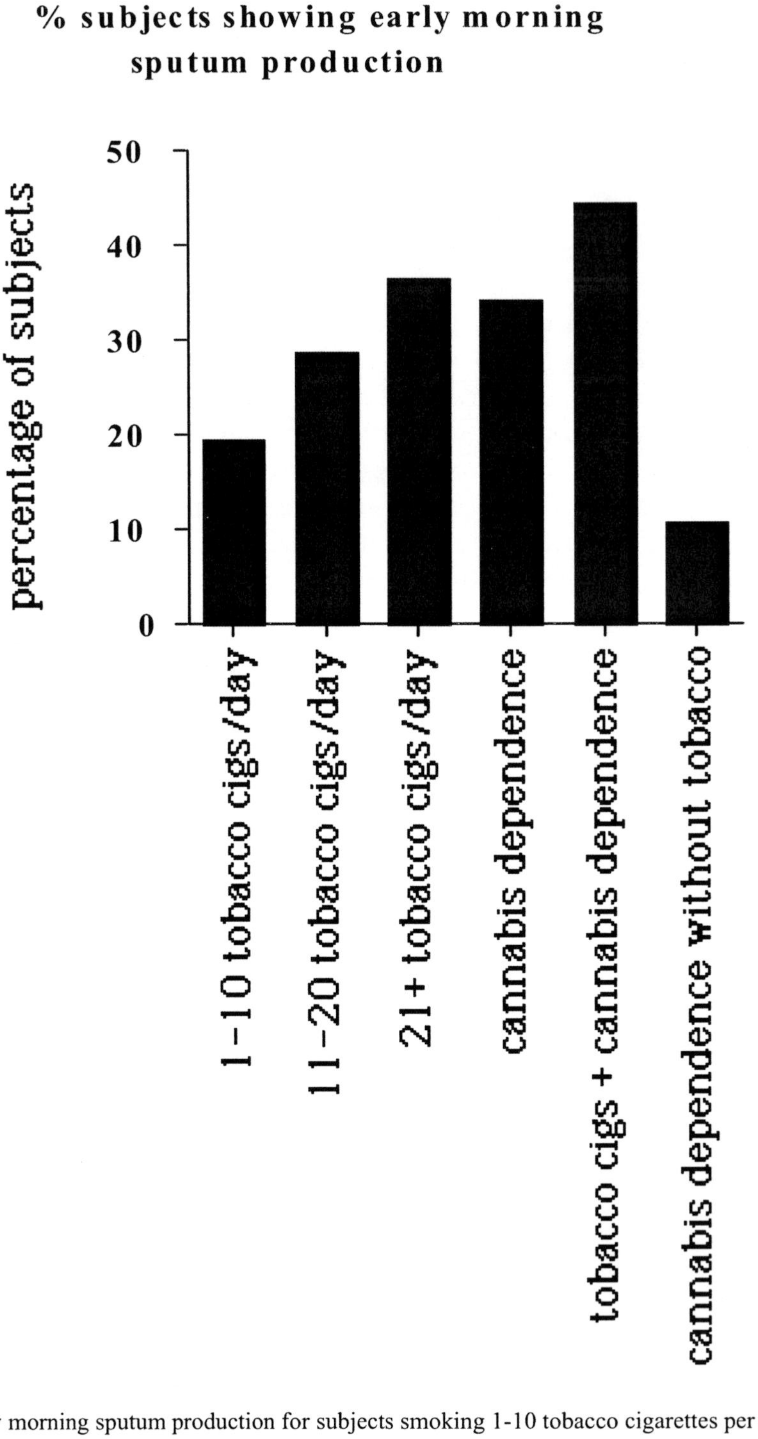

Fig. 1: Early morning sputum production for subjects smoking 1-10 tobacco cigarettes per day, 11-20 tobacco cigarettes per day, more than 21 tobacco cigarettes per day, who were cannabis dependent, who smoked tobacco cigarettes and were cannabis dependent, and who were cannabis dependent without tobacco use. Modified from Taylor et al. (2000).

Tashkin (2002) points out that the existence of the symptoms of chronic bronchitis and its histopathological correlates in marijuana only smokers, does not necessarily imply airway obstruction, and that for chronic obstructive pulmonary disease (COPD) to be present, there must be evidence of airway narrowing such as a reduced forced expiratory volume (FEV). Bloom et al. (1987) reported a significantly reduced ratio of FEV_1 (i.e. forced expiratory volume in one second) to forced vital capacity (FVC) in current marijuana smokers compared to non-smokers, although the values were still within the normal population limits (Tashkin, 2002). A six year follow-up study of the same cohort of subjects showed a significantly reduced FEV_1 and FEV_1 / FVC for previous marijuana smokers but not for current users, suggesting the possibility that chronic use may be necessary for these changes (Sherrill et al., 1991). However, Taylor et al. (2000) reported that 36% of cannabis dependent 21 year olds, only one third of whom had been dependent on cannabis at the age of 18, had a significantly reduced FEV_1 / FVC ratio compared to 20% of non-smokers. Furthermore, Tashkin et al. (1987) failed to find evidence of an association between chronic, heavy cannabis use (i.e. an average of more than 3 cannabis cigarettes per day for 15 years) and indices of COPD. In an attempt to resolve these apparent discrepancies between the different studies, Tashkin et al. (1997) investigated whether there was an age-related reduction in FEV_1 in heavy marijuana smokers compared to tobacco smokers and non-smokers. Tobacco smoking, but not marijuana smoking, was associated with an age-related decline in FEV_1 compared to non-smokers, suggesting that there is no significant association between habitual marijuana smoking and COPD. Van Hoozen and Cross (1997) suggest that a marijuana only smoker would need to smoke 4-5 marijuana cigarettes per day for at least 30 years in order to develop COPD.

Smoking Cannabis and the Risk of Lung Cancer

The cancer risks associated with cannabis smoking have recently been reviewed by Tashkin (2002) and Tashkin et al. (2002). Surprisingly, many cannabis users are not aware of the cancer risks associated with smoking cannabis, perhaps because they assume that these apply only if tobacco is also used in the cigarette. However, smoke from a marijuana cigarette, containing no tobacco whatsoever, contains a variety of pro-carcinogenic substances, including vinyl chloride, dimethylnitrosamine, methylethylnitrosamine, benz(α)anthracene and benzo(α)pyrene. While the levels of vinyl chloride, dimethylnitrosamine and methylethylnitrosamine are lower in a marijuana cigarette than in an equivalent size tobacco cigarette, the levels of benz(α)anthracene and benzo(α)pyrene, two polycyclic aromatic hydrocarbons, are considerably higher (Lee et al., 1976; British Medical Association, 1997; Tashkin, 2002; see Figure 2). Compared to smoking tobacco, smoking cannabis also results in a large increase in the amount of tar inhaled, and one third more tar being retained in the respiratory tract (Wu et al., 1988; Benson and Bentley, 1995; Tashkin, 2002; see Fig. 3). Benson and Bentley (1995) have estimated that compared to smoking a tobacco cigarette, smoking a cannabis cigarette results in an approximately five-fold increase in carboxyhaemoglobin, a stable compound formed between carbon monoxide and haemoglobin which limits the capacity of the blood to carry oxygen to the body tissues

(Slikker et al.,1991; see Fig. 4). Recently, Roth et al. (2001) have reported that marijuana smoke and Δ-9-THC can activate the transcription of the cytochrome P4501A1 (CYP1A1) gene which encodes the enzyme predominantly responsible for converting polycyclic aromatic hydrocarbons into carcinogens in the lungs (Tashkin, 2002).

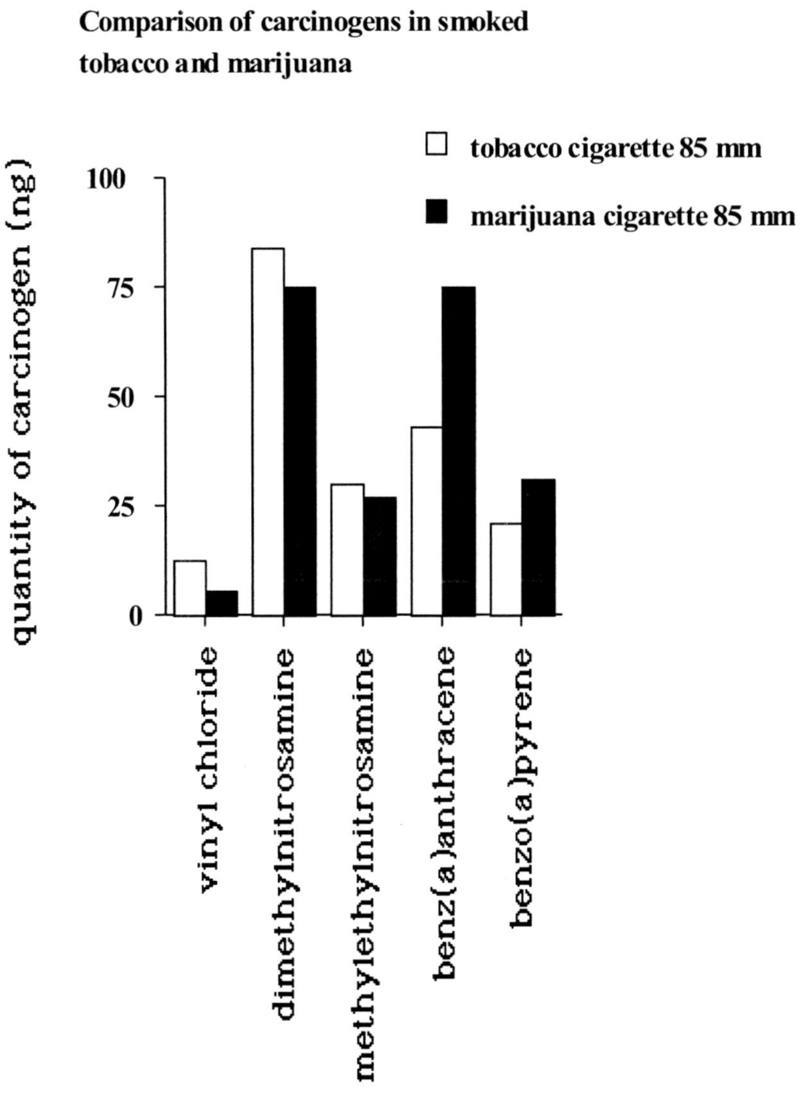

Fig. 2: Comparison of carcinogen levels in cannabis and tobacco cigarettes . The levels (in ng) of five known carcinogens (vinyl chloride, dimethylnitrosamine, methylethylnitrosamine, benz(α)anthracene and benzo(α)pyrene) are shown for equivalent size (85 mm) tobacco and marijuana cigarettes (based on data provided by the British Medical Association, 1997).

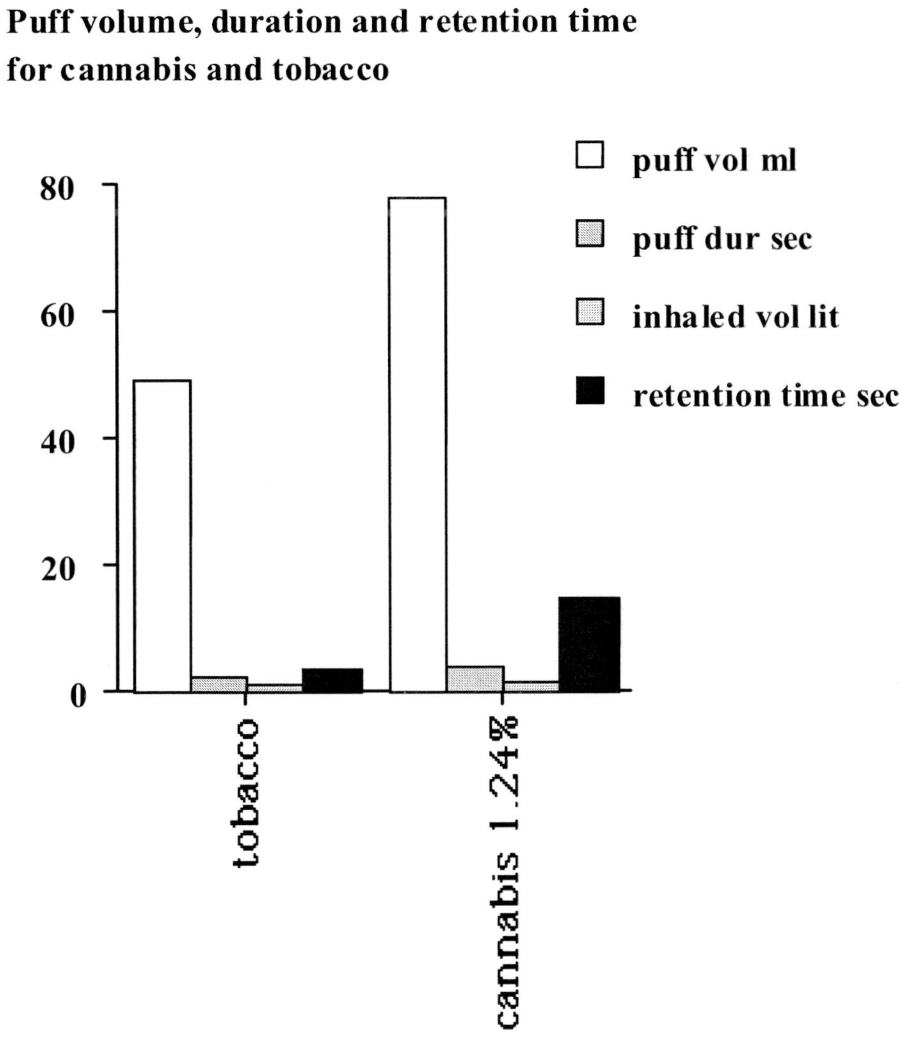

Fig 3: Average puff volume, duration, inhaled volume and retention time for subjects smoking a tobacco versus a cannabis (1.24% Δ-9-THC) cigarette. Modified from Wu et al. (1988).

The presence of carcinogenic chemicals in cannabis cigarettes does not prove conclusively that smoking cannabis can cause or contribute to the development of cancer. However, it does establish that there is a clear risk of cancer. The evidence relating to whether cannabis can actually cause cancer is divided into *in vitro* studies, *in vivo* animal studies and human epidemiological and experimental studies.

Early *in vitro* studies employed the Ames *Salmonella*/microsome test and showed that tar from marijuana smoke can induce genetic mutations to the same extent as tobacco tar (Busch et al., 1979; Wehner et al., 1980). Hamster lung explants exposed to marijuana smoke repeatedly over 2 years also showed genetic changes and malignant transformations (Leuchtenberger and Leuchtenberger, 1976). More recent *in vitro* studies using endothelial cell lines have shown that exposure to marijuana smoke can stimulate the production of reactive oxygen species in a manner that is dependent upon the Δ-9-THC concentration

(Sarafian et al., 1999). Despite these studies, there is evidence that some natural cannabinoids can inhibit the development of malignant gliomas as well as breast and prostate cancer cells when they are administered by means other than in smoke or tar (see Guzman et al., 2001 for review).

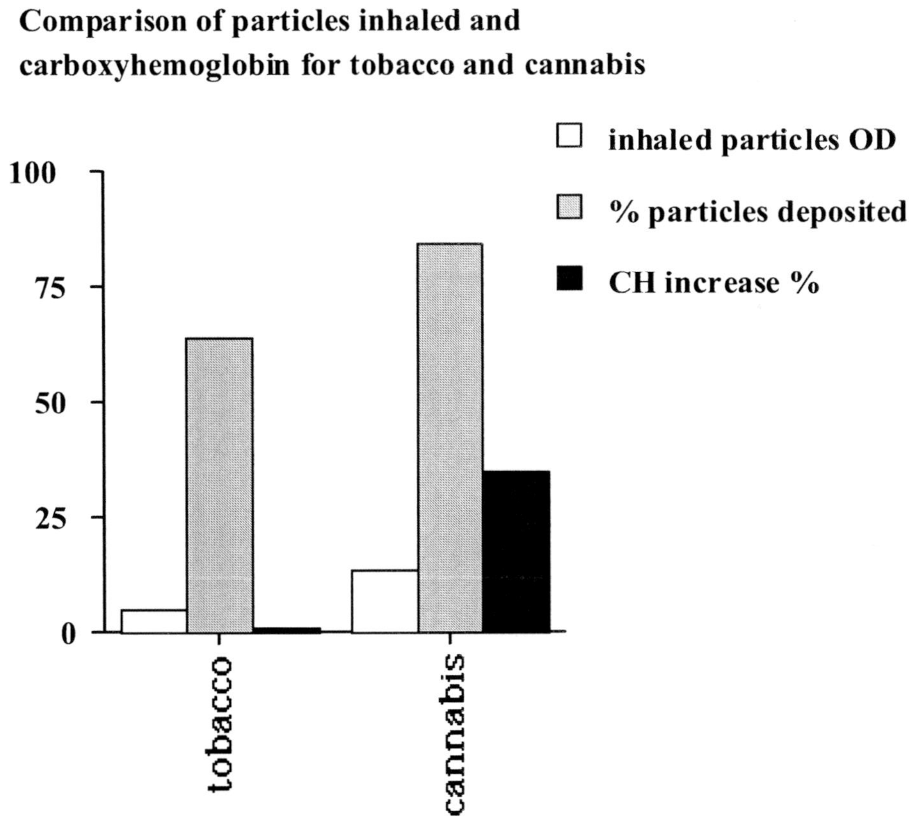

Fig. 4: The optical density (OD) of particulate matter inhaled, the % of particulate matter deposited and % increase in carboxyhaemoglobin (CH) for subjects smoking a tobacco versus cannabis (1.24% Δ-9-THC) cigarette. Modified from Wu et al. (1988).

Surprisingly few *in vivo* animal studies have been conducted which examine the effects of cannabis smoke on tumour development. However, one such study by Cottrell et al. (1973), reported that the application of tar from marijuana cigarettes onto the skin of mice resulted in the development of tumours. There are, however, a number of *in vivo* human studies that have investigated pre-cancerous pathological changes in the lungs of cannabis smokers. Using bronchial wall biopsies in 40 marijuana only smokers, Fligiel et al. (1997) found evidence of hyperplasia, metaplasia and dysplasia. Barsky et al. (1998) compared the results of bronchial biopsies with non-smokers, and found that marijuana-only smokers showed exaggerated growth of basal cells, goblet cells and squamous cells, as well as abnormal cellular components, including variations in the size of cell nuclei (see Fig. 5). There was also increased expression of the cellular proliferation marker, Ki-67, and the integral membrane protein, epidermal growth factor receptor (EGRF) (see Fig. 6). However, abnormalities in the tumour suppressor protein, p53, were seen only in tobacco smokers who also smoked either marijuana or cocaine. These pathological and molecular changes strongly suggest that marijuana-only smokers are likely to develop some of the necessary conditions for cancer to develop (Tashkin, 2002; Tashkin et al., 2002). Analyses of lymphocytes from marijuana only smokers suggest that they have a 3-fold higher incidence of mutant lymphocytes compared to non-smokers, and cord blood lymphocytes from pregnant marijuana smokers also show a higher incidence of mutant lymphocytes (Ammenheuser et al., 1998).

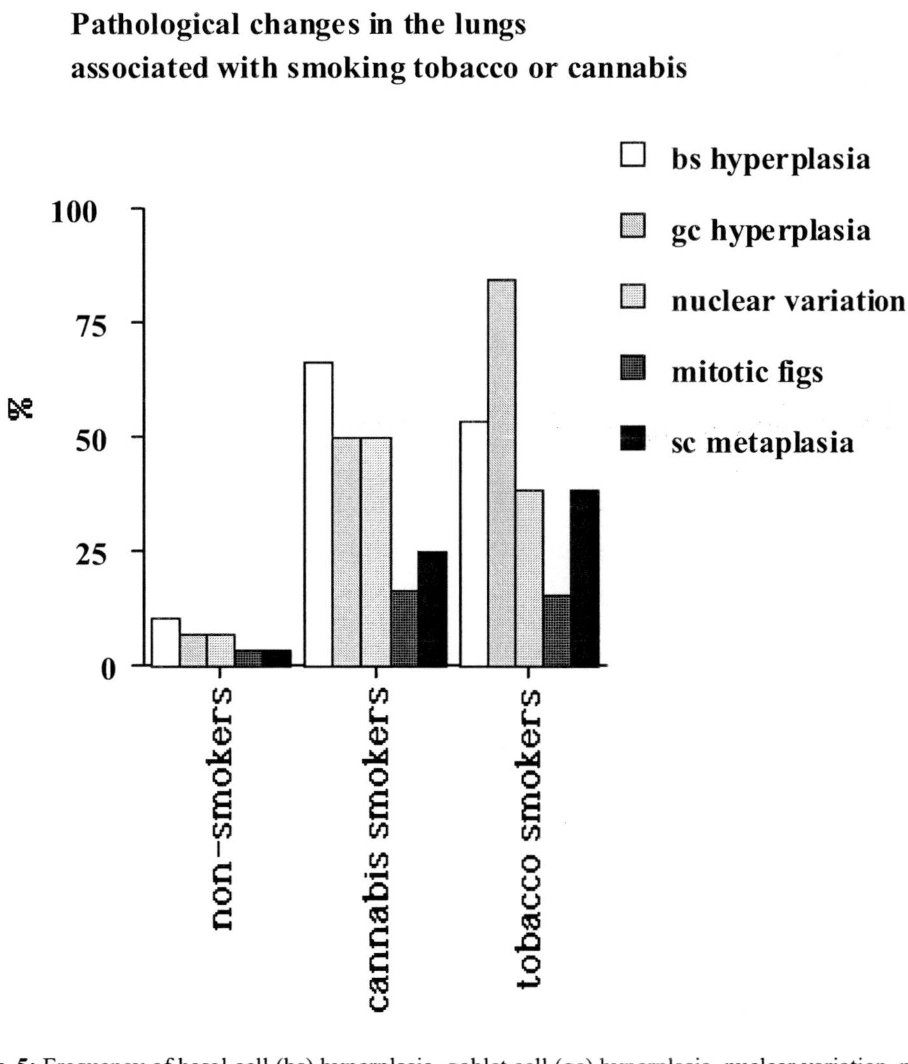

Fig. 5: Frequency of basal cell (bs) hyperplasia, goblet cell (gc) hyperplasia, nuclear variation, mitotic figures and squamous cell (sc) metaplasia in bronchial biopsies from non-smokers, cannabis only smokers and tobacco only smokers. Modified from Barsky et al. (1998).

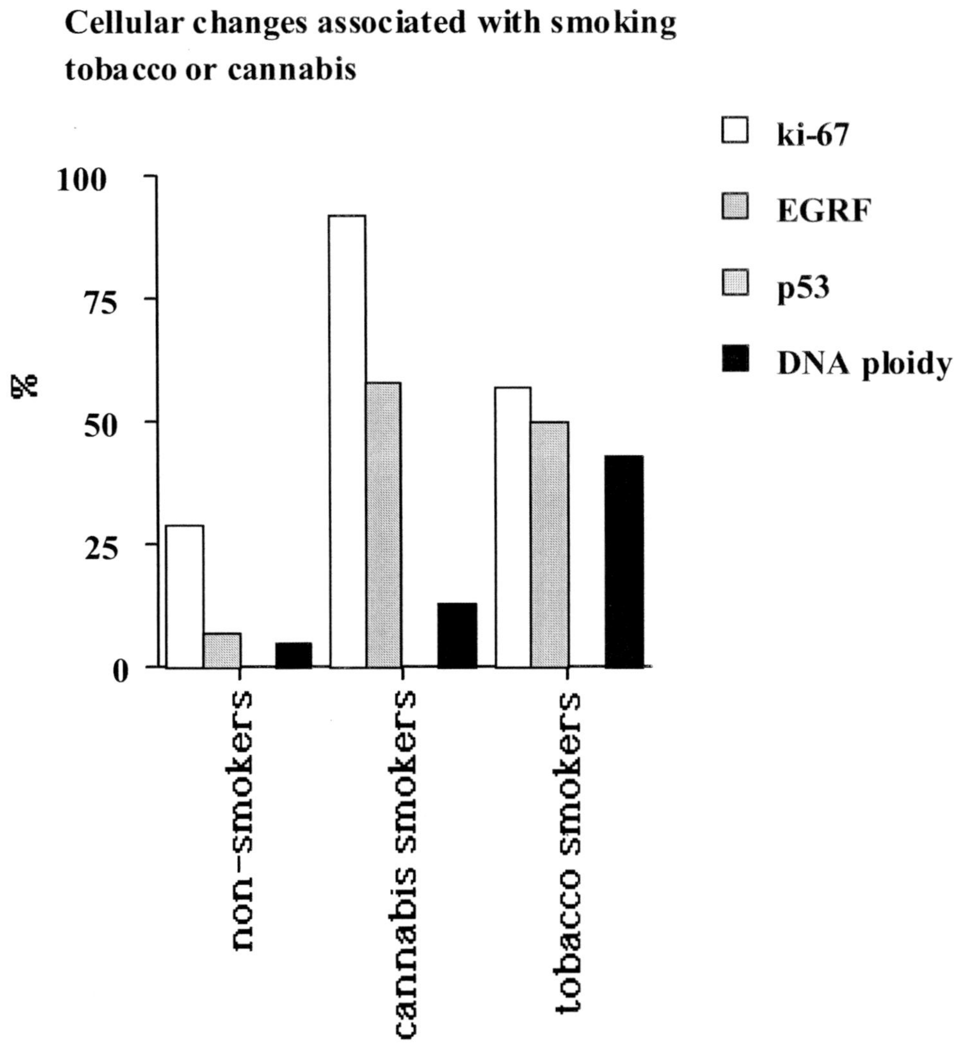

Fig. 6: Frequency of changes in Ki-67, EGRF, p53 expression and DNA ploidy in bronchial biopsies from non-smokers, cannabis only smokers and tobacco only smokers. Modified from Barsky et al. (1998).

Notwithstanding the evidence that some cannabinoids can inhibit tumour proliferation (Guzman et al., 2001), there is also reason to think that the immunosuppressive effects of cannabinoids might contribute to tumour growth in some circumstances (Tashkin, 2002). For example, Δ-9-THC has been shown to facilitate tumour growth in some murine models of cancer, and this effect is blocked by a selective cannabinoid CB2 receptor antagonist (Zhu et al., 2000). This, together with evidence that cannabinoids can inhibit the ability of alveolar macrophages to produce cytokines and destroy tumour cells (Baldwin et al., 1997), raises the possibility that smoking cannabis may undermine the lungs' own immune response against tumour development (Tashkin, 2002).

So far, no large systematic, controlled studies of cancer in cannabis smokers have been published. As Hashibe et al. (2002) and Tashkin (2002) have noted, there are a number of case studies that indicate that head, neck and lung cancers are over-represented in marijuana smokers (Taylor, 1988; Donald, 1991; Sridhar et al., 1994). However, other epidemiological studies have provided conflicting results. Using a cohort of 65,000 people in California, Sidney et al. (1997) found no significant effect of lifetime or current marijuana use on the risk of developing tobacco-related cancers. On the other hand, Zhang et al. (1999) compared 173 newly diagnosed cancer patients with 176 cancer-free subjects matched for both age and gender and found that cannabis use was associated with a significantly higher risk of head and neck cancers; the increased risk was multiplicative for smokers of both marijuana and tobacco.

A number of factors make direct causal evidence linking cannabis smoking and lung cancer difficult to obtain. First, tobacco use and other potential causes of cancer must be excluded, and many cannabis smokers also smoke tobacco or combine tobacco with marijuana. Second, it is generally accepted that there is a 15-30 year latency between the onset of tobacco smoking and the development of lung and other related cancers and therefore cancer caused by cannabis smoking may take a long time to develop (Hall, 1998). Third, it is very difficult to control for the way that cannabis is smoked, since there is no 'standard' cannabis cigarette with known Δ-9-THC and tar levels, and some cannabis smokers use pipes or other delivery devices (Hall, 1998).

Discussion

Cannabinoids are known to have various central nervous system actions that may be therapeutically useful. On the basis of currently available evidence, chief amongst these are their anti-nauseant, anti-emetic and appetite-stimulating effects that can be exploited in the treatment of cancer and AIDS. Other therapeutic possibilities for cannabinoids, such as their use as analgesics and anti-spastic agents, have yet to be fully investigated in controlled clinical trials. Recent studies in these areas using conventional medications for comparison have either shown that cannabinoids are no more effective than currently available drugs or that they are less effective and associated with more adverse side effects (e.g., Campbell et al., 2001; Tramer et al., 2001; Killestein et al., 2002). Clearly, more clinical studies are urgently needed to obtain definitive evidence on these issues, but in the interim caution must be exercised. Of particular concern is that even in the absence of convincing evidence obtained under controlled conditions, many patients with chronic pain and spasticity continue to smoke cannabis in the belief that it does alleviate their symptoms. For example, Consroe et al. (1997) reported that many patients with multiple sclerosis believe that smoking cannabis relieves their spasticity and pain. In some cases this use is encouraged by doctors who believe that no more effective treatments exist (Hall, 1998). Aside from the circumstance of terminal illness in which the adverse effects of smoking cannabis may not have time to accumulate, there must be concern about the possibility that smoking cannabis to relieve spasticity and pain may ultimately cause more harm than good. Although advocates of cannabis smoking often argue that it may be less harmful than tobacco because cannabis is used less frequently (Zimmer and Morgan, 1997), someone who uses cannabis for therapeutic purposes may in fact need to use it on a daily basis (Smith, 2003).

The respiratory studies reviewed in this chapter clearly demonstrate that people who smoke cannabis only exhibit an increased frequency of chronic cough, chronic sputum production, wheeze and acute bronchitis, as well as a proliferation of alveolar macrophages with a reduced capacity to mount immune responses. Nonetheless, the majority of the evidence to date indicates that chronic cannabis smoking does not necessarily lead to airway obstruction and COPD. The strongest case for cannabis smoking resulting in an increased risk of lung and other related cancers can be summarized as follows: 1) cannabis smoke contains potent carcinogens; 2) Δ-9-THC activates the CYP1A1 gene that facilitates the conversion of aromatic hydrocarbons in cannabis smoke into carcinogens; 3) more tar is inhaled and retained in the respiratory tract in smoking cannabis than in smoking tobacco; 4) carboxyhaemoglobin levels are higher after smoking cannabis than after smoking tobacco, resulting in poor oxygenation of the body tissues; 5) pre-cancerous pathological changes have been found in the lungs of people who smoke cannabis only; and 6) the immunosuppressive effects of cannabinoids may undermine the capacity of the immune system to destroy tumours in their early stages of development. At this stage the epidemiological evidence that cannabis smoking causes cancer is contentious and not convincing; however, this may be because of the long latency for cannabis smoke to induce tumours and also variability in the way that cannabis is smoked (e.g., cigarettes versus pipes). On the basis of the available evidence it seems very likely that smoking cannabis will contribute to the development of cancer.

Clearly, the safest way for cannabinoids to be used clinically, if and when they are proven to be effective and safe, is for them to be delivered by a route that does not involve smoking. Synthetic cannabinoids such as dronabinol and nabilone are already administered orally for clinical purposes. While it has been argued that smoking cannabis may be more effective because high blood and brain levels of Δ-9-THC are achieved rapidly, there are other ways of obtaining this advantage. GW Pharmaceuticals in the UK have been investigating the use of an aerosol spray that can be used sublingually to achieve high blood levels of cannabinoids rapidly (Smith, 2003). Although the results of these clinical trials are not yet published, it seems clear that the sublingual route of administration offers many advantages. Spray delivery of the sort used for asthma medications (e.g., salbutamol) is also possible and would achieve the fast delivery of cannabinoids not possible using oral or rectal administration. Ultimately, there is no reason why smoking must be used in order to obtain any therapeutic benefit that cannabis has to offer.

Another point worth making here is that smoking cannabis commits the user to administering Δ-9-THC which is, after all, a broad spectrum cannabinoid receptor agonist that activates both CB1 and CB2 cannabinoid receptors in many parts of the body. Many cannabinoid pharmacologists believe that the best way to exploit the therapeutic potential of cannabis will be to synthesize selective agonists that will target discrete populations of cannabinoid receptors in the brain, and such drugs will probably be delivered either orally or by aerosol spray.

REFERENCES

Ammenheuser, M.M., Berenson, A.B., Babiak, A.E., Singleton, C.R. and Whorton, E.B. Jr. (1998) Frequencies of hprt mutant lymphocytes in marijuana-smoking mothers and their newborns. *Mutation Research.* 403(1-2), pp. 55-64.

Baldwin, G.C., Tashkin, D.P., Buckley, D.M., Park, A.N., Dubinett, S.M. and Roth, M.D. (1997) Marijuana and cocaine impair alveolar macrophage function and cytokine production. *American Journal of Respiratory and Critical Care Medicine.* 156(5), pp. 1606-1613.

Barbers, R.G., Gong, H. Jr., Tashkin, D.P., et al. (1987) Differential examination of bronchoalveolar lavage cells in tobacco cigarette and marijuana smokers. *American Review of Respiratory Disease,* 135, pp. 1271-1275.

Barsky, S.H., Roth, M.D., Kleerup, E.C., Simmons, M. and Tashkin, D.P. (1998) Histopathological and molecular alterations in bronchial epithelium in habitual smokers of marijuana, cocaine and/or tobacco. *Journal of the National Cancer Institute,* 90, pp. 1198-1205.

Benson, M. and Bentley, A.M. (1995) Lung disease induced by drug addiction. *Thorax,* 50, pp. 1125-11237.

Bloom, J.W., Kaltenhorn, W.T., Paoletti, P., Camilli, A. and Leibwitz, M.D. (1987) Respiratory effects of non-tobacco cigarettes. *British Medical Journal.* 295(6612), pp. 1516-1518.

British Medical Association (1997) *Therapeutic Uses Of Cannabis.* Harwood Academic Publishers, Netherlands.

Busch, F.W., Seid, D.A. and Wei, E.T. (1979) Mutagenic activity of marijuana smoke condensates. *Cancer Letters.* 6(6), pp. 319-324.

Campbell, F.A., Tramer, M.R., Caroll, D., Reynolds, D.J., Moore, R.A. and McQuay, H.J. (2001) Are cannabinoids an effective and safe treatment option in the management of pain? A qualitative systematic review. *Brit. Med. J.* 323, pp. 13-16.

Consroe, P., Musty, R., Rein, J., Tillery, W. and Pertwee, R. (1997) The perceived effects of smoked cannabis on patients with multiple sclerosis. *Eur. Neurol.* 38, pp. 44-48.

Cottrell, J.S., Sohn, S.S. and Vogel, W.H. (1973) Toxic effects of marijuana tar on mouse skin. *Archives of Environmental Health.* 26(5), pp. 277-278.

Donald, P.J. (1991) Advanced malignancy in the young marijuana smoker. *Advances in Experimental Medicine and Biology.* 288, pp. 33-56.

Fligiel, S.E.G., Beals, T.F., Venkat, H. et al. (1988) Pulmonary pathology in marijuana smokers. in: Chesher, G.P., Consroe, P. and Musty, R. (eds.), *Marijuana: An International Research Report.* National Campaign Against Drug Abuse, Monograph No. 7, Canberra, Australian Government Publishing service, pp. 43-48.

Fligiel, S.E.G., Roth, M.D., Kellerup, E.C., Barsky, S.H. and Tashkin, D.P. (1997) Trachiobronchial histopathology in habitual smokers of cocaine, marijuana and/or tobacco. *Chest,* 112 (2), pp. 319-326.

Guzman M., Sanchez, C. and Galve-Roperh, I. (2001) Control of the cell survival/death decision by cannabinoids. *Journal of Molecular Medicine.* 78(11), pp. 613-625.

Hall, W. (1998) The respiratory risks of cannabis smoking. *Addiction,* 93, pp. 1461-1463.

Hashibe, M., Ford, D.E. and Zhang, Z.F. (2002) Marijuana smoking and head and neck cancer. *Journal of Clinical Pharmacology*. 42(Suppl. 11), pp. 103S-107S.

Killestein, J., Hoogervorst, E.L.J., Reif, M., et al. (2002) Safety, tolerability and efficacy of orally administered cannabinoids in MS. *Neurol.* 58, pp. 1404-1407.

Lee, M.L., Novotny, M and Bartle, K.D. (1976) Gas chromatography/mass spectrometric and nuclear magnetic resonance spectromatic studies of carcinogenic polynuclear aromatic hydrocarbons in tobacco and marijuana smoke condensates. *Analytical Chemistry*. 48(2), pp. 405-416.

Leuchtenberger, C. and Leuchtenberger, R. Cytological and cytochemical studies of the effects of fresh marijuana cigarette smoke on growth and DNA metabolism of animal and human lung cultures. In Braude, M.C. and Szara, S. (Eds.), *The Pharmacology of Marijuana.* New York, Raven Press, 1976, pp. 595-612.

Roth, M.D., Arora, A., Barsky, S.H., et al. (1998) Airway inflammation in young marijuana and tobacco smokers. *American Journal of Respiratory and Critical Care Medicine,* 157, pp. 928-937.

Roth, M.D., Marques-Magallanes, J.A., Yuan, M., Sun, W., Tashkin, D.P. and Hankinson, O. (2001) Induction and regulation of the carcinogen-metabolizing enzyme CYP1A1 by marijuana smoke and delta-(9)-tetrahydrocannabinol. *American Journal of Respiratory Cell and Molecular Biology*. 24(3), pp. 339-344.

Sarafian, T.A., Magallanes, J.A., Shau, H., Tashkin, D.P. and Roth, M.D. (1999) Oxidative stress produced by marijuana smoke. An adverse effect enhanced by cannabinoids. *American Journal of Respiratory Cell and Molecular Biology*. 20(6), pp. 1286-1293.

Sherman, M.P., Aeberhard, E.E., Wong, V.Z., et al. (1995) Effects of smoking marijuana, tobacco or cocaine alone or in combination on DNA damage in human alveolar macrophages. *Life Sciences,* 56, pp. 2201-2207.

Sherrill D.L., Krzyzanowski, M., Bloom, J.W. and Leibowitz, M.D. (1991) Respiratory effects of nontobacco cigarettes: A longitudinal study in general population. *Journal of Epidemiology*. 20(1), pp. 132-137.

Sidney, S., Beck, J.E., Tekawa, I.S. and Quesenberry, C.P. Jr. (1997) Marijuana use and cancer incidence. *American Journal of Public Health.* 8(5), pp. 585-590.

Slikker, W. Jr., Paule, M.G., Ali, S.F., et al. (1991) Chronic marijuana smoke exposure in the rhesus monkey. I. Plasma cannabinoid and blood carboxyhemoglobin concentrations and clinical chemistry parameters. *Fundamental and Applied Toxicology,* 17, pp. 321-334.

Sridhar, K.S., Raub, W.A., Weatherby, N.L., Metsch, L.R., Surratt, H.L., Inciardi, J.A., Duncan, R.C., Anwyl, R.S. and McCoy, C.B. (1994) Possible role of marijuana smoking as a carcinogen in the development of lung cancer at a young age. *Journal of Psychoactive Drugs*. 26(3), pp. 285-288.

Smith, P.F. *Cannabis On The Brain.* Dunmore Press, Palmerston North, 2002.

Smith, P.F. (2003) Cannabinoids for the treatment of multiple sclerosis: No smoke without fire? *Expert Review of Neurotherapeutics* 3, pp. 89-96.

Tashkin, D.P. (2001) Airway effects of marijuana, cocaine and other inhaled illicit agents. *Current Opinion in Pulmonary Medicine.* 7(2), pp. 43-61.

Tashkin, D.P. (2002) Respiratory risks from marijuana smoking. In F. Grotenhermen and E. Russo (Eds), *Cannabis and Cannabinoids. Pharmacology, Toxicology and Therapeutic Potential.* The Haworth Press, Inc. New York, pp. 325-335.

Tashkin, D.P., Baldwin, G.C., Sarafian, T., Dubinett, S. and Roth, M.D. (2002) Respiratory and immunologic consequences of marijuana smoking. *Journal of Clinical Pharmacology.* 42(Suppl. 11), pp. 71S-81S.

Tashkin, D.P., Coulson, A.H., Clark, V.A., Simmons, M., Bourque, L.B., Duann, S., Spivey, G.H. and Gong, H. (1987) Respiratory symptoms and lung function in habitual, heavy smokers of marijuana alone, smokers of marijuana and tobacco, smokers of tobacco alone, and non-smokers. *American Review of Respiratory Disease.* 135(1). pp. 209-216.

Tashkin, D.P., Simmons, M., Sherrill, D. and Coulson, A.H. (1997) Heavy habitual marijuana smoking does not cause an accelerated decline in FEV_1 with age: A longitudinal study. *American Journal of Respiratory and Critical Care Medicine.* 155(1), pp. 141-148.

Taylor, F.M. (1988) Marijuana as a potential respiratory tract carcinogen: A retrospective analysis of a community hospital population. *Southern Medical Journal.* 81(10), pp. 1213-1216.

Taylor, D.R., Poulton, R., Moffitt, T.E., et al. (2000) The respiratory effects of cannabis dependence in young adults. *Addiction,* 95, pp. 1669-1677.

Tramer, M.R., Caroll, D., Campbell, F.A., et al. (2001) Cannabinoids for control of chemotherapy-induced nausea and vomiting: quantitative systematic review. *British Medical Journal,* 323, pp. 16-21.

Van Hoozen, B.E. and Cross, C.E. (1997) Marijuana. Respiratory tract effects. *Clinical Reviews in Allergy and Immunology.* 15(3), pp. 243-269.

Voth, E.A. and Schwartz, R.H. (1997) Medicinal applications of delta-9-tetrahydrocannabinol and marijuana. *Annals of Internal Medicine,* 126, pp. 791-798.

Wehner, F.C., Van Rensburg, S.J. and Thiel, P.C. (1980) Mutagenicity of marijuana and Trnaskei tobacco smoke condensates in the Salmonella/microsome assay. *Mutation Research.* 77(2) 135-142.

Wu, T-C., Tashkin, D.P., Djahed, B. et al. (1988) Pulmonary hazards of smoking marijuana as compared with tobacco. *The New England Journal of Medicine,* 318, pp. 347-351.

Zhang, Z-F., Morgenstern, H., Spitz, M.R., Tashkin, D.P., Yu, G-P., Marshall, J.R., Hsu, T.C. and Schantz, S.P. (1999) Marijuana use and increased risk of squamous cell carcinoma of the head and neck. *Cancer Epidemiology, Biomarkers and Prevention.* 8(12), pp. 1071-1078.

Zhu, L.X., Sharma, S., Stolina, M., Gardner, B., Roth, M.D., Tashkin, D.P. and Dubinett, S.M. (2000) Delta-9-tetrahydrocannabinol inhibits antitumour immunity by a CB2 receptor-mediated, cytokine-dependent pathway. *Journal of Immunology.* 165(1), pp. 373-380.

Zimmer, L. and Morgan, J.P. (1997) *Marijuana Myths Marijuana Facts.* The Lindesmith Center, New York and San Francisco.

INDEX

A

B

C

D

E

F

I

K

L

M

N

O

P

Q

R

S

T